Grief, Loss and Bereavement

Evidence and practice for health
and social care practitioners

**Edited by Peter Wimpenny
and John Costello**

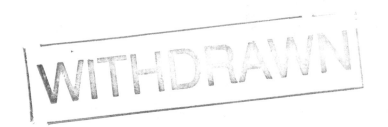

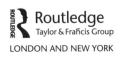 **Routledge**
Taylor & Francis Group

LONDON AND NEW YORK

First published 2012
by Routledge
2 Park Square, Milton Park, Abingdon, Oxon OX14 4RN

Simultaneously published in the USA and Canada
by Routledge
711 Third Avenue, New York, NY 10017

Routledge is an imprint of the Taylor & Francis Group, an informa business

British Library Cataloguing in Publication Data
A catalogue record for this book is available from the British Library

Library of Congress Cataloging in Publication Data
A catalog record for this book has been requested

ISBN13: 978-0-415-46750-6 (hbk)
ISBN13: 978-0-415-46751-3 (pbk)
ISBN13: 978-0-203-80575-6 (ebk)

Typeset in Baskerville
by Prepress Projects Ltd, Perth, UK

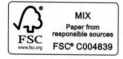

Printed and bound in Great Britain by the MPG Books Group

Grief, Loss and Bereavement

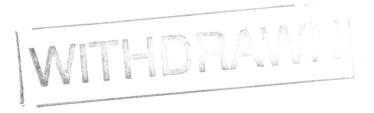

Dealing with the social experience of grief, loss and bereavement provides challenges for everyone, including health and social care practitioners, who are often well placed to offer help and support to the bereaved. This book draws together a comprehensive range of worldwide evidence for understanding and supporting the bereaved in a variety of health and social care contexts. It can be used by practitioners from a wide range of backgrounds in both health and social care to gain an appreciation of bereavement and its associated support and care. Additionally, it can be used for personal and professional development by practitioners who want to enhance their own and others' practice with the bereaved in specific contexts or organisations. The book may also be of value to those undertaking postgraduate study, who want to gain a wider understanding of the evidence related to bereavement and bereavement care practice in health and social care, and may be seeking to add to the body of evidence in this field.

Peter Wimpenny is a lecturer at the Robert Gordon University in Aberdeen. He is a member of the National Framework Group for Bereavement Care in Scotland. He has also been active in evidence informed practice through the Joanna Briggs Institute and SIGN (Scottish Intercollegiate Guidelines Network).

John Costello is an experienced teacher. He has published extensively on topics related to his research on the social experience of death and dying as well as in areas related to teaching and learning. John is a counsellor and an educational consultant to the Chernobyl Children's Project (CCP), a UK charity focused on promoting palliative care in Belarus and other areas of Eastern Europe.

To Colin Murray Parkes, who has been, and continues to be, an inspiration to all of those who work in the field of bereavement and bereavement care

Contents

List of figures   viii
List of tables   ix
List of boxes   x
List of contributors   xii
Acknowledgements   xv

Introduction   1

1   Background to bereavement and bereavement care   5
    JOHN COSTELLO

PART I
Bereavement across the lifespan   **17**

2   Bereavement in children and young people   19
    KIM MORRIS

3   Parental and family bereavement   36
    FIONA WORK AND SYLVIA WILCOCK

4   Bereavement and older people   55
    AUDREY STEPHEN

PART II
Contexts of bereavement   **69**

5   End of life care and bereavement   71
    JOHN COSTELLO

6   Mental health, trauma and bereavement   91
    DAVID ALEXANDER AND SUSAN KLEIN

7 Bereavement and primary care   111
   SALLY LAWTON AND KEN LAWTON

8 Acute care and bereavement   123
   PETER WIMPENNY

9 Children's deaths and bereavement   139
   BROTHER FRANCIS

10 Perinatal bereavement   160
   ELAINE DICK AND PETER WIMPENNY

11 Bereavement in care homes   175
   PAUL DEMPSTER

12 Bereavement and people with learning difficulties   191
   BARRY GAULT

13 HIV/AIDS and bereavement   202
   RACHEL UNWIN

14 Bereavement and occupational health   215
   ROSEMARY SHAW

PART III
**Education, interventions and organisation of
bereavement care**   **225**

15 Professional development for health and social care
   practitioners   227
   PETER WIMPENNY

16 Interventions, organisation of care and on-going support for
   the bereaved   244
   PETER WIMPENNY

   Index   259

Figures

1.1 The dual process model of coping with bereavement 10
4.1 The wheel of loss 58
5.1 Bereavement risk assessment tool 83
7.1 Influencing factors on the response to death 112
8.1 A model for bereavement support in an acute hospital 126
9.1 *My Perfect World or Death and the Child* 146
9.2 Detail from *My Perfect World or Death and the Child* 147
15.1 Tiered model of educational provision 238
15.2 Tiered levels of support for bereaved 239
16.1 Tiered provision of service provision for the bereaved 251
16.2 Stage(s) of involvement in bereavement care 253

Tables

4.1	Reaction type, contributing factors and intervention	65
5.1	Differences between anticipatory and post-death grief	74
5.2	Styles of grieving	78
5.3	A three-component model of bereavement support	86
9.1	End of life and bereavement planning	149
13.1	Stigma	204
15.1	Core components of educational programmes	233
15.2	Some identified educational programmes to assist volunteers and practitioners	236
15.3	Bereavement table	238
15.4	Principles of support	240

Boxes

1.1 Different perspectives on grief and bereavement   13
2.1 Indications of successful adaptation   31
2.2 Indications of poor adaptation   32
5.1 Factors affecting the impact of loss on bereavement   76
5.2 Risk factors in bereavement   81

The Dead

They walk with you
the dead.
Some skip along in front
some walk beside
some, like naughty children,
drag behind.
Others walk on top of you
crush you into nothing
or demand to be carried
like shopping.
A few slip like loose change
into pockets.
And one or two
lie curled together,
stitched into the lining of your heart.
Pauline Prior-Pitt
Disappearing Out, 2008

Pauline is a poet and performer living on the island of North Uist. She has written five collections of poetry, published by Spike Press, and three poetry pamphlets. *North Uist Sea Poems* won the 2006 Callum Macdonald Award for Pamphlet Poetry. For details and to read more poems, visit www.pauline-prior-pitt.com.

Contributors

Professor David A. Alexander MA(Hons), PhD, CPsychol, FBPS, FRSM, (Hon)FRCPsych. David is Director of the Aberdeen Centre for Trauma Research (Faculty of Health and Social Care, Robert Gordon University, Aberdeen, UK). He is Honorary Consultant Clinical Psychologist to the regional health board and Consultant to the Scottish Police College, where he teaches in trauma and hostage negotiation. He has been appointed as a clinical adviser by various organisations including the Royal College of Psychiatrists in the wake of a number of major incidents worldwide. He is a Fellow of the British Psychological Society, a Fellow of the Royal Society of Medicine and an Honorary Fellow of the Royal College of Psychiatrists.

John Costello RGN, PhD. John is a senior lecturer in palliative care nursing at the University of Manchester, School of Nursing, Midwifery and Social Work. His teaching role focuses on communication and ethical decision making in a clinical context. His research interests and publications include the social management of death, dying and bereavement, and the role of families, carers and professionals in helping to maintain the dying person's quality of life. John is an active contributor to the Children's Chernobyl Project, a UK charity focused on enabling children, adults and families in Belarus to come to terms with life-threatening medical illness.

Paul G. Dempster BD(Hons), DPS, DipMin, DipSW, DipAppSocStud, PhD. Paul is a Research Fellow at the Leeds Institute for Health Sciences and holds an honorary post at the University of Wisconsin–Madison. With a background in pastoral care and social work, his research interests include looking at the impact of death, dying and bereavement for workers in care homes. His current work focuses on applied health research and applications of qualitative methodology, especially using computer software.

Elaine Dick RGN, RM. Elaine is a midwife at Aberdeen Maternity Hospital. She has been a qualified midwife for 16 years, working as a rotational midwife in a large tertiary unit. For the last 5 years Elaine has specialised in pregnancy loss, working in a unit that provides care for women experiencing loss in all stages of pregnancy (Rubislaw Ward). She has developed an interest in early pregnancy ultrasound and now incorporates this into her practice to enhance her midwifery care.

Brother Francis RGN, RSCN, BSc(Hons), ENB 934 and 240. Francis was Nurse Consultant in Children's and Young People's Palliative Care for the north of Scotland. He has 25 years of experience, gained in a wide variety of clinical and counselling settings, with both children and adults. He has been recognised at international, national and local levels for his community-based service for children dying from cancer and was awarded the 'National Well Child Award' in 2007.

Barry Gault PhD, MSc, BSc(Soc), CQSW. Barry is a registered social worker, who has worked in both social work and nursing education. He is now an independent researcher with an interest in the promotion and facilitation of self-advocacy for people who are labelled as having a 'learning difficulty'. He acts as an adviser to People First (Fraserburgh).

Susan Klein MA(Hons), PhD, Cert COSCA. Susan is a Reader in trauma research at the Aberdeen Centre for Trauma Research (ACTR) and a principal member of the Institute for Health & Welfare Research (IHWR) at Robert Gordon University. She is responsible for managing the wide-based research portfolio for the ACTR and is theme leader for Neurological and Mental Health for the IHWR. She is a World Health Organization-accredited trainer of trainers, Deputy Chair of the Sudden Trauma Information Service Helpline (STISH) and a member of the UK Psychological Trauma Society and the European Society for Traumatic Stress.

Ken Lawton MB ChB FRCGP. Ken has been a GP in Aberdeen for more than 20 years. He is a clinical senior lecturer at the Centre for Academic Primary Care at the University of Aberdeen, an Associate Advisor with NHS Education Scotland and currently Chair of the Scottish Council of the Royal College of General Practitioners. His interests include mental health, depression and clinical education.

Sally Lawton RGN, DNCert, MA, PhD, LLM. Sally has been Senior Lecturer in Palliative Care (Nursing) for NHS Grampian for 6 years, following many years of working within higher education. She holds an honorary senior lecturer's post at the Centre for Advanced Studies in Nursing at the University of Aberdeen. Her interests include palliative care nursing in both primary and secondary care settings and continuing professional development.

Kim Morris RGN, BSc. Kim has worked in palliative care for more than 20 years, most recently as a Community Macmillan Specialist Nurse. Her particular area of interest is the care of children who are bereaved and she was instrumental in the establishment of a children's grief and bereavement literature resource at Roxburghe House, NHS Grampian.

Rosemary Shaw RGN, SCM, DN, PT, HV, BA, PGCertTLT. Rosemary is the Course Leader for the BA Occupational Health Practice course at Robert Gordon University in Aberdeen. She has an interest in how grief and bereavement affect work and how colleagues deal with bereaved individuals in the context of work. This subject has been of personal interest, and in highlighting the issues she hopes it may encourage people to interact in a positive way with bereaved colleagues.

Audrey Stephen MSc, BSc, RGN. Audrey's background is in general adult nursing and health services research. She has been involved in a variety of qualitative and quantitative projects, including a mapping study of bereavement and bereavement care in Scotland. She is currently a Research Training Fellow funded by the Chief Scientist Office of the Scottish Government. Her project (also for PhD) is a qualitative research study about developing bereavement care practice for older people in hospital wards, general practices and care homes.

Sylvia Wilcock BA(Hons), PhD. Sylvia is a senior lecturer at the School of Nursing and Midwifery and Lead for Knowledge Transfer at the Institute for Health and Welfare Research at Robert Gordon University, Aberdeen. In her role as Director of the Scottish Centre for Evidence-based Multi-professional Practice, Sylvia participated in the Centre's investigations into bereavement and bereavement care.

Peter Wimpenny RGN, BSc(Hons), Cert Ed, PhD. Peter is a lecturer at the School of Nursing and Midwifery at Robert Gordon University (RGU) in Aberdeen. He has been involved in a range of evidence-informed practice work, including membership of SIGN (Scottish Intercollegiate Guidelines Network) Council and the Joanna Briggs Collaborating Centre at RGU. He is currently a member of the National Framework Group for Bereavement Care in Scotland.

Fiona Work RGN, RMN, BA, BA, PHN, PGCertTLT. Fiona is a lecturer at the School of Nursing and Midwifery at Robert Gordon University (RGU) in Aberdeen. She has an interest in evidence-informed practice work, related to bereavement through the Joanna Briggs Collaborating Centre at RGU. As a former grief counsellor and lecturer, she is particularly interested in the field of grief, death, dying and bereavement, particularly in relation to the subject of male grief.

Acknowledgements

We are grateful to Colin Maclean, Librarian, RGU Library Service, for his unfailing willingness to assist us in seeking evidence in an ever-expanding world of information.

Grateful thanks go to all the authors of the chapters in this book, who completed their tasks with enthusiasm and a desire to illuminate bereavement and bereavement care and enhance understanding and provision of services. Without their skill and expertise there would be no book.

Without the love of Clare and Marie, our long suffering partners, and our children, Hattie, Mimi, George and Fred, and Joe, Robert and Ryan we would not have had the necessary support to complete this work.

Introduction

If you are reading this as a health care professional, then you may already have considered a need to engage with and enhance care for the bereaved. You may, on the other hand, just be curious to know more about bereavement and bereavement care. Bereavement is part of all our lives and is something we shall encounter at both personal and professional levels. However, although it is a common experience, for each of us it may be unique in the manner in which we grieve and our responses to loss will vary. Providing individualised bereavement care is therefore challenging within any health and social care context. This book seeks to provide you with available evidence that could assist your practice.

The title *Grief, Loss and Bereavement: evidence and practice for health and social care practitioners* is our attempt to provide coverage of a broad range of contexts and to increase awareness and understanding of the evidence base in this field, and so enhance care. We prefer to think of the work as 'evidence informed' rather than 'evidence based', to better illustrate that practice cannot necessarily be overridden by evidence, but that it should form a part of the overall approach to practice that includes the context in which it occurs and the individual who is receiving care, features of the original evidence-based medicine movement (Sackett *et al.* 1996).

The idea for this book came from a systematic literature review carried out for the Scottish Government Health Department (Wimpenny *et al.* 2007). Bereavement had been brought more fully to the attention of policy makers in the 1990s through organ retention scandals, increasing numbers of complaints and an increasing awareness that more could be done to enhance practice at this crucial time in people's lives. However, carrying out the review was particularly challenging as the amount and range of evidence related to bereavement and bereavement care was considerable. We also identified a lack of good-quality research to support many of the perspectives and approaches to care currently available, although this does not mean that practice can remain on hold until we have all the necessary research! Despite this paucity there are some valuable and consistent messages about bereavement and how care could be provided to the bereaved. Such work may already be carried out regularly by health and social care practitioners, although the extent of best practice is not known. We therefore hope that the book will not only seek to inform you and other practitioners about bereavement and bereavement care but also assist in reducing variations in practice and stimulate further questions that may contribute to future developments.

We were confronted, at the outset, with the challenge of knowing where bereavement begins and where it ends for health and social care workers. We were also struck by the amount of evidence related to bereavement and bereavement care in palliative care (cancer and hospice based) literature. This raised concerns about the extent to which cancer and palliative care might have an overbearing influence in this area even though the majority of deaths occur in general hospital settings (approximately 55–60 per cent). It might also be the case that such a focus inadvertently links bereavement care to these specific contexts, reducing responses in other areas. There is little doubt that cancer and palliative care, through the hospice movement, has enhanced individuals' care and introduced the concept of a 'good death'. This has been hugely influential in end of life care and such ideas are permeating into general health and social care settings (Department of Health 2008). However, to enhance bereavement care, greater emphasis is needed on development in all health and social care settings, so that, for example, those who are bereaved through acute or sudden death, or in care homes or at work, are as likely to receive appropriate support as those in palliative care.

The book opens with a chapter examining the background to bereavement and bereavement care. Following this, the book consists of three distinct but related parts.

Part I deals with bereavement across the lifespan. The purpose is to develop a general understanding of bereavement and how it affects children, families and older people. Although there will be some common factors across the lifespan, there are also notable differences which can influence care.

Part II deals with a range of specific contexts where death occurs. We are aware that this section of the book may not cover all contexts. We have sought to illuminate evidence and practice in a broad range of health and social care contexts where death occurs and care for the bereaved takes place. The majority of deaths in Western society will occur in hospital settings; however, it is equally important to ensure that the bereaved receive appropriate attention wherever death takes place. We have therefore sought to include bereavement care and support in primary, secondary and tertiary care settings, and have included chapters on bereavement and bereavement care related to children, HIV, mental health and trauma, learning disability, the workplace and maternity services.

Part III reviews evidence related to professional development, education, training, interventions and organisation of services for the bereaved. This final section of the book deals with some strategic issues in respect of bereavement and bereavement care, and seeks to provide a view of factors that need to be considered if provision at a national, organisational or local level is to be understood and enhanced.

The chapters are written by a variety of practitioners and include key messages, questions and case studies in an attempt to help you, as the reader, reflect on your own experiences and practice, or to illustrate or illuminate the evidence more fully. Our intention is to raise awareness and develop greater understanding of the outcomes of bereavement and to encourage the reader to consider ways in which care may be enhanced. You may, even at this stage, want to consider how, at a local level, you might contribute to the development of bereavement care services through practice, education or research.

References

Department of Health (2008) *End of life care strategy: promoting high quality care for all adults at the end of life.* London: Department of Health.

Sackett DL, Rosenberg W, Gray JA, Haynes RB and Richardson WS (1996) Evidence based medicine: what it is and what it isn't. *British Medical Journal* 312(7023): 71–72.

Wimpenny P, Unwin R, Dempster P, Grundy M, Work F, Brown A and Wilcock S (2007) A literature review on bereavement and bereavement care. Developing evidence-based practice in Scotland. *Bereavement Care* 26(1): 7–10.

1 Background to bereavement and bereavement care

John Costello

Key messages

- Historical and traditional perspectives on grief and bereavement influence our understanding of the experience of loss and its assessment.
- Contemporary theories of grief and bereavement are different from traditional approaches and tend to reflect changes in society.
- It is important not to become too prescriptive about grief reactions and their effect on bereavement.
- Bereavement is also influenced by social factors, such as the age of the mourner, the circumstances of the death, the social background of the bereaved and the extent to which mourning takes place.
- It is important to highlight from the evidence that bereavement is a process, affected by things such as religious and cultural beliefs.
- Most people experience bereavement as a normal healthy process and to become prescriptive about grief reactions can influence our thinking and cause us to label or *pathologise* bereavement as an illness.
- Both traditional and contemporary understandings of grief have a role to play in helping us provide effective quality support to those in crisis who become vulnerable as a result of experiencing bereavement.

Introduction

The purpose of this chapter is to examine traditional and cultural perspectives related to grief and bereavement, contrasting these with contemporary understandings. It provides background material for subsequent chapters and stimulates the reader to contextualise contemporary thinking and practice about bereavement based on a review of available evidence.

The chapter examines traditional perspectives from Freud (1957 [1917]) to more contemporary explanations such as continuing bonds theory (Klass *et al.* 1996) and Stroebe and Schut's (1999) dual process model. In reviewing some of the contemporary perspectives, the chapter examines their influence on thinking about bereavement care. The purpose is to highlight both how explanations and

understandings have altered over time as a result of societal changes and fundamental understandings about individual and group behaviour. In doing so, the
chapter considers more of the theoretical developments than subsequent chapters,
although each chapter has its own balance between theory and practice, with the
latter being prevalent throughout the book.

One of the key themes emerging from the available evidence is that the process
of grief can be restorative. In this sense, as the dual process model highlights (see
later in this chapter), mourners are enabled to make the necessary psychological
adjustments to help them think and feel more positively, whilst also acknowledging
the emotional impact of the loss and its influence on future well-being. Ultimately,
the 'key message' of the chapter is that understanding perspectives of grief and
loss is important but that we should view these as assisting our thinking about
bereavement and bereavement care, rather than as restrictive models that may run
the risk of labelling and *pathologising grief* as a condition instead of a normal process
that all of us will experience at some point in our lives.

What do we mean by loss, grief and bereavement?

Loss may be defined as being deprived of something we value (Stroebe 1992).
In tangible terms this includes the material loss experienced by repossession of
a home, the loss of a loved one or household pet. Conversely, it could include
the loss of respect, independence or even virginity! In many cases, there is an
expectation that responses to loss involve varying degrees of grief. Grief consists
of physical changes as well as psychological feelings and can include emotional
expression, crying, loss of sleep anxiety and a wide range of symptoms, such as
anorexia, restlessness, agitation and somatic disturbance. The evidence does not
clearly inform us when these symptoms occur in relation to the loss. There is, however, an abundance of evidence associated with the extent to which these somatic
and psychological experiences, if prolonged and sustained, may lead others to
suspect abnormality.

Grief is often reported as a response to loss, which is then followed by a period of
bereavement. The latter is influenced by the extent to which mourning, the social/
cultural behaviour associated with death, occurs (Parkes 1993). Bereavement may
be seen as the social fact of loss, which obliges the observer to offer condolences
and expressions of sympathy to the mourner. This may however, be considered
culture bound and varies according to the rules and norms adopted by the cultural
context in which grief takes place. We can argue therefore that an understanding
of the behaviour associated with loss can help us focus on what the mourner is
feeling, although how they express their emotions depends on the cultural context
as well as the perspective taken by the person listening to them. Because of this,
health and social care practitioners supporting the bereaved need to be aware not
only of the cultural significance of grief, but also about the theoretical concepts
which seek to explain it. By doing this, practice is informed and the decisions that
are made are more likely to be in the best interests of the bereaved.

Traditional perspectives on grief and bereavement

Grief and bereavement have been experienced since the beginning of time, although as a reference point, this chapter traces their origins from the early twentieth century by looking at the seminal work of Sigmund Freud (1957 [1917]), *Mourning and melancholy*, as a starting point. Evidence on bereavement is based on Freud's seminal work on the talking therapies. By examining the historical developments up until modern times, the chapter contrasts traditional approaches with what Klass and colleagues (1996) call 'newer understandings of grief' that emphasise mourners taking a more active role in their bereavement. Culturally, I begin by addressing some assumptions about important areas of life such as the universal nature of loss and grief and why bereavement is often seen as a process experienced in stages or phases. The chapter also considers bereavement in terms of a continuing spiritual experience with the deceased. Initially, the question I ask is 'Are grief and bereavement universal?'

To grieve over the loss of a loved person or object appears to be a natural phenomenon, or what sociologists called a 'truism', at the same time acknowledging its cultural diversity. Historically, the experience of grief is arguably something that will be encountered by people from all cultures, although the way grief is expressed is shaped by the religion, traditions, values and social norms of that particular cultural group. Firth (2000) points out that it is important for health and social care workers to understand the religious beliefs and cultural traditions of different ethnic communities. For example, in some Eastern cultures there is a tradition of expressing grief in a very demonstrable way using self-flagellation, and adhering to explicit periods of grief, such as 40 days and nights for some cultural groups (Firth 2000). In contrast, in the UK, Queen Victoria dressed in black for the entire 6-year period of mourning after the death of her husband, Prince Albert, in the nineteenth century. The wearing of black is a legacy that continues today, although to a lesser extent, and highlights how rituals may also be shaped by events and may change over time.

Working through grief

Historically and traditionally, approaches to bereavement were expressed through a range of ideas, attitudes and values that can be traced to the early work of Freud (1957 [1917]). These ideas, based on psychoanalytical outcomes from therapy, have been supported by further work from psychiatrists such as Lindemann (1944), Bowlby (1963), Kübler-Ross (1969) and Parkes (1972). Collectively, the views have laid the foundations for what many refer to as the grievin and represent a dominant part of what may be regarded as a cult bereavement, with more people becoming interested in th associated with death and dying (Walter 1999).

The historical literature on grief highlights an abu gest that talking about loss is a helpful way to resolve

Freud's (1957 [1917]) work spawned the notion of the *talking therapy*, which essentially argues that talking about loss is beneficial to bereavement resolution (Walter 1994). Freud argued that those who experienced loss needed to work through this and eventually emotionally detach themselves from the deceased in order to achieve successful grief resolution. This involved a process known as *cathecting* the expression of emotions such as love for the deceased and releasing emotional energy in the form of varied grief reactions – and then *decathecting* – emotionally detaching from the deceased. This view dominated understandings of bereavement, especially in psychoanalytical terms, for many decades and became known as the *grief work hypothesis* (Stroebe and Stroebe 1991).

Working through grief is seen as an ultimate goal by many bereavement counsellors who subscribe to the view that mourners should acknowledge the permanent absence of the deceased by initial expression of emotion, focusing on past memories and by being encouraged not to suppress feelings. This rather formulaic approach to explaining emotional expression after loss almost *prescribes grief* through recognition of the reality of the loss, working through feelings and 'moving on', or, as Worden (1991) points out, 'emotionally relocating'. The latter is an important part of grief work and involves severing the emotional bond with the deceased (or decathecting). This is often a painful process and involves letting go emotionally, moving on and relinquishing any future hopes of a relationship. Freud believed that to continue to have any on-going emotional connection with the deceased was pathological (Rando 1995; Davies 2004).

Closely aligned to, and following, a similar psychodynamic approach, the work of the American psychiatrist Lindemann (1944) supported Freud's grief work hypothesis, expressing the view that grief may be seen as an acute illness episode with clear symptoms and a pathological focus. Lindemann's study, which focused on a clinic for survivors and others from a nightclub fire in Boston, began to categorise grief into 'normal' and 'abnormal'. Lindemann identified that grief could be seen in terms of its symptomatology and management. His study was notable for, amongst other things, suggesting a medicalisation of grief.

Developments in the 1960s and 1970s

In the 1960s, Bowlby (1963) outlined his early work on childhood attachment, which underpinned much of what Freud and others had been arguing for in terms of grief reactions. In 1969, following the assassinations of JF Kennedy and Martin Luther King, Elizabeth Kübler-Ross (1969) published findings from her work in a New York hospital with 250 patients diagnosed with cancer. Her notion of grief being experienced as a series of stages, published as a book, *On death and dying*, was a best seller and sold a million copies in the first year. However, unlike her predecessors, Kübler-Ross worked not with mourners after death but with those facing impending death from cancer. In this sense she was working clinically with the living, and drawing conclusions about their reaction to their cancer diagnosis.

Building on the work of Freud, Bowlby and Kübler-Ross, Parkes's (1972) semi-work *Bereavement: studies of grief in adult life* was largely based on retrospective analysis of case studies of patients who presented with depression. This work is regarded as a classic and, together with Kübler-Ross's study, led to what has become known as stage-based theories or approaches to grief and bereavement.

The idea of experiencing grief and bereavement in stages or phases was developed by Parkes (1972, 1991) in the UK and by an American psychoanalyst, William Worden, in the USA. Parkes's work indicated that grief was experienced as a series of phases, beginning with shock and anger, and leading to pining and yearning behaviour. He also stressed the importance of it being seen as a process and that counsellors could identify aspects of grief as normal or abnormal. His early writings held that retained emotional links with the deceased could be seen as pathological, although subsequent reprints modified this view. Parkes argued that many of the emotions experienced by the bereaved varied in intensity, were not constant and were likely to be felt as 'pangs of grief' (1991: 60), depending on a number of factors, such as the relationship of attachment between the mourner and the deceased. Worden (2001), somewhat later, identified grief as occurring in stages, with the bereaved behaving as an active participant in their grief, undertaking four emotional tasks and not becoming a passive recipient of grief as an illness. Worden identified that, in order to successfully resolve grief, mourners are required to accept the reality of the loss, experience the pain of grief, adjust to an environment where the deceased is missing and, finally, emotionally relocate.

Developments from the 1990s onwards

In the 1990s growing disillusionment with stage theories and the grief work hypothesis, and the lack of clarity about what constitutes healthy bereavement, led Stroebe and Schut (1999) to construct a model of bereavement based on research, which examined the ways that spouses coped with the loss after the death of their partner. Their dual process model has become applicable in describing coping in more diverse groups of mourners. Unlike other models, the dual process model identifies and includes stressors associated with bereavement, as well as how people cope with loss using a variety of cognitive strategies. The key feature of the model, however, is its focus on explaining the process by which mourners oscillate between activity oriented to the loss and restorative behaviour (Figure 1.1).

The central argument of the model is that mourners can be observed demonstrating various behaviours (dependent on individual and cultural idiosyncrasies), that can be considered as either restorative or loss-focused coping behaviour. Figure 1.1 illustrates taxonomy descriptors for each coping behaviour. The model incorporates earlier observations of mourners who engaged themselves in activity focused on the loss, such as planning the funeral, as well as restorative behaviour, such as planning a holiday. The model is described as a taxonomy of the ways in which people come to terms with the loss of a loved one (Wimpenny 2007). As such, it stands apart from previous stage-based models because it highlights differences in observed behaviour and demonstrates how mourners are not focused only on coping with the loss. Moreover, it may be argued that the model is more practice based and less reliant on theoretical

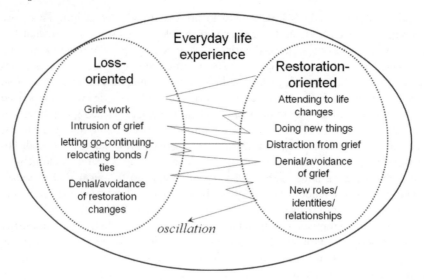

Figure 1.1 The dual process model of coping with bereavement (Stroebe and Schut 1999).

constructs. The model attempts to explain how everyday experiences of the mourner's time are necessarily focused on socialising with others, doing things such as shopping, watching television, reading and planning other activities not related to the death of their partner. The bereaved find themselves oscillating between activities that may be related to loss (loss oriented), such as denial, letting go or relocating bonds, and other restoration-oriented activity, such as planning holidays and establishing new roles and relationships. In this sense, the bereaved can be observed moving between behaviour which is loss oriented and that focused on enabling them to adapt and restore order, integrity and harmony to their lives. Mallon (2008) points out that when the bereaved engage in one form of behaviour to the exclusion of all others, they can become fixated or obsessed with one way of thinking, which can lead to difficulties. She argues that, in terms of bereavement support, some mourners, primarily women, need to be encouraged to develop more restorative forms of behaviour, whereas some men need to be encouraged to get better in touch with their emotions, a view supported by others, such as Doka and Martin (2002).

Patterns of bereavement

Despite the various explanations for loss and grief, the way we grieve and the patterns of bereavement that evolve within society depend greatly on social norms and cultural values. The literature is replete with advice and concepts drawn from psychiatry and psychology about models of grief and bereavement. What are we to make of this dominance by those professionals who seek to explain behaviour using cases of people who have had adverse experiences of loss? Parkes (1972) focuses attention on grief from a pathological perspective using case studies of his own patients.

In contrast to the belief that talking about loss has therapeutic value, there is other evidence to suggest that not all cultural groups conform to this view. Bowen (2002: 137) has pointed out that 'chief amongst all taboo subjects is death' and that talking about death is something that some cultures adopt in order to protect what may be seen as a pollutant effect. There are cultural groups in many parts of the world which have adopted such an approach. For example, Mandelbaum (1959) reported on how the North American Indian Hopi tribe in Arizona urged people to forget about the dead as soon as possible after death. It is explained that this is not for purposes of denying the pain of loss, as it is felt, but that no attempt is made to overtly express signs of grief. Similarly, in the UK, Williams (1990) describes the way older Aberdonians express grief, which contrasts with contemporary approaches that place emphasis on 'talking about the deceased' (p. 78), and expressing how much you miss and loved them. Some older Aberdonians may consider this abnormal and frown upon those who talk of the dead. For this cultural group, talking about death and the deceased can be considered socially inappropriate.

Is it good to talk about grief?

I summarise the traditional perspective on grief and bereavement by examining the influence and dominance of the psychoanalytical concept of grief work. There is clear evidence that much education and training about bereavement counselling is based on the work of Freud, Bowlby, Parkes, Worden and others, who all appear to subscribe to the idea of the grief work hypothesis. The traditional approach may be embedded in behaviourist beliefs which set out to prescribe grief behaviour and confine it to a series of stages, phases or tasks. There seems to be a link between the traditional understanding of grief and the need to break the emotional bond. Parkes (1972: 49) describes the way in which his study of widows in London revealed that interaction with the thoughts, ideas and feelings associated with the deceased, the 'inner representation', was important in helping to establish a new identity during the early stages of grief, but points out that:

> It seems odd that identification with the lost person is one of the methods that bereaved people adopt to avoid the painful reality of loss. The sense of the husband 'inside' is a transient phenomenon . . . allowing a sense of comfortable closeness followed by periods of grieving and loneliness.

Parkes acknowledges that widows did seem to emerge and develop a different identity from their altered life situations and that this involved some rumination on their past life and their relationship with the deceased, but that although this was a part of grief it needed to culminate in a breaking of the emotional bond in order for a healthy response to be made (p. 51). Parkes's (1972) study goes on to say that preoccupation with the deceased is an almost necessary phase that widows experience and that hallucinations of an auditory or visual kind are symptoms of what he calls 'searching behaviour' (p. 49), which if persistent can lead to pathological problems such as delayed grief.

We can summarise from this that Parkes's theory of grief, based on the London widows study, was ethological grief and can be understood as a pre-programmed set of behaviours made in response to loss. There is always the danger that all grief may be seen as an illness, and in this sense we may become prescriptive about our observations of the bereaved rather than interpreting behaviour as symptomatic of a clearly identified set of symptoms. The role of practitioners may therefore change from listening, expressing empathy and compassion without making judgements and trying to understand, to looking for a set of symptoms to occur that lead us to conclude that the person is in fact suffering from an illness. Many of us have encountered others who are said to be 'in denial' or 'stuck in the anger/shock stage' of their bereavement. There is also the popular view that it is 'good to talk' about our problems and that the old adage 'a problem shared is a problem halved' infers that ventilating our feelings, particularly when they are troublesome, has therapeutic value. Perhaps the fundamental principle of talking about our feelings is beneficial, if not always culturally appropriate. However, if we examine some of the contemporary models (the dual process model, for example) which seek to explain grief and bereavement, we are able to develop a more individualised and less prescriptive understanding of the complexity of grief and the implications this has for bereavement care.

Severing the relationship with the deceased

Traditional understandings of grief and bereavement inform us that the key to successful resolution of bereavement is to work through grief and break the emotional bond we have with the deceased and emotionally relocate. This model had been accepted for most of the twentieth century and remains influential today in shaping opinion and practice of bereavement care. It is perhaps noteworthy that, with the exception of Kübler-Ross (1969), who claimed there was no linear relationship to her five stages, since the 1980s, theoretical grief models have continued to perpetuate the view that grief work needs to be completed in a more or less linear fashion to successfully resolve the grief (Rothaupt and Becker 2007). A number of writers, researchers and counsellors have highlighted discrepancies in stage- and phased-based approaches, including Walter (1994), who draws attention to the fact that there have been over 30 academic papers criticising stage-/phase-based models.

Kübler-Ross's five stages have even been satirised in the American television series *The Simpsons* (the blowfish episode), in which Homer visits a Chinese restaurant, eats poisoned fish and, after being taken to the hospital, is told he has 24 hours to live. After experiencing death anxiety, Homer rapidly experiences the five stages of denial, anger, bargaining, depression and acceptance, satirically portrayed as occurring in a linear fashion and experienced in minutes! One of the earliest writers to offer an alternative explanation for grief reactions was the American researcher Teresa Rando (1985, 1986). Rando conducted a study on parental bereavement, which found that parents grieved not only for the loss of the child, but also for the loss of future aspirations and hopes of what the child could have achieved. Many others have highlighted issues where the bereaved have experienced different grief reactions which indicate that the deceased and the bereaved have an emotional link after death, without there being any evidence that they were not aware of the reality of the loss (Attig 1991; Stroebe 1992; Silverman and Klass 1996; Stroebe *et al.* 1996; Gamino *et al.* 2000; Costello and Kendrick 2000; Field *et al.* 2003).

Some of the groundbreaking research revealing the importance of emotional links between the deceased and the mourner questions the psychoanalytical view that mourners need to break emotional bonds with the deceased and comes from the Tubingen longitudinal study (Stroebe and Stroebe 1989, 1991; Stroebe *et al.* 1996). This study of young widows and widowers revealed that, 2 years after the death of their spouse, two-thirds of the sample reported that they wished to continue with their pre-loss relationship and continue to have a relationship with the deceased. Only 17 per cent reported that they were seeking a new partner. These indications of a desire to remain linked with the past call into question the reliability of the grief work hypothesis.

Other studies of children's grief (Silverman and Worden 1993) have confirmed the view that the bereaved wish to retain memories of their past lives and relationships with their deceased parent or spouse, connecting with them in an emotional way, visiting the grave, talking to them, keeping mementoes and ensuring that their memory is kept alive. These studies reveal that, rather than relinquishing their ties with the deceased or working through their grief, there is strong evidence that mourners wish to revisit their previous lives, retaining the things they hold dear in the knowledge that the previous relationship has changed. The significant memories and symbolic images of their relationships are retained, nurtured and held to be important in helping the bereaved to continue with their future lives.

Box 1.1 summarises the main developments in perspectives on loss and grief that have been described in this chapter. It has, by necessity, covered the work succinctly and you would be encouraged to undertake follow-up reading on the models and work covered.

Box 1.1 Different perspectives on grief and bereavement

1944	Lindemann: *Symptomatology and management of acute grief*
1957 [1917]	Freud: *Mourning and melancholia*
1969	Kübler-Ross: *On death and dying*
1972	Parkes: *Studies of grief in adult life*
1989	Wortman and Silver: *Coping with irrevocable loss*
1991	Worden: *Grief counselling and grief therapy*
1996	Klass and colleagues; *Continuing bonds: newer understanding of grief*
1996	Stroebe and Schut: *Dual process model of coping with bereavement*

Conclusion

It is clear that the explanations for grief and bereavement have changed over time and will continue to change as we gain further understanding through research. This chapter has considered the historical and traditional perspectives on grief and bereavement, as well as newer explanations for grief, and has included a brief examination of the dominant grief theories (alluded to as the grief work hypothesis). The key messages of the chapter are twofold:

- It is important that when we consider and review the evidence pertaining to grief and bereavement we caution ourselves not to become too prescriptive about grief reactions and their effect on bereavement.
- It is important to highlight from the evidence that bereavement is a process, affected by, for example, religious and cultural beliefs. Moreover, it is also influenced by social factors such as the age of the mourner, the circumstances of the death, the social background of the bereaved and the extent to which mourning, as the public face of grief, takes place. In general, bereavement involves a series of adaptations, or to use Parkes's (1991) phrase 'psychosocial transitions'. This involves gradual change until a point is reached where the mourner may be said (by others) to have come to terms with their loss. In practice, the intensity of the mourner's emotions diminishes to a point where the observer cannot discern an obvious cause for concern. We should perhaps also remind ourselves that most people experience bereavement as a normal, healthy process, and to become prescriptive about grief reactions can influence our thinking and cause us to label or pathologise bereavement as an illness. Finally, in reviewing different perspectives, we should consider that both traditional and contemporary understandings of grief have a role to play in helping us provide effective quality support to those in a crisis who become vulnerable as a result of experiencing bereavement.

Subsequent chapters deal with a wide range of issues relating to grief and bereavement care. Each has its own particular focus, although the overarching themes of the book are to inform the reader, using a review of the evidence as support, on how practice may be improved by considering the wider implications of bereavement. It is hoped that this chapter has provided some food for thought regarding some of the main theoretical and cultural issues. Subsequent chapters enable the reader to interact with the text through the use of reflective questions as well as case study presentations, facilitating the integration of theory to practice. Group support and other methods for people with learning difficulties, older people and those who experience mental health problems are also covered in the book.

References

Attig T (1991) The importance of conceiving of grief as an active process. *Death Studies* 15(4): 385–393.

Bowen M (2002) *Family therapy in clinical practice.* London: Aronson.

Bowlby J (1963) Pathological mourning and childhood mourning. *Journal of the American Psychoanalytical Association* 11: 500–541.

Costello J and Kendrick KD (2000) Grief and older people: the making and breaking of emotional bonds following partner loss in later life. *Journal of Advanced Nursing* 32(6): 1374–1382.

Davies R (2004) New understandings of parental grief: literature review. *Journal of Advanced Nursing* 46(5): 506–513.

Doka KD and Martin T (2002) Masculine and feminine grieving. In: Doka KJ (ed.) *Disenfranchised grief: recognising hidden sorrows.* Lexington, MA: Lexington Books.

Field NP, Gal-Oz E and Bonanno GA (2003) Continuing bonds and adjustment at 5 years after the death of a spouse. *Journal of Consulting and Clinical Psychology* 71: 110–117.

Firth S (2000) Cross cultural perspectives on bereavement. In: Dickinson D, Johnson M and Katz JS (eds) *Death, dying and bereavement.* Sage: London.

Freud S (1957 [1917]) *Mourning and melancholia.* In: Strachey J. (ed. and trans.) *The standard edition of the complete psychological works of Sigmund Freud*, vol. 14. New York: Basic Books.

Gamino LA, Sewell KW and Easterling LW (2000) Scott and White Grief Study – Phase 2: toward an adaptive model of grief. *Death Studies* 24(7): 633–660.

Klass D, Silverman P and Nickman SL (1996) *Continuing bonds: newer understanding of grief.* Washington DC: Taylor & Francis.

Kübler-Ross E (1969) *On death and dying.* London: Macmillan.

Lindemann E (1944) Symptomatology and management of acute grief. *American Journal of Psychiatry* 191: 141–148.

Mallon B (2008) *Dying, death and grief.* London: Sage.

Mandelbaum DG (1959) The social uses of funeral rites. In: Kalish RA (ed.) *Death and dyings: views from many cultures.* Amityville, NY: Baywood Publishing.

Parkes CM (1972) *Bereavement: studies of grief in adult life.* New York: International Universities Press.

Parkes CM (2001) *Bereavement: studies of grief in adult life.* Penguin: London.

Rando TA (1985) Bereaved parents: particular difficulties, unique factors and treatment issues. *Social Work* 30: 19–24.

Rando TA (1986) *Parental loss of a child.* Champaign, IL: Research.

Rando TA (1995) Grief and mourning: accommodating to loss. In: Wass H and Neimeyer R (eds) *Dying: facing the facts.* Washington DC: Taylor & Francis.

Rothaupt JW and Becker K (2007) A literature review of western bereavement theory: from decathecting to continuing bonds. *The Family Journal: Counseling and Therapy for Couples and Families* 15(1): 6–15.

Silverman PR and Klass W (1996) What's the problem? In: Klass D, Silverman PR and Nickman SL (eds) *Continuing bonds: newer understanding of grief.* Philadelphia: Taylor & Francis.

Silverman PR and Worden WJ (1993) Children's reactions to the death of a parent. In: Stroebe M, Stroebe W and Hansson RO (eds) *Handbook of bereavement: theory, research and intervention.* New York: Cambridge University Press.

Stroebe M (1992) Coping with bereavement: a review of the grief work hypothesis. *Omega* 40: 351–374.

Stroebe M and Schut H (1999) The dual process model of coping with bereavement: rationale and description. *Death Studies* 23: 197–224.

Stroebe M and Stroebe W (1989) Who participates in bereavement research? A review and empirical study. *Omega* 20: 1–29.

Stroebe M and Stroebe W (1991) Does grief work work? *Journal of Consulting and Clinical Psychology* 59: 479–482.

Stroebe M, Gergen M, Gergen K and Stroebe W (1996) Broken hearts or broken bonds? In: Klass D, Silverman PR and Nickman SL (eds) *Continuing bonds: newer understanding of grief*. Washington DC: Taylor & Francis.

Walter T (1994) *The revival of death*. Routledge: London.

Walter T (1999) *On bereavement: the culture of grief*. Buckingham: Open University Press.

Williams R (1990) *A protestant legacy: attitudes towards death and illness in older Aberdonians*. Oxford: Oxford University Press.

Wimpenny P (2007) A literature review on bereavement and bereavement care: developing evidence-based practice in Scotland. *Bereavement Care* 26(1): 7–10.

Worden JW (2001) *Grief counselling and grief therapy*, 3rd edn. New York: Springer.

Worden WJ (1991) *Grief counselling and grief therapy: a handbook for the mental health practitioner*, 3rd edn. New York: Springer.

Wortman CB and Silver RC (1989) The myths of coping with loss. *Journal of Consulting and Clinical Psychology* 57(3): 349–357.

Part I

Bereavement across the lifespan

2 Bereavement in children and young people

Kim Morris

Key messages

Practitioners need to:

- Recognise the normality of grieving and the importance of allowing the natural process to evolve and when extra informal support will be appropriate.
- Know about the importance of rituals and leave-taking rituals associated with death.
- Provide reassurance that many of the feelings are relatively normal. In this sense it is important to give the young person permission to express thoughts, feelings, questions and worries and acknowledge the normality of grief.
- Give opportunities to explore the young person's questions of why and their subsequent feelings of injustice.
- Provide reassurance that the young person did not cause the death and that sometimes things happen for reasons that cannot be explained.
- Acknowledge and recognise the young person's individual relationship with the deceased.
- Facilitate opportunities for the young person to talk to others if they are finding it hard to talk to those close to them.
- Know that as a listener they can contain their emotions and that the person will not normally be hurt by anything that they say.

Introduction

The purpose of this chapter is to examine issues surrounding grief and bereavement in children and adolescents. In doing so the chapter examines the experience of young people's grief and how this may be influenced by the nature and the context of the death. Moreover, the impact of loss at the beginning of life can have an adverse impact on a young person's future, especially if the death was perceived in a negative way and there was a lack of support. Case illustrations taken from my professional experience are included to highlight particular aspects of young people's bereavement. It is important when working with young people that they receive clear information, explanation and discussion from practitioners who can clarify some of the complex explanations that often accompany death and bereavement. Children and young people experience grief differently from adults. Their grieving can seem more like leaping in and out of puddles. First reactions may range from great distress to seeming not to be interested. One minute they may be sobbing, the next they are asking 'What's for tea?' It does not mean they care any less about what has happened.

According to the Childhood Bereavement Network (2007) there are no official statistics on the number of children bereaved; however, samples suggest that around one in 25 children and young people aged 5–16 have experienced the death of a parent or sibling. Many more are bereaved of a grandparent, school friend or other relative or significant person.

Theorists regarding children's experiences and reactions to loss generally agree that children grieve regardless of age. However, a child's understanding of death is influenced by age, verbal ability, cognitive development and other factors, such as the circumstances of the death. Their understanding continues to grow over time as the child develops cognitively (Bunce and Rickards 2004). In terms of understanding, The Child Bereavement Charity (2008) advises that children under 5 years of age have no conception of the permanence of death and think that dead could mean less alive. At 5–8 years of age, young people are developing the idea of the permanence of death but may relate death to a consequence of violence or aggression. At this age they can become intensely interested in the rituals and the practicalities around death. From age 9 onwards young people are able to understand the concept of death and may become fearful about the inevitability and finality of death.

Children often express their grief intermittently for many years because of their difficulty in articulating their feelings and thoughts at a younger age. As children grow, their intellectual abilities increase and they need new information and new ways to express their feelings about death. Despite attempts to provide age-appropriate explanations, children will continue to ask questions repeatedly. This is not to gain new or different information but almost to check up on their understanding of the situation (Rando 1984).

Children are able to cope with death, dying and funerals better than many adults anticipate but they require information to be handled sensitively. Explanation needs to be without the use of euphemisms, avoiding the use of words such as 'lost' or 'gone away'. Children need to know what caused the death, that death is irreversible and universal, that the body no longer works, feels or moves, and that the body will decompose. They need to know that bad things happen to good people.

If children are given honest and clear information they may be more able to make informed choices about such things as whether to attend a funeral. The more pre-funeral information they are given, the less likely it is that they become overwhelmed by the experience. A child may be curious about what the body looks like, what the coffin is like, where the body is resting, what graves are and the role of the church or crematorium. It is crucial that the adult takes nothing for granted and is truthful with the child, in a manner appropriate to the child's age (Granot 2005). Some parents may be anxious about seeing children very upset. It is important for children to be given the opportunity to say goodbye and to be involved in ending rituals by being part of the family's grieving process.

A death in the family impacts on every member, affecting the foundations, the expectations and the dynamics of all within, yet children who receive compassion, understanding and early acknowledgement of their feelings can, it is contended, heal and grow from their bereavement experience (Auman 2007).

Bereavement for young people

Bereavement is a normal and painful process that takes time to work through for adults, adolescents and children, although in different ways, with different challenges. Although this makes determining outcomes difficult, Auman (2007) considers that adults often mistakenly assume that all children will bounce back after a short period of mourning. However, evidence illustrates that even in stable, caring family situations, about 20 per cent of young people will have complicated bereavement symptoms extending beyond one year after the death of a parent (Dowdney 2000; Christ *et al.* 2006).

A gentle mild-mannered 16-year-old boy (Tom), 2 months following the death of his father, described himself as being crazy and 'trashing' his room. He was overwhelmed with anger and resentment and identified that he did not get the chance to say goodbye to his dad. He felt that he had been lied to by his family, who assured him that his dad would be okay and encouraged him to continue studying for his exams.

What should parents and other adults do? Caring and shielding by adults can be misconstrued by the child as being lied to and manipulated. It can prove challenging to forgive the survivors.

The death of Tom's father evoked an emotional response that resulted in uncontrollable anger. Anger, although considered a normal response to death, can be overpowering (Kübler-Ross 1991). Tom was shielded by the other significant adults in his life to 'protect him', whilst being encouraged to keep studying hard for his exams and look towards the future. In grief the pressure can became immense and Tom felt that he was now unable to trust or believe his family or to communicate his feelings of anguish and loss. Bunce and Rickards (2004) highlight that sometimes young people find it hard to explain how they are feeling (alexithymia) because they do not fully understand what is happening – their lives have become so muddled. They may not have all the information about what has happened or they may have been told inconsistent stories and so struggle to discern the truth.

Anticipating the death of a parent

Although a sudden death is shocking, living with a dying parent for weeks, months or years can also be very difficult for a child and puts stress on the entire family. In this case, support must include the use of anticipatory bereavement approaches

(Christ *et al.* 2006). This would take the form of gentle preparation by exploring feelings, fears and understanding expressed by parents or a trusted professional.

> An 8-year-old boy, John, had been cared for by a procession of friends and neighbours for 5 years whilst his mum sought curative treatment abroad, with his dad accompanying her. John was a ghost-like figure on the periphery of the situation during his mum's illness and following her death. Most of his life had revolved around sickness and death and was dominated by anxiety. There was a deeply oppressive feel in the house with no discussion about John's grief.

Siegel and colleagues (1996) studied children whose parents were in the terminal stages of illness. His findings suggest that when parental death follows a lengthy terminal illness a child's distress can precede the death itself. Unfortunately, John was lost amongst the activity of dying and death. There was neither preparation for death nor encouragement of sharing and exploring his grief because of the high level of anguish of those around him. Studies of bereaved children highlight misunderstanding and guilt surrounding the parent's deteriorating condition and terminal illness. Children and adolescents report that they value open communication with both parents about the illness and death, with research suggesting that it helps them during their bereavement (Siegel *et al.* 1996). This was illustrated through an experience of working with a young mum, Mary, who was preparing for her own death. Mary broke the news to her children (aged 7 and 5), explaining that she was going to die and what would happen to them. The eldest child thanked her mum, saying that it would have been terrible for her to die without them knowing as she intended to make every day special with her until she died. In preparation, the family were able to draw on their own spiritual and cultural beliefs together.

Although this was an emotionally charged, anguished time, Mary was able to say her goodbyes openly until she died and her children were able to show their love and create memories to sustain them into adulthood. When death is imminent, health professionals can help prepare parents by providing specific, concrete information and practical advice to facilitate coping and meeting children's needs at this very stressful, emotional time.

On the death of a parent

Kiernan (1992), using data from the UK National Child Development Study for children at age 16, found that 5.5 per cent had experienced family disruption through the death of a parent. The figures are still appropriate today and highlight the extent of this form of bereavement.

A parent who is struggling with their own depressive symptoms following spousal death will pose a risk factor for their bereaved child. One of the many fears following the death of a spouse can be financial, including the impact of loss of earnings, paying the mortgage or rent and provision of quality child care. Financial hardship affects the ways in which a family can cope with a death (Corden *et al.* 2008), as does the presence of other stressful life events going on in tandem within the family. Bereaved children need love and boundaries; however, it is likely that the person providing love and structure might offer less as a result of their own bereavement experience (Dowdney 2000; Trickey 2008).

Children affected by these additional stressors will warrant more careful monitoring, and the offer of support for their grieving parents is likely to be an important part of the recovery of the surviving parent and young person (Cerel *et al.* 2006). Health and social care professionals need to be aware of the propensity towards this type of bereavement response. Siblings can and do experience, and display, different responses to the same death. Consequently, they may have different needs (MacPherson and Emeleus 2007), so children may need to be monitored or assessed on an individual basis rather than as part of a unit.

Some adults experiencing loss and grief withdraw and neglect their children or may misuse harmful substances, particularly alcohol. Obviously this is not an appropriate method of coping to display to a child and can result in children interacting or adapting inappropriately themselves, not only initially but also later in their lives. This could mean that these children are unable to share with others or understand and identify how they are feeling. Children have good reasons for having strong emotions which, if not understood, can result in severe behavioural and mental health problems in the future. The responsible adult needs to be able to cope with the child's needs.

However, parents may not be able to cope with their own grief to the extent that their parenting capacity is diminished or their personal circumstances prior to the loss rule them out as alternative carers for the child. If the child has no surviving or capable parent, there may be times when the extended family helps; if not, an alternative carer needs to be identified. In such cases there may be an on-going responsibility to ensure that the emotional health of children who are separated from their primary carers is promoted and that they have the opportunity to form positive attachments to alternative carers. Given the long-term effects of lack of attachment (Parkes *et al.* 1991), the influence of an alternative carer is crucial as children need on-going relationships to continue their growth and development. The well-being of the child's future includes a consideration of their need to be able to grieve the separation from their significant others. Unresolved separations are known to interfere with the formation of new relationships in later life. The alternative carer will need optimum support to enable them to manage the physical, emotional, psychological and spiritual effect of bereavement on the young person. Although the alternative carer may be a friend or family member, they may also be a health and social care professional (see Chapter 9).

The experience of death for adolescents

Adolescence is a bewildering time of biological, psychological and social change due to puberty, cognitive changes in thinking, changes in self-esteem and social changes with parents and peers (Schultz 2007). Adolescence is a particularly difficult time both for children and for those dealing with them, even without the added dimension of bereavement. If bereavement occurs, the confusion in their lives may become heightened.

It is common for teenagers to question thoughts around the meaning of life, and this may be intensified by the experience of the death of someone close to them (Trickey 2008). Teenagers respond to their bereavement experience (as do other age groups), in a variety of ways, grieving similarly to adults with feelings of sadness, confusion, anger and depression. They may find that these very intense emotions are difficult to manage. Evidence from available literature suggests that it is difficult to differentiate between the direct impact of the bereavement and its consequences (Dowdney 2000; Trickey 2008). An example of this is the differences in the quality of parenting, which may shift, with resultant disruption of home life, hopes and fears.

Distress as part of the grieving response can be displayed as behavioural problems, temper tantrums, bullying, concentration issues, sleep problems and regression (Ribbens-McCarthy and Jessop 2005). This is normal and reactions generally decrease over time. Some reactions may increase over time: for example, social withdrawal, social problems, low self-esteem and anxiety, difficulty in coping with schoolwork, fear of leaving the house in case something bad happens, health fears for others, anger and violence. Adolescents can appear unemotional and may avoid discussion of the deceased in order to control powerful emotions. Adolescents may also be very busy living their lives and become independent outside their families, appearing to be burying their feelings about the loss (Trickey 2008). Sharing their emotions with adults is especially difficult at a time when they are trying to establish their own identity and break away from the family hold (Sweetland 2005). Some may revert to childish behaviours whereas others may act grown up and feel responsible for other family members.

Some adolescents may engage in risk-taking behaviour, such as drug taking or alcohol abuse, and self-harm may also be used as a way of gaining control or dealing with grief. These maladaptive coping strategies may not appear instantly but may develop over time. These young people require guidance to adopt safer, more appropriate ways of managing their bereavement. These responses and others are typical of how an adolescent might cope with bereavement as well as being part of the emotional maturation process. Sometimes it is difficult to differentiate between them.

There may be an expectation within families that after the death of a parent, a teenager will take on adult roles within a family, exerting even greater pressure on them to grow up quickly. Social support for adults can help to bring about a less distressing grief experience; however, adolescents don't like to be different and bereaved adolescents tend to become socially withdrawn (Worden 1996). They may often make efforts to appear normal despite their loss so they will not stand out amongst their peers. Adolescents can crave solitude and anonymity and so often respond well to 'faceless' support chat lines on websites. Friends may be of less help as they have little experience of bereavement (Sweetland 2005) and may not understand the torrents of emotional labour that surround the bereaved adolescent.

Adolescents may also find it hard to relate to their peers for fear of being perceived as different, and may worry about being asked questions for which they do not have answers or in response to which they may not want to disclose specific information regarding the death. They may also worry about being teased by their peers if they display their emotions, such as crying, or worry that they will not be believed or taken seriously when talking about their experience.

Like many young people, adolescents sometimes benefit from limits and boundaries and become aware that the adults around them are still able to protect them. They require the reassurance that they are loved and cared about when faced with life-changing experiences. They also need information and access to support when they feel they require it and this needs to be on their own terms. It is as important for adolescents as for anyone else experiencing the grieving process to tell their story.

The experience of sibling death

The experiences of bereavement that young people are most likely to encounter are the death of an infant sibling followed by the death of a male friend or sibling aged 15–24 (Charlton 1996). The death of a sibling, according to Christian (2007), is likely to have a longstanding impact on the character development of a surviving child. Dead siblings are frequently more important rivals than live ones, and the death of a sibling may reactivate feelings of rivalry, guilt and resentment as well as feelings of anger, sadness and sorrow, with the deceased being idealised in the minds of surviving family members.

Because the grieving process is both an individual and a family one, a child's death disrupts the way the family functions and alters the way parents and surviving siblings relate to each other (Detmer and Lamberti 1991). The sibling loss is a double loss for the child – not only the death of the sibling but often the loss of their parents' support. Parents often do not have the emotional energy left to support their remaining children because of their own grief.

A young person's fear and grief may be compounded by witnessing their parent's distress and vulnerability along with the emotive nature of their parent's feelings. The parent's distress is often so intense that bereaved young people protect their parents by not mentioning the deceased, believing it will upset them even more. Having opportunity outwith the family to grieve may be appropriate. Potts and colleagues (1999) discuss the value of a 'treasure weekend' as one through which bereaved siblings can express their grief, remember their sister or brother and potentially move on. Such events may then have a positive impact on family functioning.

A young girl (Jenny), whose brother died following a lengthy illness, had become used to taking second place during his illness. Following the death of her brother, Jenny's time was spent supporting her parents by 'being good', keeping emotions and anguish to herself to protect her parents.

Young people often attribute their parents' behaviour to some fault or failing of their own; seeing a grief-stricken parent sink into a state of mourning may have implications for the child's future, in terms of growing up and leaving the family home (Horsley and Patterson 2006). Marital strain may also accompany the loss of a child. Difficulties in the parents' relationship can become an added burden on surviving children who, because of the parents' state of mind, may operate in a state of constant vigilant awareness.

Conversely, parents who have lost a child can react with excessive anxiety over surviving children, particularly in response to any ailments or signs of illness, which in turn can affect the coping strategies of the survivors. Open communication in a supportive environment within the family is crucial following a sibling death. If the trauma of the loss cannot be worked through, it may become stagnant, emerging later in the child's life when activated by similar losses or events that represent loss (Christian 2007).

A literature review by Huntzinger (1995) has two recurrent threads that are linked to this: one that is focused on the relationship between the siblings and the consequences of the loss, and a second focusing on the loss of attention because of the parent's own grief reactions (McCown and Davies 1995; Potts *et al.* 1999).

The role of the surviving child may change, as might the relationships within the family, and this should be considered when dealing with sibling loss. More aggressive behaviour in the surviving child has been identified, particularly in younger children, and has been interpreted as a need for attention (McCown and Davies 1995). A similar analysis carried out by Birenbaum (2000) highlights the need for better assessment of children to establish the problems associated with the death of a sibling.

Bereavement by suicide

Suicide is now one of the leading causes of death in men in the 15- to 44-year-old age group, and it is towards the younger end of the spectrum that rates are increasing. This makes it a particular area of concern for children and young people's bereavement as many fathers may be included in this age group. The issues surrounding bereavement through suicide are discussed more fully in Chapter 6; however, it is worthy of further consideration here in respect of children and young people.

The World Health Organization (http://www.who.int/mental_health/prevention/suicide/suicideprevent/en/) reports that in the year 2000 approximately 1,000,000 people died from suicide – that is, one death every 40 seconds. In Great Britain, 6,000 suicides were reported in 2004 (Brock *et al.* 2006). Scotland has the highest suicide rate in Great Britain (Brock *et al.* 2006). In men, the highest suicide rate was found in the 15–44 age group, whilst in women it was found to be in those over 75 years of age.

Most people find suicide difficult to understand. It might be even harder for children bereaved through suicide to be able to think about positive memories or good things relating to the person who died, particularly if the child has been living with a parent with mental health problems for a prolonged period. The young person may worry about developing their own mental health problems or that they might commit suicide too (Bunce and Rickards 2004; Trickey 2005). This can be heightened by news stories, such as the suicide of Sylvia Plath's son, when questions of a genetic predisposition to suicide were raised.

Children who are survivors of parental suicide need to try to cope with the death and the stigma. They tend to experience even higher rates of anxiety, depression, poor school performance and decreased social adjustments than children whose parents died of natural causes (Mitchell *et al.* 2006). Guilt inevitably will surround the death; children and adults assume that the suicide was their fault or that they could have prevented it. Children bereaved by suicide suffer more shame and may assume that the deceased's rejection of life is in some way also a rejection of them. For teenagers there is an increased risk of drug and alcohol misuse following bereavement by suicide as these substances have a numbing effect. This can mean that by the time the young person displays an overt reaction to grief, everyone has assumed that they are doing fine and support is no longer offered (Trickey 2005).

A number of studies focus on the effects of psychotherapeutic interventions to help child survivors of parental suicide cope with their loss. Results concentrate on realistic and accurate communication so that young people can effectively grieve the loss of their parent. One of the ways in which people make sense of their experiences is to talk them through with those around them. When discussing suicide with children, communication needs to be as clear and honest as possible. However, there continues to be a particular stigma attached to suicide so it is talked about less than other deaths (Trickey 2005). The absence of discussion, often to hide shame and guilt, means that children can be denied opportunities to make sense of the death.

The death of a pet

Although the above sections have covered loss related to parents, siblings and others, pet loss is often a child's first experience of death. Kaufman and Kaufman (2006) and Tuzeo-Jarolmen (2007) consider that the death of a pet evokes all the same symptoms in a young person as if they had suffered a human loss and encourage parents not to trivialise a young person's grief. Greene (2003) even proposes that the grief experienced on losing a pet is similar to that on losing a family member or close friend. Anecdotally, it is considered that the death of a pet can prepare a child for the deaths of significant others in the future. From this viewpoint, it is crucial that the young person is enabled to work through and experience grief at their own pace in a loving supportive environment.

There is often an emotional impact when a pet dies (Harris 2003), which it is suggested can have a devastating effect and could lead to mental health issues. This may be different between boys and girls; studies that compare attachment styles suggest that girls usually develop stronger attachments to pets and so will suffer more when a pet dies (Brown 1996; Reynolds 1999; Wrobel and Dye 2003). However, there appears to be little evidence to substantiate this claim.

Advice such as that by Ironside (1994), who suggests techniques for coping with the death of a pet, and Sharkin and Knox (2003), in a guide for psychologists, pays special attention to how young people are affected by the death of a pet. When considering subsequent bereavements it may be that the experience of pet loss has a significantly greater impact than we might realise, particularly as loss of a family member is increasingly occurring later in life.

Support in school

School is a place where pet bereavement and other losses may be seen to impact on children and young people. Ribbens-McCarthy's and Jessop's (2005) research illustrates that schools have the potential to play a significant part in supporting a child in bereavement. One estimate suggests that 70 per cent of schools may be dealing with a bereaved child at any one time (Holland 1997).

However, Lowton and Higginson (2003) consider that there is inequity in the UK regarding bereavement services and policies within schools, which may be echoed globally. They identify a lack of provision for bereavement education and training for teachers to enable them to provide school-based counselling. They highlight concerns expressed by teachers that there is limited on-going communication between health and social care agencies and schools.

Holland (1997) discusses a survey based in schools in Humberside, UK, which highlighted that teachers were aware of problems in bereaved children and so recognised a need for training and guidelines. Similar findings are reported in other cultures (Papadatou *et al.* 2002 in Greece; Servaty-Seib *et al.* 2003 in the USA) although there are also distinct educational, ritual and family oriented factors which may not be present in the UK. As a result of findings, Holland (2003) went on to develop and introduce a structured interactive training package 'Lost for Words'. This has resulted in teachers in one area being trained in dealing with loss and bereavement issues through a structured training programme, thus empowering teachers to be able to handle sensitive issues such as grief. This has also led to the introduction of policies on bereavement in schools where training has taken place.

In support of such programmes Lowton and Higginson (2003) and Servaty-Seib and Hayslip (2003) identify numerous practical approaches that can be used by teachers and schools to deal with bereavement. These range from methods and approaches to improve communication with children and families to ensuring involvement of pupils in decision making. There is certainly a wide range of web-based, video/DVD and printed material which may be helpful.

Many schools offer the *Seasons for Growth* programme. Introduced in 1996, this is a grief education course involving small group work, whose vision is 'A healthy society where grief and loss are recognised as a normal part of life and appropriate support is available to all' (www.seasonsforgrowth.co.uk). This is a well-established programme in Australia, New Zealand, Ireland and the UK. It is run in small groups of five to seven participants, facilitated by a trained companion, and promotes the recognition of normal emotions encouraging expression of grief with peer support. The aim is for participants to support, understand and manage their grief experience caused by loss through death, separation or divorce. Whereas teachers need to be trained in bereavement skills, children also need the offer of provision of bereavement services from external agencies if required (Lowton and Higginson 2003).

It is crucial that the young person's school be informed when bereavement has occurred or is expected to occur. One of the places where children may indicate how they are feeling is at school. Unlike everywhere else, it may be the one place that has not altered following bereavement. Consequently, school may be viewed as a safe place for young people to either not talk about what is happening or alternatively express their worries.

Areas to consider in terms of a child's bereavement response and school are that the child may worry about attending school in case something happens at home whilst they are away. This will result in them finding it hard to concentrate on lessons or find it to contain their emotions throughout the school day. Alternatively, the young person may become highly focused on achievement and being 'good' as a way of forgetting their grief. Their behaviour may in fact mask how a child is truly feeling. This may be seen as an example of hidden grief (Doka 2002).

School administrators must be made aware of the burden that pupils carry when they experience a traumatic loss and of their need for individual, informal bereavement assessment. School nurses and guidance teachers are ideally situated to participate in supportive care if they are aware of factors that affect childhood grief (Auman 2007).

This should extend to higher education, with Balk (2001) suggesting that universities should also have a centre to deal with the support of students who are bereaved. Such a centre, he suggests, should also have a responsibility for undertaking research into grief and bereavement. He believes that students are hidden grievers who will not make use of pastoral care and may view counselling as an indication that they are not coping and are perhaps in need of mental health support. His argument is persuasive when considering that the potential number of students who may be recently bereaved is high and the extent to which their bereavement may impact on retention and completion of their course.

Mementos/resources for adaptation

Although there is limited evidence of their effectiveness, remembrance and commemoration can be very important, not only for the initial bereavement experience but also as the child grows and matures into adulthood. Memories sustain children through adolescence into adulthood. The child can make a memory box to include the deceased's perfume or aftershave, photos, trinkets, letters or items which are significantly personal to that relationship. Memory boxes can be created by parents who know they are dying and left for a child. These can take the form of making a recording on video or DVD, creating a biography, writing letters for significant future events or leaving memories of special times or occasions.

I remember a child of 9 (Flora) having a plaster of Paris mould of her mum's handprint. She used it to place her hand into her mum's when she needed to feel close. In preparation for her expected death, her mum prepared this during a play time with her child. Making a plaster of Paris mould of a parent's hand can be a creative activity to share with the person who is ill, and in bereavement to have the hand print of the parent can create a much-needed connection.

There is a great deal of literature available which can be a very powerful, yet gentle, resource to support children. Books and leaflets are available to support parents preparing their child for a death and for parents supporting a bereaved child in terms of what to expect behaviourally and what sort of language to use. Corr (2000) identifies a range of death-related literature which he considers useful to be read with or by children. He considers that this can assist in raising and answering some crucial questions.

Bereavement activity books for both children and adolescents to use are extremely useful and are designed to explore emotions, changes and memories. Such books discuss ways of coping and introduce ideas to ponder and explore. This allows exploration of feelings in a non-challenging way that can be carried out at the child's own pace. The child is able to revisit these books over the years as their development and maturity grows. There are many leaflets and types of literature available to help parents support their child. Health and social care professionals need to be aware of how to gain access to them. This requirement is supported by Schuurman (2004), who identifies selected literature for professionals and parents to assist them in supporting bereaved children. A number of formalised bereavement service providers exist to help parents and their children. Childhood bereavement services such as Winston's Wish and Compassionate Friends are instrumental in this process and offer a spectrum of bereavement services for young people in the UK. There is also a diverse range of service provision and interventions available within individual communities.

The role of health and social care in childhood bereavement

It is important to remember that not every child is in need of external support or will necessarily experience problems. Bereavement care must certainly be available to young people, but if possible it should be provided by the parents or close family members. Grief is an intensely personal journey and is shaped by our culture, beliefs and family. The person ideally suited to support a child through grief is someone from within that family or who plays a part in their spiritual, cultural and religious background.

Health and social care support needs to be about facilitating the family to grieve together and, primarily, supporting the surviving adult or significant adult in the child's life to allow them to support their child. The family live the culture, they talk the language used, and they have come through the previous happy or challenging experiences of the family. Only that family has a lifetime of knowing each other. The professional role must be to advise and support parents on what is a 'normal' bereavement process and what can be expected, in order for them to recognise when a child is developing a complicated bereavement response that requires professional intervention. Health and social carers also need to be aware of what resources are appropriate and available within their area and who would benefit from them.

Parents often find it difficult to understand and respond to their children's unique, developmentally specific, expressions of grief, which may seem unconcerned, callous or indifferent and at times inappropriate by adult standards (Christ *et al.* 2006), so health and social carers professionals need to be well informed and understanding in their response to a bereaved child or to the parent supporting that child and in identifying distressed or disturbed families in need of more formal support.

Box 2.1 can be used to reinforce and highlight the sort of behaviour that indicates that the young person is successfully adapting to their loss, and therefore draws together the different scenarios of death and bereavement that have been discussed so far.

Conversely, behaviour which may indicate that the young person requires additional, focused bereavement support is identified in Box 2.2. Adults should be conscious of certain tell-tale modes of behaviour that might indicate distress.

Although the above may seem self-explanatory, it must be remembered that, for children and young people, bereavement may have an impact that will remain with them into adulthood. Addressing their needs more fully may, it is concluded, help to produce greater benefits in the future.

As can be seen in Box 2.2, there are a considerable number of behaviours that could be attributable to factors other than bereavement. However, it illustrates the degree to which some children may be affected by a death and how this may impact on their lives and on the lives of those around them. In using Box 2.2 it is advisable to take into account the age of the young person and the length of time that they are 'stuck' in this behaviour.

Box 2.1 Indications of successful adaptation (Granot 2005)

- Returns to a normal eating and sleeping pattern
- Activity, enquiring mind and energy return alongside enthusiasm
- Returns to planning activities and renewing social contacts and activities
- Able to form new healthy relationships
- Regains the level of independence enjoyed prior to the loss
- Spends less time in the close proximity of adults and spends time playing with friends
- Understands the finality and irreversibility of new circumstances
- Conforming with changed reality

Box 2.2 Indications of poor adaptation (Granot 2005)

- Absolute disregard and complete denial of the death and its implications
- On-going consistent intense anxiety, fear and panic
- Complaints of illness or pain with no medical evidence to support the claim
- On-going feelings of guilt
- Chronic depression and apathy
- Chronic anger and aggressive behaviour
- Frequent offensive temper tantrums
- Openly displays an abusive manner
- Initiates fights
- Exhibits disobedience and acts in a rebellious way despite disturbing those around
- Drastic behaviour change and instability for a prolonged period of time
- Decline in schoolwork
- Keeping a distance from friends and family for a prolonged period
- Dramatic changes to sleep pattern or eating habits
- Bedwetting and/or poor bowel control
- Abuse of alcohol and or drugs
- Suicidal thoughts and/or actions including the taking of exaggerated risks
- Clashes with authority figures
- Adolescents exhibiting inappropriate sexual behaviour

Conclusion

The adaptation to bereavement of children and young people is significant but often unknown, assumed and poorly supported. It is clear that effective information, explanation and discussion from practitioners and others (for example, teachers) can help to clarify some of the complex explanations that often accompany death. Recognising the normality of grief and enabling practitioners to access knowledge about death, dying and bereavement is an important goal. Doing so can help to influence practice principles by giving young people permission to express thoughts, feelings, questions and worries. This chapter has raised the issue of the normality of grief for young people and the need to allow them time and the opportunity to find out what they want to know. Crucially, it is also important to allow opportunities for young people to explore their questions about death and be provided with the reassurance that they did not cause the death and that sometimes things happen for reasons that cannot be explained. Moreover, practitioners will come to learn to acknowledge and recognise the young person's unique, individual relationship with the deceased.

References

Auman MJ (2007) Bereavement support for children. *Journal of School Nursing* 23(1): 34–39.

Balk DE (2001) College student bereavement, scholarship and the university: a call for university engagement. *Death Studies* 25(1): 67–84.

Birenbaum LK (2000) Assessing children's and teenagers' bereavement when a sibling dies from cancer: a secondary analysis. *Child Care Health and Development* 26(5): 381–400.

Brock A, Baker A and Griffiths C (2006) *Suicide trends and geographical variations in the United Kingdom. Health Statistics Quarterly* 31: 6–22.

Brown B (1996) Pet bonding and pet bereavement among adolescents *Journal of Counselling and Development* 74(5): 505–509.

Bunce M and Rickards A (2004) Working with bereaved children: a guide. Available at: http://www.essex.ac.uk/armedcon/unit/projects/wwbc_guide/ (accessed 2011).

Cerel J, Fristad MA, Verducci J, Weller RA and Weller EB (2006) Childhood bereavement: psychopathology in the 2 years post parental death. *Journal of the American Academy of Child and Adolescent Psychiatry* 45(6): 681–690.

Charlton J (1996) Trends in all cause mortality: 1841–1994. In: Charlton J and Murphy M (eds) *The health of adult Britain 1941–1994*, Vol. 1. London: HMSO.

Child Bereavement Charity (2008) When your partner dies: supporting your children. Available at: http://www.childbereavement.org.uk/support_information/cbc_shop/free_downloadable_resources/when_a_parent_dies_supporting_your_children (accessed 21 June 2011).

Childhood Bereavement Network (2007) Grief matters for kids campaign. Available at: http://www.childhoodbereavementnetwork.org.uk/griefMatters.htm (accessed 21 June 2011).

Christ GH and Christ AE (2006) Current approaches to helping children cope with a parent's terminal illness. *Cancer Journal for Clinicians* 56(4): 197–212.

Christian C (2007) Sibling loss guilt and reparation: a case study. *International Journal of Psychoanalysis* 88(1): 41–54.

Corden A, Hirst M and Nice K (2008) Financial implications of the death of a partner. York: SPRU, University of York. Available at: http://www.york.ac.uk/spru/pubs/1148/ (accessed 21 June 2011).

Corr CA (2000) Using books to help children and adolescents cope with death: guidelines and bibliography. In: Doka KJ (ed.) *Living with grief: children, adolescents and loss.* Washington, DC: Hospice Foundation of America.

Detmer CM and Lamberti JW (1991) Family grief. *Death Studies* 15(4): 363–374.

Doka KJ (ed.) (2002) *Disenfranchised grief: recognising hidden sorrows.* Lexington, MA: Lexington Books.

Dowdney L (2000) Annotation: childhood bereavement following parental death. *Journal of Child Psychology and Psychiatry* 41(7): 819–830.

Granot T (2005) *Without you: children and young people growing up with loss and its effects.* London: Jessica Kingsley Publishers

Greene LA (2003) *Saying goodbye to the pet you love: a complete resource to help you heal.* Oakland, CA: New Harbinger.

Harris JA (2003*) Pet loss: a spiritual guide.* New York: Lantern Books.

Holland J (1997) Child bereavement in Humberside schools. *Bereavement Care* 16(1): 8–10.

Holland J (2003) Supporting schools with loss: lost for words in Hull. *British Journal of Special Education* 30(2): 76–78.

Horsley H and Patterson T (2006) The effects of a parent guidance intervention on communication among adolescents who have experienced the sudden death of a sibling. *American Journal of Family Therapy* 34(2): 119–137.

Huntzinger NW (1995) A selective review and discussion of the literature on early sibling loss. *Depression and Stress* 1(2): 133–163.

Ironside V (1994) *Goodbye dear friend: coming to terms with the death of a pet*. London: Robson Books.

Kiernan KE (1992) The impact of family disruption in childhood and transitions made in young adult life. *Population Studies* 46(2): 213–234.

Kübler-Ross E (1991) *On death and dying*. London: Macmillan.

Lowton K and Higginson I (2003) Managing bereavement in the classroom: a conspiracy of silence? *Death Studies* 27(8): 717–741.

Kaufman K and Kaufman N (2006) And then the dog died. *Death Studies* 30(1): 61–76.

McCown DE and Davies B (1995) Patterns of grief in young children following the death of a sibling. *Death Studies* 19(1): 41–53.

MacPherson C and Emeleus M (2007) Children's needs when facing the death of a parent from cancer: part two. *International Journal of Palliative Nursing* 13(12): 590–597.

Mitchell AM, Wesner S, Brownson L, Dysart-Gale D, Garland L and Havill A (2006) Effective communication with bereaved child survivors of suicide. *Journal of Child and Adolescent Psychiatric Nursing* 19(3): 130–136.

Papadatou D, Metallinou O, Hatzichristou C and Pavlida L (2002) Supporting the bereaved child: a teacher's perceptions and experiences in Greece. *Mortality* 7(3): 324–339.

Parkes CM, Stevenson-Hinde J and Marris P (1991) *Attachment across the life cycle*. London: Routledge.

Potts S, Farrell M and O'Toole J (1999) Treasure weekend: supporting bereaved siblings. *Palliative Medicine* 13(1): 51–56.

Rando T (1984) *Grief dying and death: clinical interventions for caregivers*. Champaign, IL: Research Press Company.

Reynolds TE (1999) Pet bonding and pet bereavement as a function of culture and gender differences among adolescents. University of Sarasota, FL, EdD thesis.

Ribbens-McCarthy J and Jessop J (2005) *Young people, bereavement and loss: disruptive transitions?* London: National Children's Bureau for the Joseph Rowntree Foundation.

Schultz LE (2007) The influence of maternal loss on young women's experience of identity development in emerging adulthood. *Death Studies* 31(1): 17–43.

Schuurman DL (2004) Literature for adults to assist them in helping bereaved children. *Omega* 48(4): 415–424.

Seasons for Growth (1986) Available at: http://www.seasonsforgrowth.co.uk (accessed 1 November 2008).

Servaty-Seib H and Hayslip B (2003) Post-loss adjustment and funeral perceptions of parentally bereaved adolescents and adults. *Omega* 46(3): 251–261.

Sharkin B and Knox D (2003) Pet loss: issues and implications for the psychologist. *Research and Practice* 34(4): 414–421.

Siegel K, Karus D and Raveis VH (1996) Adjustment of children facing the death of a parent due to cancer. *Journal of the American Academy of Child and Adolescent Psychiatry* 35(4): 442–450.

Sweetland C (2005) The palliative care nurse's role in supporting the adolescent child of a dying patient. *International Journal of Palliative Nursing* 11(6): 294–298.

Trickey D (2005) Young people bereaved by suicide: what hinders and what helps. *Bereavement Care* 24(1): 11–13.

Trickey D (2008) Grief and adolescence. Available at: http://www.traumaticstress.org.uk (accessed 11 March 2008).

Tuzeo-Jarolmen JA (2007) *When a family pet dies: a guide to dealing with children's loss.* London: Jessica Kingsley.

Worden WJ (1996) *Children and grief: when a parent dies.* New York: Guilford Press.

Wrobel T and Dye A (2003) Grieving pet death: normative, gender and attachment issues. *Omega* 47(4): 385–393.

3   Parental and family bereavement

Fiona Work and Sylvia Wilcock

Key messages

- Professionals supporting bereaved families need to consider patterns of family cohesion and the different influences on family dynamics caused by a death.
- There is evidence of a range of factors which influence grief and bereavement in parents that need to be assessed and addressed by all professional groups who may deal with death and dying in children.
- Co-ordinated interventions using validated programmes of support and trained staff may make a difference to the trajectories of normal grief and reduce the likelihood of complicated grief.
- Professionals working with families may be able to predict which individuals will require most support, from their knowledge of the family dynamics and their awareness of a range of risk and protective factors.
- Although grief is not sex specific, males and females demonstrate different grieving styles.
- Parents need effective information about the impact of loss on children in order to be able to offer support and meet their needs as well as those of other family members.

Introduction

The purpose of this chapter is to provide a broad overview of a number of related topics focused on parental and family bereavement. The quantity of literature available is quite large, although the quality is often not robust (Wimpenny *et al.* 2007).

As parental grief will have an impact on the family unit as a whole, parental and family bereavement are discussed together. A considerable amount of available literature on parental bereavement exists in the context of palliative care, which will be alluded to in this chapter, although the focus of much of the discussion will include spousal and parental bereavement with an additional focus on gender differences in grieving. The chapter is supplemented by authentic case studies taken from one author's clinical practice.

The family unit

Kissane and Bloch (1994) defined family bereavement as a loss of one of its members, whether a nuclear or extended family unit, such that those who are bereaved will influence and be influenced by the others. Even with divorce rates falling in Britain in 2008, about one-quarter of the couples divorcing had at least one child under the age of 16 (Office for National Statistics 2009). In addition, some children are born to single parents or same-sex parents; thus the family unit today is a broad contextual statement with multifaceted definitions. However, defining the make-up of a family unit from an anthropological, biological or sociological stance is not particularly important to families after a death. Moreover, for health and social care professionals, it is necessary to be able to offer a non-judgemental, deep sense of caring and personal involvement (Fetus and Newborn Committee and Canadian Paediatric Society 2001). Additionally, holistic care of a family unit as a whole is complex, as anthropological nature, ethnicity and religious affiliation may have a strong influence on the family grieving responses and process (Kissane and Bloch 1994).

Traylor and colleagues (2003), in their American study of 61 individuals who had experienced parental or spousal bereavement, found that the family structure was of less importance than the cohesiveness of the family unit. Their findings indicated that families who were more cohesive in terms of the way they worked together, and shared ideas and feelings, reported fewer adverse grief symptoms over time. Families able to express their emotions with one another reported less intense grief over time compared with what were described as stoic families. Fletcher (2002) labels this process *reunification*, whereby the family communicate with each other, sharing ideas, information, values and beliefs in an attempt to reduce isolation within the family and restore the family unit. Kissane and Bloch (1994) add that family interaction can be more pronounced in cases of distressing illness, such as those observed in families where a member has died of cancer or by suicide. Another area requiring additional support was for individuals and families who experienced a loss due to circumstances described as clandestine.

Doka (1999) describes situations like these, where relationships are not overt, such as people who have extramarital affairs or cases of sexual relations with same-sex partners. In such circumstances, the wider community is often unaware of the true nature of the relationship. When the death of a partner in such cases occurs, Doka (1989, 1999) calls this *disenfranchised* grief because its true nature is hidden. Such secret relationships have been known to cause the family great distress because they are not publicly recognised. Such grief reactions can occur in a number of ways:

Jane lived with Bob for 7 years; Bob had three children from a previous relationship, but they had no children of their own. Bob had previously been married to Susan and had never divorced, and although he had not lived with her for almost 7 years he continued to maintain and pay for the marital home. Jane had a good relationship with Bob's children but they had ignored her at the funeral at their mother's request. On Bob's gravestone it said: 'Bob, loving husband of Susan'.

Jane found visiting the grave challenging and felt she had nowhere else to go to remember him. The words on the gravestone were hurtful and made her feel isolated and resentful when she visited. She felt excluded from his former life, even though she had nursed him until he died peacefully at home, with her. His children appeared to cut her out and the family she felt she had appeared to die with Bob. Jane came to counselling to share her frustration and pain of feeling 'the other woman' forever, and the pain of losing her family. After only a few sessions, Jane decided that she would make a new life for herself and re-established a relationship with Bob's children. Jane built a memorial bush in her garden that she shared with Bob. She bought a special garden seat which she placed beside the bush, where she sat in the summer months, and talked about Bob when his children came to visit. These visits were valuable for both Jane and the children. Jane never visited his grave again as she felt that it was not here that she remembered him. He loved her garden when he was alive and the garden was full of happy memories.

The above case illustrates the need for professionals to have some knowledge of family dynamics (Traylor *et al.* 2003) in order to work effectively with the bereaved. In this way they could potentially identify those members of the family unit who may require additional support.

Identifying family members who require support

Identifying families in need of some form of intervention is important and the use of screening tools such as the 12-item brief version of the family relationship tool, known as the family relationship index (Moos and Moos 1981), could potentially aid assessment of family cohesion, conflict and expressiveness (Kissane *et al.* 1998).

Kissane and colleagues (1996) also identify five family types that could be helpful for determining needs in bereavement care: supportive, conflict-resolving, intermediate, sullen and hostile.

- *Supportive* families demonstrated high levels of cohesiveness, showed minimal conflict with each other and had an ability to be openly expressive.
- *Conflict-resolving* families demonstrated ability to handle conflict effectively through expressiveness and cohesion.
- *Intermediate* families demonstrated moderate cohesiveness, but were regarded as being prone to psychological morbidity.
- *Sullen*-type families demonstrated moderate levels of conflict, cohesiveness and expressiveness.

- *Hostile* families demonstrated high conflict, low cohesiveness and moderate expressiveness.

Half of the families reported by Kissane and colleagues (1998) appeared to be functioning well together and it was suggested that in well-functioning families, grief waned over 13 months and bereavement outcomes were positive. In contrast, one-third of the families in the study described demonstrated a poor outcome after bereavement. Hostile families were particularly chaotic in their adaptation and sullen families reported a high incidence of depression.

Kissane and colleagues (1998) also suggest that practitioners could identify dysfunctional families through using tools such as the Family Relationship Index (FRI), enabling them to proactively improve the psychosocial outcomes of grief. By examining family patterns of grief in this way, together with the identification of other issues, such as type of loss, circumstances and social support, 'at risk' families can be identified. Conducting assessments such as the FRI or the Family Adaptability and Cohesion Evaluation Scale (FACES) (BrintzenhofeSzoc *et al.* 2001) could provide information that will have a positive impact on current health status but will also play a valuable role in reducing the morbidity of the population as a whole (Kissane and Bloch 1994). However, not all families will require this degree of assessment, as most experience 'normal' grief, in which relationships within the family remain relatively intact after the loss experience (Prigerson 2004). The majority of families, after loss, demonstrate evidence of cohesiveness, mutual support, clear communication and emotional expressiveness, and have the ability to work through and deal with conflict (Wimpenny *et al.* 2007). This is demonstrated by their working together to organise the funeral and helping with practical arrangements, such as 'clearing the wardrobe' type activities and being mutually supportive of each other. In such cases, there may be no need for additional support services. Subsequently, professionals working with these families may be able to predict, from their knowledge of the family dynamics, individuals requiring most support.

The nature of family loss

The nature of family loss and the setting in which death takes place can influence the support requested by families. Bereaved family and friends of Dutch cancer patients who died from euthanasia appeared to cope better in terms of the severity of grief symptoms and post-traumatic stress reactions than families bereaved through cancer (Swarte *et al.* 2003). Perhaps a significant factor is also the openness of communication in such deaths, in terms of family members having the opportunity to say goodbye and talk about death when their family member was still aware they were present. This is illuminated by Teno and colleagues (2001), who found that families experiencing loss in a hospice setting reported fewer problems with care than those in acute hospital settings. Therefore, the place where a family member dies and the care provided can have an impact on the family as a whole or on individual family members. Often family members prefer the death to be at home (Brazil *et al.* 2002), although Higginson and Priest (1996) found no significant difference in anxiety levels among relatives of those who died in hospital, at home or in a hospice. Most anxiety was caused by age differences, for example when the deceased was aged less than 45 years, or if they were disabled. Additionally, anxiety was experienced by the spouse of the deceased. Important predictors of anxiety were whether the family member was a spouse, had a diagnosis of breast cancer, was of a young age, died soon after the diagnosis and had reduced mobility. However, Higginson and Priest (1996) did report less anxiety when there had been early referral to palliative care.

Other issues impinging on the experience of grief include the financial burden of, for example, caring for a family member (Corden *et al.* 2002a,b). As the family regroups after the death, family members carry the cost of caring for a terminally ill family member and meeting funeral costs. Social security benefits, which reduce by as much as 72 per cent after a child has died, can also have a serious impact on the remaining family. Finding employment soon after the death, after previously claiming social security benefits whilst caring for the dying, can be a stressful process. However, retrospectively, some find returning to work soon after the death to be a positive decision for them (Corden *et al.* 2002a,b). As families are vulnerable at such a challenging time, financial support and advice should be an integral aspect of caring for the bereaved family, although this is often forgotten as the focus is on end of life care of a physical and psychological nature.

Spousal bereavement

The word 'spouse' usually refers to a husband or wife through marriage; however, within this chapter it will be used interchangeably as a term for an unmarried partner, in light of multifaceted family units. Literature exploring spousal bereavement has a strong bias towards widows, with less focus on exploring widowers' experiences. Gay conjugal relationships or long-term clandestine relationships are also highlighted in the literature. No firm conclusions about who suffers more, widows or widowers, were made by Wimpenny and colleagues (2007) in their systematic literature review when looking at spousal loss. However, Stroebe and colleagues (2001a) suggest that bereaved men are more at risk of developing post-bereavement grief problems than bereaved women (compared with married women).

Conjugal bereavement has been identified as one of the most stressful events in an individual's life. Studies have demonstrated that most widows and widowers grieve over the death of their spouse (Avis *et al.* 1991; Zisook and Shuchter 1991a,b; Kaunonen *et al.* 1999; Bonanno *et al.* 2005a). Symptoms of grief in the surviving partner are reported to decrease over time. Such grief has been reported as being at its most intense immediately after the death, giving validation to the statement 'time heals'. There is a consensus in the evidence that sudden or unexpected death was related to more intense grief at an early stage of the bereavement but this had reduced by the 7-month stage (Avis *et al.* 1991; Zisook and Shuchter 1991b; Lieberman and Yalom 1992; Hyrkas *et al.* 1997).

Given the strong bias towards widows in most studies, it is difficult to draw conclusions about whether gender is influential in spousal loss and if one sex suffers more as a result of loss. It is interesting to note that and question why more widows than widowers agree to participate in spousal bereavement studies. Some studies clearly suggest that spousal loss has a stronger effect on mortality and/or morbidity for widowers than it does for widows (Martikainen and Valkonen 1996, 1998; Bauer and Bonanno 2001). In contrast, Manor and Eisenbach (2003) found a 10 per cent increase in mortality for widows in the first and second year post bereavement. However, it is generally agreed that the younger widow or widower is more vulnerable (Zisook and Shuchter 1991a; Powers and Wampold 1994; Bauer and Bonanno 2001) as are individuals at the lower end of the social spectrum (Martikainen and Valkonen 1998). Younger widows and widowers can exhibit greater psychopathy than those in the older age groups (Zisook and Shuchter 1991a). Perhaps this is in part a result of death being an inevitable event and a more frequent and accepted experience in the older age group (International Working Group on Death, Dying and Bereavement 2000).

Kaunonen and colleagues (2000) reported variations in responses from widows and widowers. Whereas 26 per cent of widows and widowers worried about survival, 18 per cent of widows worried about illness and death compared with 10 per cent of widowers. Loneliness was felt by 17 per cent of widows and 26 per cent of widowers, and the loss of their relationship and the life they would have had with the deceased worried 12 per cent of widows and 9 per cent of widowers. Statistically, the only difference reported was the increased incidence of panic behaviour felt by widows, especially related to undertaking and performing new tasks such as managing their financial affairs. There appears to be a dearth of information and practical support generally for young widows and widowers, although a new voluntary group, the WAY Foundation, has recently set out to address this (WAY Foundation 2010). Funeral directors often provide valuable practical support and advice but this is limited to a short period soon after the death.

Zisook and Shuchter (1991a) presented similar findings in their study, reporting that widows demonstrated more anxiety than widowers. The nature of the attachment between the mourner and the deceased seemed to have an impact on response to loss. The evidence suggests that individuals who appeared stable, balanced and secure reminisced about the deceased more than so-called insecure people. The authors concluded that attachment style had an effect on spousal grief.

Bonanno and colleagues (2002) added to this by suggesting that the clearest predictor of adverse grief symptoms was excessive dependency in the relationship. However, no significant differences were found relating to conflict and ambivalence towards the spouse in most of the groups in the study. The chronically depressed group in the study were reported as being less positive about their spouse and marriage. The evidence again seems to indicate that having knowledge of family dynamics can help health professionals predict families or family members who may need additional support after a death.

Waskowic and Chartier (2003) reported that if the widow or widower felt more securely attached to the spouse prior to death, subsequently they were less angry, felt less socially isolated and less guilty, with less death anxiety and fewer somatic symptoms, as well as less despair, depersonalisation and rumination about the deceased. Secure people reminisced more about the deceased than insecure people and it was therefore again suggested that attachment style had an effect on the partner's grief.

Continuing bond relationships

The concept of continuing bonds and relationships with the dead, described in Chapter 1, is that of an enduring spiritual relationship between the mourner and the deceased. A study by Field and colleagues (2003) on spousal loss found that the greater the continuing bond between mourner and deceased after the death, the greater the severity of the grief. When participants reported a greater satisfaction with the relationship prior to death, the authors concluded that it was predictive of a higher continuing bond with the deceased. Some of the continuing bonds remained evident long after the death.

Hyrkas and colleagues (1997), in a study of Finnish widows and widowers, suggested that widowers who had lost their spouse more than 2 years previously displayed more feelings of blame and anger than did widows. In contrast, Manor and Eisenbach (2003) found no differences between widows and widowers in their longitudinal mortality study in Israel, which again possibly highlights the impact of cultural and religious factors and their impact on the grief experience.

Depression and distress

In a consideration of the extent to which loss causes depression and distress, a number of authors and research studies identify complicated grief reactions linked to the severity of certain symptoms. The chapter on mental health and trauma (Chapter 6) also discusses complicated grief reactions although here we will highlight links between spousal loss and complicated grief or chronic grief. Zisook and Shuchter (1991a) found that most of the widows and widowers had a depressive episode at some time during the 7 months after their bereavement and that this episode did not begin until some time after the first months of bereavement. A quarter of their sample met the DSM-III (Diagnostic and Statistical Manual of Mental Disorders) category for diagnosing clinical depression. Bonanno and colleagues (2004) found nearly half of their sample presented few or no depressive symptoms and that 10 per cent actually showed an improvement in their mental health following their loss; the remainder showed low levels of depression even before the bereavement. Therefore, it appears that before 'diagnosing' complicated or chronic grief after spousal loss, it is important for the practitioner to acknowledge that the depressive symptoms may have commenced before the bereavement (Bonanno *et al.* 2002). This may also pose a challenge to practitioners in the diagnosis of complicated or chronic grief without a holistic mental health assessment.

Bonnano and colleagues (2002) also found, in their prospective longitudinal study of widowers and widows, that most of the sample (90 per cent) were captured in five conceptually relevant patterns: common grief (11 per cent), chronic grief (16 per cent), resilient (46 per cent), chronic depression (8 per cent) and depressed-improved (10 per cent). Overall, the most frequent bereavement pattern was the low depression resilient type. Each group reported at least some grief symptoms at 6 months post loss, which demonstrated a decline with time; however resilient individuals had fewer grief symptoms than others, with the exception of the depressed-improved. However, by 18 months post loss the resilient, common and depressed-improved groups did not differ from each other, although the chronic depressed and chronic grievers (who did not differ significantly from each other), showed more signs of grief than all other groups. One of the clearest predictors of complicated or chronic grief was an excessive dependency on their spouse.

Individuals with complicated or chronic grief presented as one of the smallest groups overall, although, as Bonnanno and colleagues (2002) indicate, they have the greatest need for intervention and, as described in Chapter 16, will probably benefit most from professional interventions. In addition, as already highlighted by Field and colleagues (2003), the greater the continuing bonds the widow or widower had with the deceased after death, the greater the complicated or chronic grief pattern.

Finally, Nolen-Hoeksema and colleagues (1997) studied gay widowers and reported that those men who evidenced more negative ruminative thoughts showed greater psychological distress. Men who engaged in increased analysis of themselves and the meaning of their loss reported greater positive morale at 1 month after the loss; however, this was counterbalanced with more persistent depression and absence of a positive state of mind over the 12 months since their loss. Social friction on the other hand was related to enduring depressive symptoms, highlighting the potential challenges to addressing bereavement in homosexual relationships.

The importance of social support

Social support throughout most of the studies appeared to be the most important source of help, especially that from family and friends (Duke 1998). Having to realign assumptions about self, relationships and life, which no longer fitted to their current reality (Danforth and Glass 2001), was also an important process of being widowed, which initially could bring feelings of stigmatisation (Lieberman and Yalom 1992). In exploring gender effects on social support, Thuen (1997a) concluded that social support was of benefit only in the later phases of bereavement and that female respondents receive slightly more support from friends than do males. However, it is difficult to quantify as women were found to naturally have a wider and more active social network before and after widowhood. This may be the key influencing factor within this assumption (Antonucci 1990; Umberson *et al.* 1992). Stroebe and colleagues (2001a) reported similar findings, in that the widowers tend to have lower levels of social support and that the effects of depression and loneliness related to bereavement appear to be stronger in men. However, they also concluded that although there was evidence of gender differences in bereavement outcomes and social support, there was no evidence that social support influences those differences. In contrast, Caserta and Lund (1996) found that men were as likely as women to engage in social contact with other members outwith social group meetings. In exploring the timing of the social support, Caserta and Lund (1996) found the frequency of contact increased over time outwith the support group meetings and had no relation to attendance at the meetings. Perhaps, as Thuen (1997b) suggests, social support is beneficial to individuals only in the later phases of bereavement, which he records as 30 months or more. There is a lack of evidence exploring the implications of high- and low-risk bereaved individuals and the relationship to social support or integrated on-going evaluations to assess efficacy. Cultural and spiritual implications or nature of the loss, which may themselves have a strong bearing on social needs and support, are also not well documented in studies.

Although the evidence from the literature is mixed in this section, it appears that social support is important, particularly in the later phases of a bereavement. It also suggests that females may be in a position to benefit more from the social support as they were found to have a wider and more active social network already.

Parental bereavement

A significant component of family bereavement is the parents' response to the death of a child. Parental bereavement occurs with the loss of a child (even an adult offspring). Although some of this will be covered specifically in the chapter on perinatal bereavement and children's deaths in hospital/hospice care (Chapter 9) there is a considerable range of general writing and research in this area [mainly observational (survey, retrospective evaluations, cross-sectional studies) in nature]. This writing and research demonstrates the significant impact of children's deaths on parents, often greater in intensity than the death of a partner. The death of a juvenile child also has greater impact on the parent than the death of an older child (Murphy et al., 2002; Seecharan et al., 2004) and the death of a child can have a significant impact on parents' physical and mental well-being (Stroebe et al. 2001b; Znoj and Keller 2002). De Vries and colleagues (1994) draw upon Rando's (1986) work to highlight the range of influencing factors in determining grief responses to the death of a child, namely the untimeliness of the death, the nature and quality of the lost relationship, the role the deceased played, the characteristics of the death and the social support system. They outline a range of issues which affect each of these factors and also point out the need to examine the loss against the age of the child (infant, young child or adult child) as these impact in different ways on 'family' functioning and development, influencing family dynamics and cohesion. Murray and colleagues (2000) also identify some specific risk factors, some of which you will have already encountered above: lack of perceived social support, ambivalent relationship with the baby/infant, particularly traumatic circumstances surrounding the death, other difficult life circumstances, difficulty with coping in the past, problematic individual characteristics and unsatisfactory relationships within the nuclear family.

Janzen and colleagues (2003–2004) suggest that the sudden death of a child can also result in the parent(s) developing post-traumatic stress disorder (PTSD). Since adolescents may be seen as being at particular risk of dying from accidents and suicide (Davies 2001; Murphy *et al.* 2002), this suggests that parents of adolescents are at increased risk of responding outside the 'normal' responses to death. This may be due to concurrent emotional and relationship changes occurring both for the adolescent and within the family. However, much of the evidence offered fails to differentiate the death of adolescents as a distinct group.

Dyregrov (2003) suggests that the factor causing most concern is that of traumatic death rather than the age of the child. In addition, Murphy and colleagues (2003) conclude that the type of traumatic death is not very significant. In addition, deaths in younger children [for example from sudden infant death syndrome (SIDS)] may occur when parents are younger and have less well-established partnerships and coping skills.

Irrespective of age, it appears that parents who lose a child suffer a reduced quality of life over a long period (Dyregrov 1990). The Centre for Advancement of Health review (Genevro 2004) indicates that it can take 3–4 years for parents to accept the death of a child. It also suggests that parental health post loss is diminished, particularly for fathers over the long term. The differences between men and women in respect of grief and child loss are accompanied by a variety of explanations related to different aspects: attachment to the child, methods of coping, emotional responses and social situations (Dyregrov 1990; Murphy *et al.* 2002).

Giving meaning to family bereavement

The search for meaning and its reconstruction after the death of a child is considered an important issue in relation to keeping the memory of the child alive (Klass 1997; Wheeler 2001). Davis and colleagues (2000) question whether this search for meaning is appropriate, particularly when the events surrounding the death and the death itself shatter deeply held world views. Klass (1997) proposes that grief does not end with the severing of bonds with the child but continues through integration of the child into the parent's life in a different way from before the death. Such changing perspectives on parental bereavement are noted by Davies (2004), who indicates that models of bereavement have moved from detachment from the dead to maintaining attachment and continuing bonds in some form.

Support from professionals

In 1990 Dyregrov highlighted that the support offered to parents from health professionals was reported as variable, and the extent to which this has changed in the intervening years is questionable. Janzen and colleagues (2003–2004) used parents' experiences to illustrate their points in providing advice to professionals (police, nurses, doctors, coroners, social workers/crisis counsellors, funeral directors and clergy). They divide their guidance into three areas: instrumental assistance (e.g. providing access, allowing time, respecting decisions), provision of information (e.g. details of death, what to expect and do, rituals and memorials) and compassion and empathy (e.g. give control, actively listen, be present, respect for the child's body, respect faith). One parent stated:

> It is amazing what an impact the actions/reactions of others can have during this traumatic and very vulnerable time. I remember very clearly the things that were said and done which were comforting. I remember just as clearly, in fact, perhaps more clearly, the things that were said and done which were hurtful and upsetting.
>
> (p. 161)

This illustrates the significant impact that professionals can have at the time of death and afterwards, and the potential for better training and education across professional groups to enhance some fundamental aspects of care (Oliver *et al.* 2001). However, it is not always straightforward, as the following scenario illustrates:

Susan was a student midwife and had academic preparation for caring for a family after perinatal death, including cultural health care perspectives. However, when left alone in the delivery room with a stillborn baby and his Asian parents, Susan found it distressing to witness the overwhelmingly loud wailing of the mother. Although she was aware that this was a recognised cultural behaviour, she had not anticipated her own reaction to expressing grief in such a loud cathartic manner. Susan sat, stunned, unable to function and felt unable to meet the needs of the family.

On reflection, Susan identified that her distress stemmed from a cultural clash with her own Scottish 'Presbyterian' background, whereby grief was not overtly expressed. Having academic knowledge of a culture is not always enough. The importance of experiential learning supported by clinical supervision was essential to Susan's professional development to care effectively for such a family.

Interventions

Although interventions are considered more fully in both the children's deaths in hospital/hospice and perinatal chapters (Chapters 9 and 10) and also more generally in the chapter on interventions (Chapter 16), it is useful to introduce some general evidence here that relates to families/parents. Murray and colleagues (2000) describe an intervention to assist parents to adjust to loss ('normal' grief) of a child using an Australian programme known as *An Ache in Their Hearts*. This well considered controlled study using a trained grief worker and validated resources demonstrated that parents do benefit from such intervention and, again, those at most risk are likely to benefit most. Differences in time for benefit were noted between mothers and fathers, with mothers benefiting earlier than fathers, again suggesting different patterns of grief. As you may now be aware, and as Rowa-Dewar (2002), in a review of interventions for parental bereavement, indicates, interventions should be targeted at parents who are at high risk, taking account of individual and gender issues, rather than applied with blanket coverage.

Generally we may consider that men may benefit from interventions that help them to express their grief, although women are more likely to attend grief support groups (Laasko and Paunonen-Ilmonen 2002; Schut *et al.* 2001). In addition interventions that provide social support, of all types, can have an impact on bereavement (Thuen 1997a,b).

Studies by Laasko and Paunonen-Ilmonen (2002) and Thuen (1997a) remind us that cultural differences exist and that, therefore, we should consider the setting for research and the impact this may have on any comparison of results (many other cultural differences and similarities exist; see, for example, Malkinson and Bar-Tur 1999; Bonanno *et al.* 2005b).

Self-help groups for widows have, for some time, demonstrated positive outcomes (Vachon *et al.* 1980), and, similarly, Dent and colleagues (1996), in a UK-based study, found that parents want to interact with others who have suffered the same loss (Klass 1997). There are now a range of self-help groups that cover the spectrum of bereavement in families. Geron and colleagues (2003) evaluated the value of group interventions for bereaved parents run by the Ministry of Defence in Israel, and concluded that these are most beneficial for those seeking to form relations with others in the same situation. Groups, they suggest, offer identification, empathy and a sense of belonging and provide an opportunity to express feelings and learn from others. Riches and Dawson (1996) agree that support groups can offer social and cultural resources not available elsewhere. Of course, such group support may, at one time, have been more readily available within communities but is now often, but not always, more distant, by means of internet and telephone services.

Gender stereotypes

Historically, in the early Victorian period, the burden of a public show of mourning, within a middle-class family, was the responsibility of females. With that responsibility came the required etiquette; this often involved the imposed issue of fidelity (from the widow) and the wearing of suitable black mourning dress. This displayed the grief of the family as a whole. However, males in the same family could assume a different role, which was deemed equally important, and involved being responsible for resuming employment and supporting the family financially (Draper 1996). In some orthodox cultures, the role of the younger male was, if necessary, to marry his sister-in-law, to ensure financial support for the widow and children. Whether this cultural and historical influence has shaped the coping strategies in the present day is unclear, but it has been suggested that in general females are assumed to demonstrate more emotionally oriented behaviour and males more problem-oriented behaviour in their response to grief (Vingerhoets and van Heck 1990; DeRidder 2000). However, DeRidder (2000) and Vingerhoets and van Heck (1990) also state that in the uncontrollable event of a partner's death they perceive the problem-oriented approach to be less useful than an emotionally oriented approach. Martin and Doka (2000: 29) point out that there are two specific patterns of grief: 'an intuitive pattern of grief', whereby individuals express their grief in an effective way (stereotyped as female grief), and an 'instrumental pattern', whereby individuals express grief in a physical or cognitive way (stereotyped as male grief). Added to these is a third explanation, a 'blended pattern' (a combination of the intuitive and instrumental grievers), whereby the individual favours different patterns at different times during the grief process. Intuitive grievers have a need to express their feelings as a form of catharsis by seeking the support of others, but instrumental grievers engage in a more cognitive approach and may immerse themselves in some form of activity.

The blended approach resonates with the oscillation seen between loss-oriented and restoration-oriented behaviour in Stroebe and Schut's dual process model of coping with bereavement (1999) described in Chapter 1, whereby the individual moves between behaviours at different times in an attempt to adapt and restore order, integrity and harmony in their lives. Such a thesis poses that there is more than one way to effectively grieve; however, the authors do not clarify in their book whether one style is more effective than another or that they are merely different. However, it does help to dispel the grief work hypothesis (Stroebe *et al.* 2005) that unless one expresses one's feelings in an open manner, then grief is ineffective and will not be successfully resolved. Martin and Doka (2000) conclude that grievers may experience, express and adapt to grief in different ways, which seems to avoid stereotyping males or females and compartmentalising individuals into grief coping boxes. It also suggests to health and care practitioners that there are strengths and limitations to each pattern of coping with grief and, given this, we should work with the individual within a family unit and not stereotype certain members by their gender.

Consequently, we should also be aware that such variance in coping style has the potential to cause conflict after bereavement as individuals react and cope with bereavement in different ways. For example, an instrumental griever wishing to clear the family home may intimidate an intuitive griever who wants to reminiscence and vice versa. Such clashes of coping strategies within a family create the potential for conflict and may require understanding and support from health and social care practitioners, who may even be asked to take allegiances within such family battles.

Differences and similarities between men and women are explored by Wing and colleagues (2001), who identify, from the available evidence, a convergence of responses and symptoms over time. Wing and colleagues (2001) highlight the effects on couples and the value of providing therapy aimed at the couple, as much as aimed at the individual parents. The use of the Grief Experience Inventory is suggested as a useful tool to facilitate discussion (Schwab 1996) at the outset of such therapy. The impact on men and women from, for example, a child's death, may also be felt in the workplace as parents seek to cope with the demands of work to maintain economic status whilst at the same time struggling with their grief (Klass 1997). The potential impact of the work environment on the grief trajectory and of the bereaved employee on the work environment are discussed elsewhere (Chapter 14). However, it should be noted that grief may also be compounded by the male or masculine culture of work and may be experienced differently by men and women.

In general, there is a stereotypical assumption that females tend to express emotions more than men and engage in a more active manner in 'grief work':

Nancy was registered blind and had lost her mother 4 years ago. Whilst in for a routine visit, Nancy confided that she had been worried about the fact that she felt she had not grieved properly after her mother had died, as she had never really cried. She was apprehensive and had avoided family functions because she felt that if she expressed emotion at such events and began crying, she might not be able to stop. She questioned why she might be holding back and was unable to cry openly, as her older sister had done.

After a long discussion with Nancy, it was evident that, as the youngest child, she had always been with her mother and her mother had always made decisions for her, even as a single adult. Since her mother's death, she had undertaken the onerous tasks of changing the family home and had even been manually digging the large garden they shared, which had taken her several months to complete. In recent months, she had walked up Mount Kenya and even learned to water-ski on her fortieth birthday. It was evident that Nancy was a strong instrumental griever and when the practitioner explored if this could be correct, she felt an overwhelming sense of relief that she had a different coping strategy from her sister and had indeed been grieving in her own unique way for her mother. Nancy had felt an immense burden lifted that she did not have to cry uncontrollably after the death.

Nancy's story illustrates the pressure that some individuals feel when they have not been able to express grief in an expected 'normal' way, that is by crying and openly expressing emotions. Being aware of the different coping strategies of grief, as discussed under 'Gender stereotypes' above, perhaps allowed Nancy to identify for herself that she coped with the grief using her own style in her own time.

Conclusion

This chapter has considered the bereavement experiences of family members, both as a family unit and as individuals, in terms of issues such as age and gender differences. It is helpful to consider the needs and support options available to the family and its members because it is clear that individuals grieve in different ways at different times using different coping styles. Specifically, the needs of bereaved parents during their early and later adult years have been discussed and it is clear that a number of risk factors can be identified that may impact on grief and that interventions are most helpful for those with greatest risk and who have complicated grief.

It has also been made clear that the level of cohesiveness demonstrated by the family before the impact of death is an effective indicator of how they may respond to the crisis of death. Health and social care practitioners need to have some prior knowledge of family functioning in order to make an accurate assessment and formulate appropriate supportive strategies.

References

Avis NE, Brambilla DT, Vass K and McKinlay JB (1991) The effect of widowhood on health: a prospective analysis from the Massachusetts Women's Health Study. *Social Science & Medicine* 33(9): 1063–1070.

Antonucci TC (1990) Social supports and social relationships. In: Binstock RH and George LK (eds) *The handbook of aging and the social sciences.* 3rd edn. San Diego: Academic Press. Chapter 11.

Bauer JJ and Bonanno GA (2001) Doing and being well (for the most part): adaptive patterns of narrative self-evaluation during bereavement. *Journal of Personality* 69(3): 451–482.

Bonanno GA, Wortman CB, Lehman DR, Tweed RG, Haring M, Sonnega J, Carr D and Nesse RM (2002) Resilience to loss and chronic grief: a prospective study from preloss to 18-months postloss. *Journal of Personality and Social Psychology* 83(5): 1150–1164.

Bonanno GA, Wortman CB and Nesse RM (2004) Prospective patterns of resilience and maladjustment during widowhood. *Psychology and Aging* 19(2): 260–271.

Bonanno GA, Moskowitz JT, Papa A and Folkman S (2005a) Resilience to loss in bereaved spouses, bereaved parents, and bereaved gay men. *Journal of Personality and Social Psychology* 88(5): 827–843.

Bonanno GA, Papa A, Lalande K, Zhang N and Noll JG (2005b) Grief processing and deliberate grief avoidance: a prospective comparison of bereaved spouses and parents in the United States and the People's Republic of China. *Journal of Consulting and Clinical Psychology* 73(1): 86–98.

Brazil K, Bedard M and Willison K (2002) Correlates of health status for family caregivers in bereavement. *Journal of Palliative Medicine* 5(6): 849–855.

BrintzenhofeSzoc KM, Smith E and Zabora R (2001) Screening to predict complicated grief in spouses of cancer patients. *Cancer Practice* 7(5): 233–239.

Caserta MS and Lund DA (1996) Beyond bereavement support group meetings: exploring outside social contacts among the members. *Death Studies* 20(6): 537–556.

Corden A, Sainsbury R and Sloper P (2002a) When a child dies: money matters. *Illness, Crisis and Loss* 10(2): 125–137.

Corden A, Sloper P and Sainsbury R (2002b) Financial effects for families after the death of a disabled or chronically ill child: a neglected dimension of bereavement. *Child: Care, Health and Development* 28(3): 199–204.

Danforth MM and Glass CG Jr (2001) Listen to my words, give meaning to my sorrow: a study in cognitive constructs in middle-age bereaved widows. *Death Studies* 25(6): 513–529.

Davies AM (2001) Death of adolescents: parental grief and coping strategies. *British Journal of Nursing* 10(20): 1332–1342.

Davies R (2004) New understandings of parental grief: a literature review. *Journal of Advanced Nursing* 46(5): 506–513.

Davis CG, Wortman CB, Lehman DR and Silver RC (2000) Searching for meaning in loss: are clinical assumptions correct? *Death Studies* 24(6): 497–540.

de Vries B, Lana RD and Falck VT (1994) Parental bereavement over the life course: a theoretical intersection and empirical review. *Omega* 29(1): 47–69.

DeRidder D (2000) Gender, stress and coping: do women handle stressful situations differently from men? In: Sherr L and St Lawrence JS (eds) *Women, health and the mind.* Chichester: Wiley.

Dent A, Condon L, Blair P and Fleming P (1996) A study of bereavement care after a sudden and unexpected death. *Archives of Disease* 74(6): 522–526.

Doka, KJ (1989) *Disenfranchised grief: recognizing hidden sorrow.* Lexington, MA: Lexington Books.

Doka KJ (1999) Disenfranchised grief. *Bereavement Care* 18(3): 37.

Draper A (1996) But men must work and women must weep: representations of gender, mourning and bereavement in Victorian visual culture. University of London, PhD thesis.

Dyregrov A (1990) Parental reactions to the loss of an infant child: a review. *Scandinavian Journal of Psychology* 31(4): 266–280.

Dyregrov A (2003) Micro-sociological analysis of social support following traumatic bereavement: unhelpful and avoidant responses from the community. *Omega* 48(1): 23–44.

Duke S (1998) An exploration of anticipatory grief: the lived experience of people during their spouses' terminal illness and in bereavement. *Journal of Advanced Nursing* 28(4): 829–839.

Fetus and Newborn Committee and Canadian Paediatric Society (2001) Guidelines for health care professionals supporting families experiencing a perinatal loss. *Paediatric and Child Health* 6(71): 469–477.

Field NP, Gal-Oz E and Bonanno GA (2003) Continuing bonds and adjustment at 5 years after the death of a spouse. *Journal of Consulting and Clinical Psychology* 71(1): 110–117.

Fletcher PN (2002) Experiences in family bereavement. *Family and Community Health* 25(1); 57–70.

Genevro JL (2004) Report on bereavement and grief research. *Death Studies* 28(6): 491–575..

Geron Y, Ginzburg K and Solomon Z (2003) Predictors of bereaved parents' satisfaction with group support: an Israeli perspective. *Death Studies* 27(5): 405–426.

Higginson I and Priest P (1996) Predictors of family anxiety in the weeks before bereavement. *Social Science and Medicine* 43(11): 1621–1625.

Hyrkas KMNS, Kaunonen MMNS and Paunonen MME (1997) Recovering from the death of a spouse. *Journal of Advanced Nursing* 25(4): 775–779.

International Work Group on Death, Dying and Bereavement (2000) Death, dying, and bereavement in relation to older individuals. *Illness, Crisis and Loss* 8(4); 388–394.

Janzen L, Cadell S. and Westhues A (2003–2004) From death notification through the funeral: bereaved parents' experiences and their advice to professionals. *Omega* 48(2): 149–164.

Kaunonen M, Tarkka MT and Paunonen M (1999) Grief and social support after the death of a spouse. *Journal of Advanced Nursing* 30(6): 1304–1311.

Kissane DW and Bloch S (1994). Family grief. *British Journal of Psychiatry* 164(6): 728–740.

Kissane DW, Bloch S, Onghena P, McKenzie DP, Snyder RD and Dowe DL (1996) The Melbourne family grief study, II: psychosocial morbidity and grief in bereaved families. *American Journal of Psychiatry* 153(5): 659–666.

Kissane DW, Bloch S, McKenzie M, McDowall AC and Nitzan R (1998) Family grief therapy: a preliminary account of a new model to promote healthy family functioning during palliative care and bereavement. *Psycho-Oncology* 7(1): 14–25.

Klass D (1997) The deceased child in the psychic and social worlds of bereaved parents during the resolution of grief. *Death Studies* 21(2):147–176.

Laasko H and Paunonen-Ilmonen M (2002) Mothers' experience of social support following the death of a child. *Journal of Clinical Nursing* 11(2): 176–185.

Lieberman MA and Yalom I (1992) Brief group psychotherapy for the spousally bereaved: a controlled study. *International Journal of Group Psychotherapy* 42(1): 117–132.

Malkinson R and Bar-Tur L (1999) The aging of grief in Israel: a perspective of bereaved parents. *Death Studies* 23(5): 413–431.

Manor O and Eisenbach Z (2003) Mortality after spousal loss: are there socio-demographic differences? *Social Science and Medicine* 56(2): 405–413.

Martikainen P and Valkonen T (1996) Mortality after death of a spouse in relation to duration of bereavement in Finland. *Journal of Epidemiology and Community Health* 50(3): 264–268.

Martikainen P and Valkonen T (1998) Do education and income buffer the effects of death of spouse on mortality. *Epidemiology* 9(5): 530–534.

Martin TL and Doka KJ. (2000). *Men don't cry . . . women do: transcending gender stereotypes of grief.* Philadelphia: Brunner/Mazel.

Moos R and Moos B (1981) *Family environment scale manual.* Palo Alto, CA: Consulting Psychologist Press.

Murphy SA, Johnson LC and Weber NA (2002) Coping strategies following a child's violent death: how parents differ in their responses. *Omega* 45(2): 99–118.

Murphy SA, Johnson C and Lohan J (2003) Challenging the myths about parents' adjustment after the sudden, violent death of a child. *Journal of Nursing Scholarship* 35(4): 359–364.

Murray JA, Terry DJ, Vance JC, Battistutta D and Connolly Y (2000) Effects of a program of intervention on parental distress following infant death. *Death Studies* 24(4): 275–305.

Nolen-Hoeksema S, McBride A and Larson J (1997) Rumination and psychological distress among bereaved partners. *Journal of Personality and Social Psychology* 72(4): 855–862.

Office for National Statistics (2009) Divorces in England and Wales. Available at: http://www.statistics.gov.uk/statbase/Product.asp?vlnk=14124 (accessed 23 May 2011).

Oliver RC, Sturtevant JP, Scheetz JP and Fallat ME (2001) Beneficial effects of a hospital bereavement intervention program after traumatic childhood death. *Journal of Trauma, Injury, Infection and Critical Care* 50(3): 440–448.

Parkes CM (2000) Comments on Dennis Klass article 'Developing a cross-cultural model of grief'. *Omega* 41(3): 323–326.

Powers LE and Wampold BE (1994) Cognitive-behavioral factors in adjustment to adult bereavement. *Death Studies* 18(1): 1–24.

Prigerson H (2004) Complicated grief; when the path of adjustment leads to a dead end. *Bereavement Care* 23(3): 38–40.

Rando TA (1986) Parental bereavement: an exception to the general conceptualisations of mourning. In: Rando TA (ed.) *Parental loss of a child.* Champaign, IL: Research Press.

Riches G. and Dawson P (1996) Communities of feeling: the culture of bereaved parents. *Mortality* 1(2): 143–161.

Rowa-Dewar N (2002) Do interventions make a difference to bereaved parents? A systematic review of controlled studies. *International Journal of Palliative Nursing* 8(9): 452–457.

Schut H, Stroebe MS, van den Bout J and Terheggen M (2001) The efficacy of bereavement interventions: determining who benefits. In Stroebe MS, Hansson RO, Stroebe W and Schut H (eds) *Handbook of bereavement research: consequences, coping, and care*. Washington, DC: American Psychological Association.

Schut HAW, Stroebe MS, Boelen PA and Zijerveld AM (2006) Continuing relationships with the deceased: disentangling bonds and grief. *Death Studies* 30(8): 757–766.

Schwab R (1996) Gender differences in parental grief. *Death Studies* 20(2): 103–113.

Seecharan GA, Andresen EA, Norris K and Toce SS (2004) Parents' assessment of quality of care and grief following a child's death. *Archives of Pediatric & Adolescent Medicine* 158(6): 515–520.

Stroebe M and Schut H (1999) The dual process model of coping with bereavement: rationale and description. *Death Studies* 23(3): 197–224.

Stroebe M, Stroebe W and Schut H (2001a) Gender differences in adjustment to bereavement: an empirical and theoretical review. *Review of General Psychology* 5(1): 62–83.

Stroebe MS, Hansson RO, Stroebe W and Schut H (eds) (2001b) *Handbook of bereavement research: consequences, coping and care*. Washington, DC: American Psychological Association.

Stroebe W, Schut HA and Stroebe MS (2005) Grief work, disclosure and counseling: do they help the bereaved? *Clinical Psychology Review* 25(4): 395–414.

Swarte NB, van der Lee ML, van der Bom JG, van den Bout J, Heintz APM (2003) Effects of euthanasia on the bereaved family and friends: a cross sectional study. *British Medical Journal* 327(7408): 189–193.

Teno JM, Weitzen S, Fennell ML and Mor V (2001) Dying trajectory in the last year of life: does cancer trajectory fit other diseases. *Journal of Palliative Medicine* 4(4): 457–464.

Thuen F (1997a) Social support after the loss on an infant child: a long-term perspective. *Scandinavian Journal of Psychology* 38(2): 103–110.

Thuen F (1997b) Received social support from informal networks and professionals in bereavement. *Psychology Health and Medicine* 2(1): 51–63.

Traylor ES, Hayslip B, Kaminski PL and York C (2003) Relationships between grief and family system characteristics: a cross lagged longitudinal analysis. *Death Studies* 27(7): 575–601.

Umberson D, Wortman CB and Kessler RC (1992) Widowhood and depression: explaining long-term differences in vulnerability. *Journal of Health and Social Behavior* 33(1): 10–24.

Vachon ML, Lyall WA, Rogers J, Freedman-Letofsky K and Freeman SJ (1980) A controlled study of self-help interventions for widows. *American Journal of Psychiatry* 137(11): 1380–1384.

Vingerhoets A and van Heck GL (1990) Gender, coping and psychosomatic symptoms. *Psychological Medicine* 20(1): 125–135.

Waskowic TD and Chartier BM (2003) Attachment and the experience of grief following the loss of a spouse. *Omega* 47(1): 77–91.

WAY Foundation (2010) Young widowed men and women supporting each other across the UK. Available at: http://www.wayfoundation.org.uk/ (accessed 21 June 2011).

Wheeler I (2001) Parental bereavement: the crisis of meaning. *Death Studies* 25(1): 51–66.

Wimpenny P, Unwin R, Dempster P, Grundy M, Work F, Brown A and Wilcock S (2007) A literature review on bereavement and bereavement care: developing evidence-based practice in Scotland. *Bereavement Care* 26(1): 7–10.

Wing DG, Burge-Callaway K, Rose Clance P and Armistead L (2001) Understanding gender differences in bereavement following the death of an infant: implications for treatment. *Psychotherapy: Theory, Research, Practice, Training* 38(1): 60–73.

Zisook S and Shuchter SR (1991a) Early psychological reaction to the stress of widowhood. *Psychiatry* 54(4): 320–333.

Zisook S and Shuchter SR (1991b) Depression through the first year after the death of a spouse. *American Journal of Psychiatry* 148(10): 1346–1352.

Znoj H and Keller D (2002) Mourning parents: considering safeguards and their relation to health. *Death Studies* 26(7): 545–565.

4 Bereavement and older people

Audrey Stephen

Key messages

- Successful ageing involves balancing losses and gains throughout life, including adapting to bereavement.
- Diverse experiences of older people mean that they exhibit a range of responses to bereavement.
- Bereavement brings emotional and practical difficulties that require loss- and restoration-oriented coping activities.
- Common experiences are health problems, loneliness, maintaining a continued bond with the deceased and changed identity.
- Identification of patterns of bereavement reaction can indicate who could benefit from additional support.

Introduction

This chapter explores the meaning of bereavement for older people. I begin by describing the origins of my interest in the topic, formed through the kind of experiences that could be common to many health care workers, and go on to examine bereavement as it is experienced by older people and to identify common patterns of grief in older people. The ideas expressed can be used to assist in the identification of those bereaved older people who may be at risk of having difficulty coping after a death, and who may have support needs.

I first experienced caring for dying people and supporting their relatives as a newly qualified staff nurse in a medical ward in a large teaching hospital in the 1980s. My focus then was more on caring for the dying patient, and though I had an awareness of relatives being there, I relied on senior staff to take them away and talk to them. However, on one particular occasion a male patient died on an evening shift and I remember being struck with feelings of grief myself that I could not find any explanation for other than that I had really liked him and enjoyed looking after him. I remember relating better to his family than to any others in the past and feeling satisfied that I had helped them in some small way. That was a turning point that enabled me to engage with people more meaningfully in many challenging circumstances.

In later years I worked in an accident and emergency (A&E) unit, where I began to develop some understanding of the needs of relatives who had experienced the sudden death of a family member in traumatic circumstances. I found this to be a challenging aspect of A&E nursing that brought with it further realisation that what was said and done at this time made a difference to relatives. In retrospect, I did not always handle situations as well as I would have liked. However, as I gained experience of caring for relatives with diverse responses, I also experienced death in my own family, and my confidence in providing support grew. I became particularly concerned for the welfare of spouses of elderly people who were taken to the department with their collapsed husband or wife. On many occasions colleagues and I made efforts to contact another relative to come to the hospital to be with the bereaved spouse and for a fair number this was no easy task. I was often left wondering how that person coped after they left our care and what life would be like for them without their life partner. This chapter seeks to some shed light on the bereavement experiences of older people and to examine the role of health and social care staff in meeting their needs.

Ageing and loss

Ageing is a multifaceted process of physical, cognitive, psychological, social, spiritual and practical change. In later life these changes are more marked and appear to manifest in degeneration and loss of functionality. That is not to say that ageing is synonymous with decline, as often it is a time when people develop psychologically and socially (Anderson 2007). The point at which a person becomes 'old' is blurred and in recent years older people have been characterised by their ability to resist the changes associated with old age until a much later time. However, responses to ageing differ depending on the person's health, psychological and social circumstances.

The challenge of promoting old age positively has, in recent years, taken on increased importance and highlighted the need to see the older person as a valued contributor to society and not just a passive recipient of health and social care services (International Work Group on Death, Dying and Bereavement 2000). Taking a late life developmental perspective, Godfrey (2001) perceives successful ageing to involve achieving a balance of losses and gains through the setting and attainment of realistic goals.

As people age, bereavement becomes a more frequent experience (International Work Group on Death, Dying and Bereavement 2000). Older people commonly endure loss of a spouse, family members, close friends, former colleagues and associates. Bereavement particularly affects older women owing to their additional longevity over men and spousal loss being the norm. In addition, losses often impact on, or are instrumental in, the reduction of social support networks, particularly in old age. The death of someone close is a major life stressor and, along with the additional losses accumulated in later life, may lead to decreased ability to cope, health consequences and reduced capacity to self-care (Hansson and Stroebe 2007).

Jean's story, below, describes the experience of a bereaved older person that may be fairly typical. She was a 79-year-old widow who had lived alone since her husband Jim died a year previously.

Jean had a two-bedroom council house in Aberdeen. She had rheumatoid arthritis and diabetes and was slightly overweight. She enjoyed writing and had a cousin in New Zealand with whom she had regular contact. She liked to spend the evening watching TV.

Since Jim's death Jean did not go out much and felt lonely at times. Her son, James, lived in another part of Scotland and had a young family. They didn't visit often, though Jean went to see them for a few days about twice a year. At times she felt quite depressed. She didn't drive and it was a bit too far to walk to the shops. She ate for comfort and her physical symptoms got worse.

Her younger sister, Sheila, also a widow, visited twice a week, and took her shopping and to church on a Sunday. They phoned each other between times. Jean enjoyed the chance to catch up with friends and neighbours at the shops and at the church. Jean felt much closer to Sheila since Jim's death and was enjoying memories of childhood activities and growing up together. When she went to bed at night she told Jim what they had been doing.

At teatime one Saturday Jean got a phone call from Sheila's daughter, Alison, who told her that Sheila had collapsed and died at the bowling green that afternoon. Jean was grief stricken by the news and even felt guilty that this had upset her more than Jim's death. She felt that her grief went unrecognised in the days leading up to the funeral and at the funeral, when the focus was on Sheila's family.

Jean's feelings of loneliness and isolation worsened after the loss of Sheila and for a time she didn't go out or see anyone on a daily basis.

Jean's story illustrates some of the complexity of ageing and helps to explain how people may have to deal with a number of losses as well as particular physical and social difficulties. Bereavement resulted in increasing feelings of loneliness and social isolation for Jean that impacted further on her health and led to her experiencing depression. The story illustrates how bereavement can change relationships within families and with other social contacts, and portrays the experience of many older people of maintaining a bond with their dead spouse. These important issues are described later in the chapter and are common findings of research examining bereavement in older people. Jean also felt that her feelings of grief were not recognised when Sheila died. This is often called 'disenfranchised' grief (Doka 2002). Following Jim's death Jean balanced her loss with the rekindling of the relationship with Sheila and contact with her cousin in New Zealand. However, since Sheila's death losses appear to outweigh gains for Jean.

How a particular person integrates loss and change into their life is an important consideration for health and social care practitioners. Figure 4.1 illustrates the complexity and range of losses that people face as they age, into which bereavements must be integrated. Jean's experience appears to fit into all the 'spokes' in the wheel.

Bereavement is most commonly associated with distress, sadness and isolation. However, some individuals are able to make sense of their loss and adapt positively, both emotionally and socially, to their situation. This major life event is marked by personal growth and resilience for many (Dutton and Zisook 2005). In addition, cultural and individual differences manifest in diversity of grief response (Hansson and Stroebe 2007). All losses bring to mind emotions and memories, and some people will respond and work through their grief with relative ease, whereas for others it is a destructive life-changing experience (van Praagh 2000). Failure to understand diversity in reactions to loss and its meanings for older people could limit the scope of health and social care staff to respond appropriately.

In addition to emotional aspects of bereavement, older widows in particular

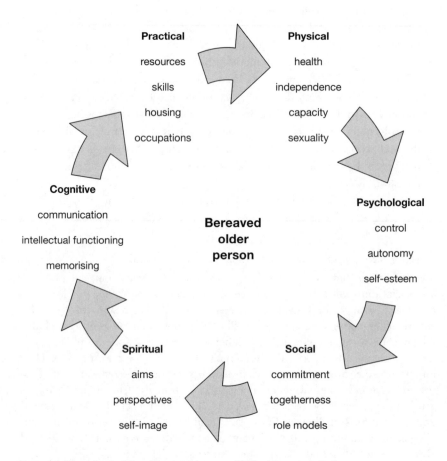

Figure 4.1 The wheel of loss (from Adriaensen 2006 with permission).

have to deal with changes in the normal division of labour within the household, such as paying bills and house maintenance, that ensured good housekeeping when they were a couple. Economic and practical challenges to daily routines are common stressors (Utz 2006). The dual process model of coping with bereavement (Stroebe and Schut 1999) proposed that adjustment to bereavement depends on oscillation between loss-oriented and restoration-oriented coping (see Chapter 1). In order to cope with widowhood and adjusting to life as a single person, both styles are necessary. Loss-oriented grieving allows the bereaved to concentrate on resolving the emotional bond severed after death and coming to terms emotionally with the loss. By oscillating to restoration-oriented coping, the bereaved person can develop strategies that allow adjustment of daily activities to accommodate the reality that the spouse is no longer there (Utz 2006). For example, a man may, for the first time, have to cook meals and a woman may have to take the car to the garage on her own.

The newly bereaved will therefore continually work through their grief by carrying out loss- and restoration-oriented grieving tasks. In most cases the support of family and friends will be sufficient for them to do this satisfactorily. However, Utz (2006) additionally suggests that intervention programmes, such as the provision of financial advice, that target secondary stressors of widowhood could be an effective way of reducing some of the psychological strain.

Bereavement experiences of older people

The available evidence pinpoints some common features of the experiences of older people; however, it is fragmented and unfortunately does not reflect the wide range of experiences. Studies of widowhood, predominantly involving older women, dominate the evidence, along with experiences of bereaved carers. Little attention has been paid to other common situations; for example, older men; experiences of sibling loss; loss of an adult son or daughter; loss of a grandchild; loss of friends and associates; sudden versus expected death; multiple losses; and experiences in non-white cultures. This may be because of the sensitive nature of bereavement research and ethical and practical issues that arise; alternatively, it may be considered so normal for older people to be bereaved that its significance is missed or hidden.

Studies of bereavement and older people in general reflect widowhood, and highlight four main areas of experience:

- health effects;
- loneliness;
- continuing bonds with the deceased;
- changed identity.

Health effects

Bereavement in older people can and does have an adverse effect on the physical and mental health of individuals, and thus should have the attention of health care practitioners and providers. For example, the risk of depression, sleep disruption, or tobacco and alcohol use is increased after bereavement. Early mortality may also be a consequence although the link to bereavement may not always be recognised by health care practitioners (Prigerson and Jacobs 2001).

High mortality rates following conjugal loss have been identified, though trends suggest that older people are at less risk of death than younger bereaved people (Hansson and Stroebe 2007). Estimated increased risk of death for bereaved older men was calculated to be 21 per cent and for older women 17 per cent in a study following up medical records for 9 years (Christakis and Allison 2006). Bereavement related mortality and morbidity research indicates increased risk of death from many causes for bereaved individuals (Stroebe *et al.* 2007). However, causes of death in the very old are more likely to be related to normal patterns of ageing with little variance being due to bereavement. Stroebe and colleagues (2006) also conclude that those with more symptoms before bereavement have the highest mortality. It may be useful, however, for health and social care providers to consider more frequent contact with older bereaved people for at least a year post bereavement. This would enable closer surveillance of health and well-being and provide opportunities to assess risks of common diseases, take preventative measures or give information about certain disease types. Who might provide such surveillance and how it may be carried out are useful questions to consider.

Bereavement in older widows is also characterised by reduced physical activity. Grimby and colleagues (2008) studied widows aged 76 years and older and found that they spent less time walking in the first year of widowhood than married women. However, the amount they walked gradually increased in the 5 years post bereavement. Other health and social issues related to not feeling well, for example, musculoskeletal and cardiac problems, having fewer than two friends and not being in formal clubs were associated with limited mobility. Reduced physical health and social isolation in the short term have also been seen as barriers to widowed women taking part in physical activity. In the long term, lower levels of activity can lead to poor health and inability to exercise. Most, however, seem to regain a certain level of activity as time since bereavement lengthens and social involvement increases. Possible intervention strategies are provision of information on health problems and facilitating increases in social activity, for example, as a member of a walking group.

In terms of mental health consequences, O'Rourke (2004) tested psychopathology and life satisfaction in 232 widowed women (mean age 60.6 years). Physical health conditions were found to contribute significantly to psychiatric distress. Additionally, Siegel and Kuykendall (1990) examined the relationship between recent death of a close family member and depression in a sample of older married and widowed men and women. Poor health, unemployment and loss of a close family member in the last 6 months were related to higher levels of depression. Widows were found to be particularly depressed and, interestingly, non-church members also scored higher for depression. Physical health status and socialising are shown to be important factors in maintenance of physical and mental health for the older bereaved.

For an older person, particularly a bereaved spouse, many changes in mental and cognitive state and physical health can lead to change in social circumstances. Nihtilä and Martikainen (2008) found that the risk of entering a nursing home following spousal bereavement dramatically increased in comparison with that for married persons. The authors conclude that loss of support makes the bereaved spouse vulnerable to physical and mental health difficulties that can lead to admission to long-term care. Long-term care may be seen as the easiest way to deal with complex ageing effects in people who find it hard to cope on their own. However, currently in health and social care there is limited capacity to place every person. Alternative arrangements for care are often made, including supported living in the person's own home, which are often viewed as preferable for the individual.

The health consequences of bereavement can mean that the older, recently bereaved will come into contact with health and social care providers in hospitals, general practice and other settings. This provides a valuable opportunity for assessing how people are coping and working through their bereavement. Those who need further support can then be either given information about services or referred on to specialists, for example, in psychiatry (Stephen *et al.* 2009). Health and social care staff may have some reluctance to discuss death and bereavement and the time taken to 'tell the story' can be considerable. However, some interaction is likely to have a beneficial outcome and it is unlikely that the bereaved person will be made to feel worse. Many older people will welcome the opportunity to talk about their spouse and their feelings since the death.

Loneliness

The experience of loneliness and social isolation following loss commonly means that the older person is less able to look after their own health. Exploration of grief experiences with bereaved spouses has found feelings of shock and disbelief, a sense of loneliness and depression, isolation and the development of an on-going dialogue with the deceased (Anderson and Dimond 1995; Costello and Kendrick 2000; Hegge and Fischer 2000). These feelings commonly persist beyond 6 months, with some resolution taking place after 12 months. Loneliness is one of the most common and often intense experience of bereavement, and it may be made worse by daily reminders of the dead spouse, anniversaries and having to learn to socialise as a single person (Anderson and Dimond 1995). Ageing and loneliness result in feelings of social isolation that are seen as part and parcel of the social experience of ageing (Costello 1999). Factors associated with more loneliness for the widowed are: strong feelings of emotional loneliness before the death; more support from the partner during marriage; talking about the death beforehand; poorer physical health; and having more reliance on support from others. Anticipated death of the partner and being able to prepare can mean that the bereaved spouse experiences less loneliness in bereavement (van Baarsen *et al.* 1999). Being able to help the spouse to prepare for the death is an important aspect of caring for older people who face the loss of a husband, wife or partner. There are many aspects that can be explored, including the care of the dying spouse, what will happen at the time of the death, practical issues regarding end of life rituals, such as funerals, and how the bereaved spouse is likely to cope. However, the reality of being a bereaved spouse is something that, no matter how much grief is anticipated, may still come as a shock and affect the widow in ways that they did not expect.

Conjugal bereavement as a social experience for older people can cause significant life changes, resulting in social disenfranchisement. Furthermore, the social structures for support appear to be less visible and available in many families and communities. Grief may go unrecognised, for example, in the case of losing a friend whose family are the main focus for sympathies. Jean's experience of losing her sister illustrated feelings of marginalisation. In general the bereaved are expected to pick themselves up and continue to function as they did before, when in reality it is often hugely difficult for them to adapt to the loss. As the story of Jean highlights, the loss may not be seen as significant by the family and others whereas it may have had a profound impact on the person concerned.

There are significant challenges for the wider social network and health and social care providers to support the older person to adapt to their new situation and to carry on living a meaningful life. An awareness of the circumstances of the death and how prepared the bereaved person is will allow those who care for bereaved older people to identify those who may have difficulties with loneliness and social isolation.

Continuing bonds

Bereaved older people, particularly those who are lonely and socially isolated, may develop an on-going emotional attachment with the deceased person. This continuing bond with the deceased is generally experienced by the bereaved individual as the presence of an on-going inner relationship (Field 2006). In recent years, researchers have argued that continuing a bond with a deceased person facilitates coping through a process of reflecting on the loss and managing reminders (Anderson and Dimond 1995). Bereaved older spouses commonly have vivid dreams of the dead spouse and sense their presence (Hegge and Fischer 2000). People find comfort in memories and being able to feel near to the dead person and to continue to include them in their lives. There is no desire to be rid of the dreams and memories. Listening to older people's stories of times with their late spouse and how their death has been amalgamated into their on-going life is more valued by the bereaved than advice about moving on or getting over their grief.

In addition, widows often look for explanations for their husbands' deaths to help them make sense of it and to cope with the loss (Costello and Kendrick 2000). They develop an inner representation of the death that aids the development of a continued dialogue with the deceased (Costello and Kendrick 2000; Bennett 2004). A key theme of their bereavement for widows is the death of the partner. Development of a story of the events that took place around the spouse's death may help to clarify events that have been unclear and confusing (Bennett and

Vidal-Hall 2000). Both widows and widowers may form an explanation for the death that is memorised for retelling to others and with the purposes of helping the widow to adjust to continuing life with, and without, the deceased spouse and to assist in the re-creation of his or her own identity (Walter 1996). Bereavement care and support interventions should give the widowed permission to retain their bond with the dead partner. They should be allowed the time and opportunity to develop an explanation for the death of their spouse, be listened to and have questions about the death answered as they search for meaning in their spouse's death. The individual's general practitioner (GP) may be the person best placed to address such needs (Walter 1996) but may have the least time available to listen.

Changed identity

Widowhood brings a major change in identity for individuals who previously experienced life as a couple. Lifestyle changes are necessary, but at the same time should allow the continued bond with the deceased to endure. Financial and practical issues often arise for the remaining partner. Older women commonly find that they are less well off and have to take on responsibility for financial arrangements. Men, on the other hand, have to learn new roles that traditionally belonged to the wife, for example cooking and shopping. Threats to the person's identity caused by role change may cause additional psychological distress for the widowed (Utz 2006).

Hockey and colleagues (2001) described the use of spaces, both private and public, as challenging for the widow and widower as they adapt to their new status. Commonly, changes include differences in use of rooms in the house, meal arrangements and taking holidays. Rearrangements could help them to deal with feelings of social isolation and loneliness associated with previously shared spaces. Such changes will be made gradually, over a period of time that the widow feels is appropriate. The support of family and friends through adjustments will be important to allow them to feel reassured that the changes made are acceptable.

Following bereavement, changes are made to more than living arrangements and spaces. Perhaps more importantly, relationships are often renegotiated in families for mutual benefit, and new commonalities with and sources of support in friends are found. However, bereavement is sometimes found to exacerbate family difficulties, adding to the stress of loss (Hockey *et al.* 2001). Relationships between family members, friends and others often change to accommodate the loss. Bereaved widows change their social worlds to minimise feelings of isolation, for example, by socialising with other widows (Anderson and Dimond 1995). Older people's concerns about changes to lifestyle and family dynamics following bereavement should be taken seriously. It is important that people are listened to, helped to make sense of what is happening to them and encouraged to explore alternative arrangements. For example, Jean lost the support and companionship of her husband, and through realignment of her social network and renewing of a kinship bond, found that she and her sister, also a widow, could form a mutually supportive relationship.

Patterns of grief reactions following spousal loss

As well as examining bereavement experiences, bereavement researchers in recent years have identified common patterns of grief in older people who have lost a spouse. It is useful to present these trajectories and examine which particular aspects of the bereaved person's health profile prior to the death, circumstances surrounding the death and reaction to the death may affect the bereavement reaction. These have important implications for the making of decisions about providing bereavement care services. The findings were the result of investigating longitudinal data from the Changing Lives of Older Couples (CLOC) study, involving 1,532 married people. Respondents were the surviving members of couples where the male partner was aged 65 years or over (Bonanno *et al.* 2002). Three common patterns of bereavement outcome for older people were identified (see also Chapter 2 for a general review of bereavement):

- short-term disruptions in functioning, for example, increased depression, cognitive problems, health problems;
- chronic disruptions in functioning;
- relative absence of grief reaction.

The study found that a large number of participants showed little evidence of intense grieving or denial. A further finding was that chronic grief was different from chronic depression. In chronic grief the level of depression increased following the partner's death and remained high for up to 18 months afterwards. Those with chronic depression had high levels of depression before the death that remained elevated throughout the bereavement. Others showed signs of depression before the death that improved afterwards. A further group displayed common grief responses with low levels of depression before the death, increased depression levels up to 6 months after the death, followed by a reduction by 18 months afterwards. An understanding of these patterns is useful as an aid to identification of those who may need support and those to whom support would be less beneficial.

More recently, Bonnano and colleagues (2004) used CLOC data to examine variables that determine the four common grief reactions identified above. Table 4.1 gives an overview of the factors found to contribute to each reaction type and suggestions for whether or not intervention is needed and what should be addressed through intervention.

Table 4.1 provides an indication of needs based on some broad differentiation of reactions to the death. In addition, Lee and Carr (2007) examined contextual factors, including gender, and assessed whether they related to physical functioning in widows. The aim was to assist practitioners to identify those most at risk of poor quality of life, chronic ill health, and even mortality, by identifying specific aspects of spousal loss that affected physical functioning. Again CLOC data were analysed 6, 18 and 48 months post loss. This study confirmed that the particular context of the loss could have long-term effects on physical functioning. Distressing

Table 4.1 Reaction type, contributing factors and intervention

Reaction	Contributing factors	Intervention
Little evidence of intense grieving	Satisfying marriage Less time thinking about the loss, searching for meaning or using avoidance strategies Finds comfort in memories	Unlikely to need or benefit
Depressed before death – improved after death	Spouse's death likely to mark end of long-term cause of stress Marriage less likely to be satisfying Spouse likely to have had poor health Unlikely to be in denial Positive memories of life with spouse	Likely to cope well and not need intervention
Chronic grief (often now included in complicated grief)	Emotional and cognitive disruption at time of the death Likely to have yearning feelings and emotional turmoil in early stages Think and talk about the death more often Search for meaning in the loss up to 18 months into bereavement	Help to process the loss and make meaning
Chronic depression	Emotional difficulties prior to the loss worsened by the loss Not influenced by time since the loss	Help to build self-esteem and deal with daily stresses

aspects of the death had negative physical effects that did not diminish over time. However, no single aspect of the death had distinct harmful or protective effects. Women were found to have similar levels of physical functioning before and after the death regardless of the nature of the death; however, men's functioning post loss varied widely. When the partner died in distressing circumstances there was little difference in physical function in bereavement for men and women. However, in less distressing conditions men fared better. This, it was explained, may be because women generally have higher levels of stress at home that include providing practical, emotional and health-related support to their husbands and responsibilities that lead to high stress even in bereavement.

The study also concluded that the adverse affects of widowhood were long term, with implications for supporting older people to be independent in the weeks, months and years after the death of the spouse. The context of the death often determined the response to the loss and, given this, factors that are important to the bereaved older person should be part of risk assessment whether carried out on a formal or an informal basis. In general, bereavement support is more likely to be offered in the first 6–12 months, when distress is most evident, but may be more helpful when continued long term.

Health and social care providers have many factors to consider when assessing a bereaved person's reaction including availability of support, the nature and quality of the spousal relationship and the circumstances of the loss. These could be considered as part of risk assessment procedures that can assist in making decisions about whether or not bereavement counselling or other interventions are required or would be beneficial. There are, of course, practical issues of staff availability, time and workload planning for health and social care practitioners in providing bereavement support. To make best use of these valuable resources, the research reviewed implies that bereavement care should be provided only to those with particular needs who have been identified through risk assessment. Intervention that is tailored to need and promotes self-care and independence in the bereaved would be most helpful for the bereaved themselves and most satisfying and cost-effective for practitioners. Older people with bereavement difficulties could, however, be signposted to other appropriate services where they are available. For example, Cruse Bereavement Care is a UK-wide voluntary organisation that provides bereavement support and counselling to help people to understand their grief and cope with their loss (Cruse Bereavement Care 2010).

Conclusion

My experiences, outlined at the beginning of the chapter, may reflect the type of interaction that health and social care staff have with bereaved older people on a regular basis. I found that as my career progressed I developed some understanding of older people's reactions and needs when someone close dies, and of the support that it was possible for me to provide. In the hospital situation opportunity to support is limited; however, simple words of sympathy, being able to listen and to provide information about the events that led to the death are useful ways of interacting with relatives.

The chapter confirms bereavement as a major life stressor that may be part of one of many losses accumulated over a number of years, and that can lead to health consequences and compromised ability to cope. Many older people show resilience to the effects of grief and, though distressed and saddened, can balance the loss against positive aspects in their life. Achieving the balance can be found through the maintenance of a bond with the deceased or by forming links with other family members that ameliorate the loss. Some of the consequences of bereavement can, however, be debilitating and detrimental to the functioning of the older person. The role of health and social care staff when dealing with bereaved older people is challenging in many ways. Care delivered at the time of a death and in the weeks and months that follow is often based on a relationship that has built up over a period of caring for the ill person and the family before the death. During this time professionals will get to know the family and should be in a position to help the family members prepare for the death and subsequently the bereavement. It may also be a time when some assessment of the coping strategies and needs of the relatives can take place. When thinking about older bereaved spouses, for example, the patterns of bereavement described by Bonanno and colleagues (2004) are useful models to use to assess a widow's or widower's support needs. Whether assessment of the bereaved is sensitive to the diversity of bereavement responses is arguable. However, as the chapter has highlighted, sharing of information about the bereaved between services and facilitated follow-ups to appropriate support agencies is likely to lead to improved services.

The identification of the important contribution made by older people to their communities could indicate that independence and self-care should be promoted following bereavement. Loss through death is not something that people recover from but something that they generally adapt to and build into their lives. Understanding how bereavement is experienced by older people should enable health and social care staff to interact with them in an empathic way.

References

Adriaensen M (2006) *Als Ouderen rouwen: oudere mensen helpen bij verlies*. Tielt: Lannoo.

Anderson MA (2007) *Caring for older adults holistically*, 4th edn. Philadelphia: FA Davis.

Anderson KL and Dimond MF (1995) The experience of bereavement in older adults. *Journal of Advanced Nursing* 22(2): 308–315.

Bennett KM (2004) Why did he die? The attributions of cause of death among women widowed in later life. *Journal of Health Psychology* 9(3): 345–353.

Bennett KM and Vidal-Hall S (2000) Narratives of death: a qualitative study of widowhood in later life. *Ageing and Society* 20(4): 413–428.

Bonanno GA, Wortman CB, Lehman DR, Tweed RG, Haring M, Sonnega J, Carr D and Nesse RM (2002) Resilience to loss and chronic grief: a prospective study from preloss to 18-months postloss. *Journal of Personality and Social Psychology* 83(5): 1150–1164.

Bonanno GA, Nesse RM and Wortman CB (2004) Prospective patterns of resilience and maladjustment during widowhood. *Psychology and Aging* 19(2): 260–271.

Christakis NA and Allison PD (2006) Mortality after the hospitalization of a spouse. *New England Journal of Medicine* 354(7): 719–730.

Costello J (1999) 'Filling the void': grief and loneliness in older adults. *Illness, Crisis and Loss* 7(3): 218–232.

Costello J and Kendrick K (2000) Grief and older people: the making or breaking of emotional bonds following partner loss in later life. *Journal of Advanced Nursing* 32(6): 1374–1382.

Cruse Bereavement Care (2006) Cruse Bereavement Care. Available at: http://www.crusebereavementcare.org.uk/ (accessed 20 April 2009).

Doka KJ (ed.) (2002) *Disenfranchised grief: new directions, challenges and strategies for practice*. Champaign, IL: Research Press.

Dutton YC and Zisook S (2005) Adaptation to bereavement. *Death Studies* 29(10): 877–903.

Field NP (2006) Unresolved grief and continuing bonds: an attachment perspective. *Death Studies* 30(8): 739–756.

Godfrey M (2001) Prevention: developing a framework for conceptualizing and evaluating outcomes of preventive services for older people. *Health & Social Care in the Community* 9(2): 89–99.

Grimby A, Johansson AK, Valter S and Grimby G (2008) Walking habits in elderly widows. *American Journal of Hospice & Palliative Care* 25(2): 81–87.

Hansson RO and Stroebe MS (2007) *Bereavement in late life*. Washington, DC: American Psychological Association.

Hegge M and Fischer C (2000) Grief responses of senior and elderly widows: practice implications. *Journal of Gerontological Nursing* 26(2): 35–43.

Hockey J, Penhale B and Sibley D (2001) Landscapes of loss: spaces of memory, times of bereavement. *Ageing and Society* 21(6): 739–757.

International Work Group on Death, Dying and Bereavement (2000) Death, dying, and bereavement in relation to older individuals. *Illness, Crisis and Loss* 8(4): 388–394.

Lee M and Carr D (2007) Does the context of spousal loss affect the physical functioning of older widowed persons? *Research on Aging* 29(5): 457–487.

Nihtilä E and Martikainen P (2008) Institutionalization of older adults after the death of a spouse. *American Journal of Public Health* 98(7): 1228–1234.

O'Rourke N (2004) Cognitive adaptation and women's adjustment to conjugal bereavement. *Journal of Women & Aging* 16(1–2): 87–104.

Prigerson HG and Jacobs SC (2001) Perspectives on care at the close of life: caring for bereaved patients: 'all the doctors just suddenly go'. *Journal of the American Medical Association* 286(11): 1369–1376.

Siegel JM and Kuykendall DH (1990) Loss, widowhood, and psychological distress among the elderly. *Journal of Consulting & Clinical Psychology* 58(5): 519–524.

Stephen AI, Wimpenny P, Unwin R, Work F, Dempster P, Macduff C, Wilcock SE and Brown A (2009) Bereavement and bereavement care in health and social care: provision and practice in Scotland. *Death Studies* 33(3): 239–261.

Stroebe M and Schut H (1999) The dual process model of coping with bereavement: rationale and description. *Death Studies* 23(3): 197–224.

Stroebe M, Schut H and Stroebe W (2006) Who benefits from disclosure? Exploration of attachment style differences in the effects of expressing emotions. *Clinical Psychology Review* 26(1): 66–85.

Stroebe M, Schut H and Stroebe W (2007) Health outcomes of bereavement. *Lancet* 370: 1960–1973.

Utz RL (2006) Economic and practical adjustments to late life spousal loss. In: Carr D, Nesse RM and Wortman CB (eds) *Spousal bereavement in late life*. New York: Springer.

Van Baarsen B, Smit JH, Snijders TAB and Knipscheer KPM (1999) Do personal conditions and circumstances surrounding partner loss explain loneliness in newly bereaved older adults? *Ageing and Society* 19(4): 441–469.

Van Praagh J (2000) *Healing grief: reclaiming life after any loss*. London: Piatkus.

Walter T (1996) A new model of grief: bereavement and biography. *Mortality* 1(1): 7–25.

Part II
Contexts of bereavement

5 End of life care and bereavement

John Costello

Key messages

- The need for supportive bereavement services after death is generally recognised as an integral part of palliative care provision.
- The families of those who need hospice and specialist palliative care services generally have better access to bereavement care both before and after death. Such bereavement care should be available to everyone.
- Implementing National Institute for Health and Clinical Excellence (NICE) guidelines for palliative care could improve bereavement services for all families of those dying from cancer but may increase inequity to those dying from other diseases. Standards/protocols for bereavement care are required for all settings.
- Cultural diversity needs to be addressed in bereavement services.
- As multiple factors may influence bereavement, it is essential to undertake assessment of risk. There is a need to identify those who are less likely to cope with and at risk of complicated grief. Formal assessment tools can be used to facilitate this process.
- All staff involved in bereavement care require appropriate education, training and supervision in order to provide optimal end of life care.
- There is a need for assessment of individuals and families in the bereavement period both before and after death, particularly to identify those at most risk, although there is a lack of consensus on how to conduct follow-up, by whom, and at what time.
- Anticipatory grieving is distinct from conventional grief in both duration and form. Often the patient and their significant others are experiencing similar emotions during a period of sustained uncertainty.

Introduction

The purpose of this chapter is to examine the increasing evidence base relating to end of life care and bereavement and to identify ways of providing optimal bereavement support based on this. Considerable discussion took place on the inclusion of a specific chapter on end of life care and bereavement. The debate revolved around whether or not palliative care should be seen separately from bereavement care, occupying a separate context, as it may be argued that it should be integral to all services. This begged the question of how it could be omitted from a book that sought to examine the evidence on bereavement, when so much had been developed within this field related to end of life care and bereavement – more than any other! The evidence reviewed in this chapter includes a range of bereavement issues. These have been elicited from evidence related to the literature on palliative care which, we would argue, can be applied equally in any health and social care setting.

Palliative care covers a multitude of medical conditions, chiefly cancer, although emphasis has now been placed on non-malignant life-threatening medical conditions (Addington-Hall and Higginson 2001). Focusing on the palliative care literature relating to bereavement specifically proved to be quite a challenge. In broad terms the review of evidence highlighted a small number of randomised controlled trials and non-systematic literature reviews and in-depth case studies from hospices. The contemporary evidence clearly indicated that palliative care needs robust bereavement support services in order to enable optimal services to be provided (Payne *et al.* 2008).

This chapter will examine three key areas related to bereavement identified in the available evidence. The first of these is the need for appropriate assessment pre bereavement, looking specifically at anticipatory grief and its role for individuals and families facing impending death. Second, related to this, is the need to examine the multiple factors influencing bereavement, notably the impact of the bad news and the context in which loss takes place. Third, the chapter considers the pre- and post-death need for bereavement risk assessment in order to highlight those features of bereavement likely to give cause for concern regarding the possibility of grief becoming complicated. The three major themes encapsulate the emerging issues from the evidence; namely, that for many individuals and families, care can be provided for an extensive period of time before death. During this time, individuals and families adjusting to changing circumstances face a range of bereavement needs which can become apparent before death owing to both the type of disease and their response to the circumstances surrounding the impending loss. In terms of promoting optimal bereavement support, the chapter also identifies the need for practitioners to implement guidelines which are likely to lead to improved standards and protocols for bereavement.

The development of bereavement support in palliative care

In the last 10–15 years, evidence of the need for good bereavement support in palliative care has been stressed by many writers. Payne and Relf (2001: 158) make the following assertion: 'The emphasis placed on family centred care means that continuing support after a patient's death is, logically, an integral component of palliative care.'

The global evidence concerning the nature and extent of bereavement services provided by hospices and specialist palliative care teams highlighted similar provision for families, especially after the death of a child (Beardsmore and Fitzmaurice 2002; DeCinque *et al.* 2004). In the UK the most common forms of bereavement support include one-to-one counselling and befriending. Other forms of bereavement care include telephone support (Field *et al.* 2004) and a range of services which included referral to other agencies, memorials, anniversary and remembrance services (such as day-after-day events) and a wide network of support group resources (Wimpenny *et al.* 2007).

The evidence from the UK literature clearly indicates disparities across the UK in the provision of bereavement services, with families of those who access hospice and specialist palliative care services having more effective bereavement experiences both before and after death. This indicates a need for greater equity of bereavement care provision to individuals and families. Moreover, it highlights a need to determine, through accurate assessment, when this type of care is likely to be required and how effective it might be. It does however, need to be recognised that conducting research with seriously ill patients is very difficult and challenging, not least because of attrition rates, missing data and a lack of willingness to make a sustained contribution to research, which is a particular problem in palliative care. Let us begin by considering when palliative care begins and how to assess the need for bereavement support.

When does palliative care begin?

The evidence carries with it an assumption that the starting point for providing palliative care is the point of diagnosis (Watson *et al.* 2005; Mount *et al.* 2006; Wee and Hughes 2007; Payne *et al.* 2008). According to the evidence, it is commonly accepted that when some people are first told their diagnosis, they begin their cancer journey (Tadman and Roberts 2006) or dying trajectory (Strauss 1984). For many this is an experience of sustained uncertainty (Walter 1999), framed by a fear that they may die (Woodhouse 2004; Mallon 2008) and an all-consuming emotional propensity to consider end of life in a spiritual sense (Cobb 2001). It may be argued, as it is by Leader (2008), that grief is a very painful process and that for mourners, bereavement can take many years to develop depending on the nature of the loss.

For many families and individuals, the disclosure of bad news sets off a chain reaction of thoughts, feelings and ideas about the future, and is less an event and more of a process (Arber and Gallagher 2003). The subsequent crisis involves worry, fear and anxiety about the patient and others, especially when children are involved. It may therefore be argued that, for some, bereavement support begins at the time the patient and family are made aware that the diagnosis does not involve cure. The breaking of bad news is described in Chapter 15, although, as Baile and colleagues (2000) point out in their SPIKES protocol, it is important for those who disclose such information that empathic responses are made which help the family to explore emotions, assess the patient's response and agree a plan or a contract for the future. This contract can include the provision of continuous support to help with their anticipatory grief (Costello 1999) and conclude with post-bereavement support. One of the concerns of this chapter is how bereavement support can be provided to families and individuals living with a life-limiting illness, and begins with assessment.

Assessment

Palliative care embraces the notion of physical, social and psychological care, which includes spirituality and a complex of psychosocial care widely reported to include bereavement support for the family and those close to the patient. Palliative care originated in the modern hospice movement and, in general terms, it is widely assumed that bereavement care is central to effective palliative and supportive care. This integral part of palliative care philosophy has been formally recognised and named as supportive care (Department of Health 2008). Supportive care is the term used to highlight the importance of providing help, advice and guidance to patients, friends and family who share many of the adverse experiences of the illness. Despite the plethora of journal articles and books on palliative care, there is a lack of empirical evidence about how and when assessment of grief reactions should be made and the type of interventions likely to provide optimal support for bereaved individuals and families. The evidence related to assessment of individual grief reactions prior to death is limited. It has been reported that anticipatory grief (grieving prior to death) occurs, although what to do about it remains unclear (Costello 1996; Rando 2000; Clukey 2008). Anticipatory grief experiences were first identified by Lindemann as early as 1944 and later described in more detail by Schoenberg and colleagues (1974) as the emotional experiences some people have before the loss of a loved one. They involve a complex range of cognitive, physical and social responses made by the dying person as well as the soon to be bereaved, prior to death. Grief experiences that take place before death are different in duration and form from those that take place after death. Table 5.1 summarises the main differences between anticipatory and post-death grief.

Anticipatory grieving is distinct from conventional grief in both duration and form. As Table 5.1 illustrates, often the patient and their significant others are experiencing similar emotions during a period of sustained uncertainty. It provides the mourner with the opportunity to carry out grief *in advance of* death but can also complicate what people refer to as the *working through process*, by enabling

Table 5.1 Differences between anticipatory and post-death grief

Anticipatory grief	Post-death grief
Experienced by both dying person and family	Grief experienced by mourners only
Grieving can begin from time of diagnosis and finishes at death	Grieving begins after death
Duration limited to time of death	May last indefinitely
Emotional intensity increases as death approaches	Emotional intensity diminishes over time

the griever to realise their emotional feelings about and towards the dying person before death. The early evidence indicates that preparation for the loss is an important part of anticipatory grief. However, as Rando (1986) points out, when the duration between diagnosis and death is prolonged, especially in younger people, there is a greater likelihood of difficulties arising. Where the loss relates to older people there are contradictions in bereavement outcome, although, in general, bereavement outcomes were considered more positive when a period of preparation allowed grieving to take place prior to death (Glick *et al.* 1974; Parkes 1974; Evans 1994). Later in the chapter, I consider the impact of sudden death and how the trauma arising from such experiences correlates with poor bereavement outcomes. One of the challenges in helping people with anticipatory grief is that it may include not only the family but, in some cases, the patient as well. Consider the following case study:

> Ken (72) was diagnosed with liver cancer and was told he might have only a few months to live. He was cared for at home by his wife Edna (74), herself an ex-nurse. In the period before his death Ken wrote down all the 'man' type things he did and explained about bills and household repairs that he took care of. He made a list of things to do and bought a cuddly dog and explained that when he was gone, if she became lonely and fed up she could give it a cuddle.

Ken's wife Edna referred herself to me for bereavement counselling. When she told me her story I asked her what was specifically bothering her? 'It doesn't feel right', she said:

> I am not very sad, I miss him of course but I feel ok, we arranged things like he said, the funeral and the scattering of the ashes went according to the plans we made. But I feel odd, unusual, everyone keeps telling me I will work through the pain but I feel fine is there something wrong with me?

Edna's story may be considered unique. There are estimated to be about 6 million carers in the UK who work hard to meet the physical and emotional needs of people with a range of long-term illnesses (Costello 2009). Edna had *worked through* a lot of grief *prior to* Ken's death. Observers of Edna's grief may often mistake her behaviour as denial because the pattern of observed grief does not follow conventional behaviour when a person has experienced anticipatory grief. Edna's conjugal bereavement is not unlike the experience of spouses who care for others with neurological diseases, such as advanced Alzheimer's disease, who encounter what is called *social death* (Sweeting and Gilhooley 1991). This is where the patient has little or no meaningful social interaction with those around them. Spouses of such patients have commented to me that *they are not the person they married*. This may be because they are unable to have any meaningful social and emotional contact.

Instead they may even be found to *look forward to the death of a loved one* as a form of release or a blessing. This, in itself, can be confusing and worrying for the carer. When death occurs their behaviour is not like that of others whose spouses die suddenly, where there may be a limited or non-existent illness trajectory to enable them to make the necessary adaptations to the impending loss.

The experience of loss

When assessing the impact of bereavement in a palliative care context, the evidence from a wide range of reports and research, including professional opinion (largely psychoanalytical), states that it is important to consider a number of key issues (summarised in Box 5.1) relating to the person and their experience of loss. These factors are useful in identifying the extent to which the bereaved's grief may become complicated; in other words, is the grief part of a normal process of adjustment to loss or are there signs that the intensity and duration of the grief is such that there are indications of pathology likely to require professional help? Emphasis should be placed on understanding and listening to the person. In many cases, grief is complex and influenced as much by the society in which a bereaved person lives as by the attitudes and expectations of those around them (Relf 2006). Much of the evidence relates to conjugal bereavement in adult heterosexual couples, with some exceptions (see, for example, Glackin and Higgins 2008). The evidence, in palliative care, widely recognises that the death of a partner represents a very significant loss, not only because of their connection with the deceased, which is significant, but also because the mourner's future dreams, hopes and plans for the future will be or are lost. These factors associated with making the adjustment to loss are taken from a broad range of evidence (Clark *et al.* 1997; Sheldon 1997; Clark and Seymour 1999; Copp 1999; Dickenson *et al.* 2000; Payne and Relf 2001; Field *et al.* 2004; Seymour 2001; Sandman 2005; Relf 2006; Mallon 2008; Glackin and Higgins 2008).

Loss history

This is the experience of previous loss. This may be tangible, such as the death of a person or a pet, house repossession or amputation. It is important to identify the connection or what is termed the quality of the *relationship of attachment*

Box 5.1 Factors affecting the impact of loss on bereavement

- Loss history
- Circumstances of the loss
- Personal grieving styles
- Social network
- Strategies for coping and supportive services

(Parkes *et al.* 1995). This is the extent to which emotion, such as love, has been invested in the relationship and can give an indication of the amount of emotional pain being experienced. Conversely, the loss can be intangible, such as the loss of self-respect arising from house repossession, loss of independence through hospitalisation or imprisonment. In some cases, as Charmaz (1980) points out, loss of self can occur, when a person experiences this as trauma such as rape, severe physical symptoms such as those arising from a road traffic accident (RTA), severe mental illness or psychological and physical abuse. The last can result in a change in the person's expressed emotions and appear to alter their personality. I once had a young woman attend a bereavement workshop who had had an RTA which resulted in severe spinal injuries necessitating 6 months in hospital. After discharge she felt that her personality had changed, she was no longer the extrovert person she once was and she worried about where her old self had gone. Other people following trauma from abuse experience intangible forms of loss that are difficult to assess and understand, and many require specialist guidance.

Circumstances of the loss

It is important to asses the circumstances as well as the relationship of attachment (ROA), with the mourners identifying likely sources of regret that may arise from the varied situations arising from stigmatised death such as suicide and murder. Despite many patients receiving palliative care in a variety of contexts, this does not preclude sudden death occurring from conditions other than the primary source. This can give rise to severe forms of grief, preventing the person from adjusting because they failed to say goodbye or because there was what Parkes (1990:148) calls *unfinished business of the relationship*. Within a palliative care scenario, it is not unusual for people to feel aggrieved by the lack of active treatment or by not being given information after the death, such as the deceased having had cancer or a Do Not Resuscitate order (DNR) placed in their medical notes without prior discussion. This once again highlights the importance of engagement with the patient and the family to identify their understanding. After the death, one of the most effective ways of responding to these issues is to actively listen to the story of the bereaved; find out what happened (the facts) as well as the associated feelings attached to the loss. Hearing is not the same as listening, as Brother Francis points out in Chapter 9. It may be useful to ask if the bereaved has any specific regrets about any of the events leading up to and including the death itself. A problem-solving approach can be used to untie the emotional knots associated with the circumstances.

Personal grieving styles

Central to promoting effective bereavement outcomes is the importance of giving meaning to the loss and recognising its effects. The contemporary literature discusses 'grieving styles', a term used to describe behavioural patterns during bereavement (Martin and Doka 2000). A widow crying every day in the immediate aftermath of the death is relatively normal, although if this persists for ever, it may raise some concerns. We all cope with crises in different ways; some cry to express themselves. *It's good to talk* is an adage that works well for some and not for others. In some cases grievers choose to use recreational or prescribed drugs, such as sedatives, to manage the loss. In a broad sense patterns or styles of grieving may be summarised as effective and ineffective (see Table 5.2).

Some people, referred to as feminine grievers (Martin and Doka 2000), express themselves and are articulate in their emotional expression. Others, referred to by Doka as masculine grievers, feel more comfortable doing tasks which can lead to them feeling better because sitting and talking is perceived as being too difficult for them. Doka points out that not all women are feminine grievers and not all men masculine grievers (see the case scenario on Nancy in Chapter 3). We all have our own coping styles and it is important to assess grief on the basis of the individual constraints, cultural rules and norms, and the environmental factors, which include family relationships. Asking a person to disclose their loss history and to describe and recall how they coped in the past and where they gained strength can help the person to recognise their own strengths and limitations. It may also help to answer some of the more complex questions about the meanings that people attach to loss.

Social network

We are all influenced in different ways by our environment and by those around us. We draw strength from our relationships, although we can also be adversely affected by negative influences. The existence of a social network of friends and family members can be a source of comfort during bereavement, although not everyone has a supportive network. Employment can be a potential strength, as some people can receive support from colleagues and to an extent become distracted by their work roles and relationships (see Chapter 14). Family members may be supportive, but this is not guaranteed because bereaved families can express their grief in a variety of ways, some by *not* talking about the loss, others constantly wishing to discuss the death, to the discomfort of others. I recall visiting

Table 5.2 Styles of grieving

Effective	Ineffective
Choosing exercise or physical and activity to discharge energy	Lack of interest in physical activity
Using small amounts of support or *dosing*	Unable to utilise existing support networks or support is fragmented
Shelving grief in order to meet responsibilities and discussing personal issues with appropriate people at certain times and dosing emotional pain when obligations have been met	Tendency to focus on loss and become distressed at different times when faced with reminders of the deceased

an elderly bereaved lady whose husband had recently died and she cautioned me that if her son were to come back we should stop the session as he did not believe in counsellors and would be upset if he were to 'catch us talking' about his father's death!

It is, however, widely assumed that family members are generally supportive of each other, and the absence of family members, close neighbours and work colleagues for reasons such as retirement, unemployment and disability can mean that a person's social network is limited and the opportunities for sharing their concerns, worries and fears are restricted. Many of my clients have others to talk to, but sometimes feel inhibited because they feel they are hogging the conversation, imposing themselves on others or being a burden (often if they are elderly), or being selfish and self-indulgent. One-to-one counselling is an important way of enabling the bereaved to respond and share their concerns in an empathic climate.

Now consider the difficulties associated with the following situation:

> Mr Hall (82) was recently diagnosed with pancreatic cancer and was not likely to live for more than a few months. He was unaware of his diagnosis and the outcome and keen to return to the nursing home, which he regarded as his home and where he was very happy. His son was told his father's diagnosis by the consultant, who adopted the principle that he did not tell patients they were dying, only next of kin. However, if the patient asked he would disclose the diagnosis. His son was aware of the diagnosis but was reluctant to discuss it with his father. How might health care staff deal with this situation?

In the above scenario, you may think it relatively straightforward to simply tell the patient that he has cancer and is going to die. The *closed awareness* principle of the consultant in not disclosing the truth to the patient acts as an impediment to promoting effective communication. This is one of the organisational issues experienced by some patients dying in hospital (Costello 2004). There are many other issues, such as the confidence, ability, knowledge and expertise of the practitioner. How many of us feel confident to have conversations with patients facing impending death?

Clukey's (2008) research indicated that supporting families facing impending death is complex and changes the nature of the relationship between family and caregiver. Further evidence of the need to consider a more integrated approach to understanding family grief reactions comes from the work of Moos (1995), who argues that family dynamics change when facing loss. She points out that it is important to develop an understanding of how families change when faced with impending death. On a personal note, a key issue for me when my father was dying had to do with the cohesion of the community nursing team and my inclusion in it, and the value of feeling part of the caring, multidisciplinary team (Costello 1990). Towards the end of his life, the family had to have a discussion with the GP about continuing treatment for a chest infection when Dad's cancer was advanced and death inevitable. We were united in allowing him to die without antibiotics and the GP was keen to treat the chest infection. As a compromise we agreed on 2 days of medication and then allowed Dad to die with dignity, which he did. It was a good compromise as it allowed a breathing space for all concerned and it felt positive to have the co-operation of the professionals in what was a very difficult situation.

Acknowledging the importance of anticipatory grief can provide a space at the end of life to *put things in order.* Knowing someone is going to die and sharing this between care providers and patients can be uplifting but also very challenging. It does allow time for a range of things to take place, such as making a will, spiritual care, sharing intimate things such as giving thanks and telling them how loved they are and what influence they had on your life.

Practitioners who are reluctant to create any distress at the start of the illness may feel a need to maintain a sense of hope and well-being, important elements of effective palliative care (Clark and Seymour 1999; Cobb 2001; Sandman 2005). However, the evidence indicates that having advance warning of the likely outcome of the disease is positively associated with good bereavement outcomes (Huber and Gibson 1990; Sweeting and Gilhooley 1991; Clukey 2008).

Strategies for coping and supportive services

Grief is multidimensional and impacts on a range of behaviours, often causing physical and psychological ill health. Following a long illness before death, some mourners are left physically exhausted and experience weight loss, lack of sleep and an inability to concentrate. Agoraphobia and a lack of desire to perform domestic tasks such as cooking, driving, going to work or doing housework, and many other routine activities, are not uncommon although my experience is that many become very houseproud and obsessively tidy! Others may experience vivid dreams and have panic attacks, breaking down in tears in public places, which causes them embarrassment and a reluctance to venture out of doors. Mentally they can appear full of anxiety and uncertain of what are the next steps. Others can become obsessed about their bodily functions.

There are a number of different strategies that can be considered in terms of providing effective bereavement support. Much depends on the situational and individual factors associated with the loss. Effective bereavement care is not always a case of one size fits all situations. Allowing the person to talk about their loved one is a common, and often very good, way to provide comfort and enable the bereaved person to express their anxieties. It may also be necessary at some time to point out that it is also OK to stop grieving and to get on with life. This approach, based on Freud's talking therapy, can be developed to include extending it to talking to and about photographs of the bereaved person's loved one, recalling the background to the photograph and what it represents. Where there is evidence of regret, perhaps due to the suddenness of the death, when things were not said and a proper goodbye did not occur, it can be useful, if the person feels it is appropriate, for them to write a letter and express themselves on paper. Writing a letter to the deceased is a way of enabling feelings to be expressed in a different form, especially when there are difficulties associated with articulating emotions. The letter can be read out, shared and passed amongst family members or become a therapeutic activity done by the person in their own home. I have used this technique on several occasions to good effect. In some cases, practical help in the form of visiting the graveside is a useful way of enabling bereaved people to make an important step after the funeral. There may be a tendency to disengage with others and become isolated. Visiting the graveside can provide time to cry and speak to the deceased. Going with others and being alone for a part of the time can be a significant step in working through the grief.

Assessing risk

Bereavement risk assessment has traditionally been undertaken in hospices, which have tended to lead the way in assessing likely grief reactions after death based on a variety of tools, often based on the pioneering work of Parkes and Weiss (1983). However, such tools can be adapted to apply across many health and social care settings. There are a number of broad risk factors that need to taken into consideration, although often the factors leading to complicated grief may be multiple and difficult to assess unless a lot is known about the bereaved and their relationship with the deceased. In health and social care contexts this can be undertaken based on knowing the family during the illness and getting to know their strengths, vulnerability and likely response to the impending death. Box 5.2 is a summary of risk factors associated with bereavement, which is not exhaustive but provides a broad basis upon which to base an initial assessment.

Risk factors, such as those in Box 5.2, give an indication of the likelihood of the mourner's grief becoming complicated, for example age, which raises the issue that younger and older people tend to be vulnerable to the impact of loss. Other factors such as poverty, low self-esteem and other simultaneous situations, such as loss

Box 5.2 Risk factors in bereavement (Parkes 1990)

- Age (death of a child)
- Poverty (financial hardship)
- Low self-esteem, anger, ambivalence towards deceased
- Multiple loss factors (death after a prolonged illness)
- Concurrent crisis (divorce, redundancy)
- Relationship difficulties prior to loss
- Perceived lack of social support
- Family/friends not seen as helpful or not in contact
- History of mental health issues
- Mode of death, sudden stigmatised death, murder, suicide, AIDS

of relationships, divorce and redundancy, influence and often accentuate the loss. Unexpected death can exacerbate feelings of loss, especially when there are any relationship issues referred to by Parkes (1990: 148) as 'unfinished business'. This can include ambivalence between the bereaved and the deceased or when there is dependency between the two. Where the patient has been cared for at home by the bereaved, over a long period, this can give rise to a sense of loss, referred to as the 'empty room syndrome' (Teel 1991). This arises because the bereaved has been used to providing active support to the deceased. Situations like this can occur with long-term illness and when the death is sudden. Mode of death can make a difference in terms of helping the bereaved make sense and give meaning to the loss. I encountered a family who refused to disclose that the son died of AIDS because of the stigma sometimes attached to such deaths. The acceptable cause reported by the family was hepatitis acquired during a trip to India. Stigmatised deaths can give rise to more long-term problems depending on the extent of social support (also see Chapter 3) (Doka 2002). The unemployed may have a more reduced social network and disabled people who find it difficult to mobilise and see others may be more at risk because of their limited social contact.

Bereavement risk assessment

The bereavement risk assessment tool illustrated in Figure 5.1 is taken and adapted from the work of Parkes (1990). Its purpose is to help professional care staff identify predictors around the time of bereavement which may adversely influence the development of complicated grief and are associated with good and bad outcomes. The risk assessment takes the form of a biographical section and a questionnaire with seven categories each with five items scored 1–5. Low-risk scores of 1–14 probably require no follow-up; scores of 15 and above should probably be followed up. However, any score of 4–5 in specific categories may require follow-up. In relation to the severity of grief reactions, the assessment of specific reactions as normal or abnormal needs to be considered in the context of what Prigerson and colleagues (2000) term 'competing views'. There are, as Klein and Alexander (2003) indicate, other criteria for establishing differences in normal/ abnormal grief reactions, such as severity of symptoms/reactions, duration of symptoms/reactions, delayed onset of symptoms/reactions and level of dysfunction related to home and work life.

Bereavement and palliative care

The consensus of evidence reviewed indicates that bereavement support has many guises and can take the form of practical help, including visiting the graveside or clearing the wardrobe and more intangible forms of help in adjusting to the loss, designed to help in coming to terms with the diagnosis (Walter 1999). In England and Wales, NICE guidance focuses on improving supportive and palliative care services for adults with cancer and specifies bereavement care (National Institute for Clinical Excellence 2004). The guidance acknowledges that families and carers provide essential support, often at the expense of their own needs for

Biographical details: name of the deceased and date of birth	
• Time, place and mode of death • Length of illness • Name of key person and contact details • Relationship to the deceased person • Any evidence of anticipatory grieving? • Any previous intervention by a counsellor/supportive person? • Would they object to any follow up? • Staff member most involved	
A: Children under 14 at home 0: None 1: One 2: Two 3: Three 4: Four 5: Five or more	**D: Anger** 1: None (or normal) 2: Mild irritation 3: Moderate, occasional outbursts 4: Severe, spoiling relationships 5: Extreme always bitter
B: Employment of key person outside the home 0: Unemployed 1: Works full time 2: Works part time 3: Retired 4: House person 5: Other	**E: Self reproach** 1: None 2: Mild – vague and general 3: Moderate, some clear self reproach 4: Severe, preoccupied with blame 5: Extreme major problem
C: Evidence of grieving 0: Never 1: Seldom 2: Moderate 3: Frequent 4: Constant 5: Constant/intense	**F: Relationship now** 1: Close intimate relationship with another person 2: Warm supportive family permitting expression of feeling 3: Family supportive but live at a distance 4: Doubtful 5: None of these

Figure 5.1 Bereavement risk assessment tool (adapted from Parkes 1990).

emotional and practical support being unrecognised, largely because they put the needs of the person/patient first (National Institute for Clinical Excellence 2004). The need for families and carers to be provided with support is particularly acute at certain times, for example around the time of diagnosis, at critical junctures when treatment is withheld or withdrawn or recurrence happens and at the end of treatment. Specifically bereavement care and support is required at the time of death and afterwards. One of the key issues arising from the NICE guidance is that professional support is not always available for families and carers who need it, despite a recommendation that improvements are needed.

Much of the advice from NICE is highly dependent on workforce development and the appointment of additional and well-educated staff to fulfil key roles within hospitals, care homes and health and social care organisations. In addition, this guidance is only extended to England and Wales, although a working party of the Scottish Partnership Agency for Palliative and Cancer Care (1998) has provided guidance within the last decade similar to the NICE recommendations, pointing out that education in palliative care for all health professionals should include cultural aspects of care and bereavement.

Follow-up for the bereaved

The need for supportive bereavement services after death appears to be generally recognised as an integral part of palliative care provision (Payne and Relf 2001). These services tend to be confined to those who have accessed hospice or specialist palliative care services while the deceased was alive. This may reflect the view that 'if you have cancer you are sorted' (Stephen *et al.* 2009). However, there appears to be a lack of bereavement services for cancer patients unable to access hospice or specialist palliative care. NICE (2004) indicates that provision of bereavement services is fragmented and often funded by the voluntary sector, although some recent attempts to develop bereavement services more widely in English acute hospital Trusts are reported by Field and colleagues (2004). It may be that a lack of contact between bereaved families and professionals results in support needs not being identified (National Institute for Clinical Excellence 2004). Contact through follow-up could provide some on-going contact that would allow support to be available after death to those who need it.

Several surveys have attempted to identify the nature and extent of follow-up bereavement services provided by hospices and specialist palliative care teams, mainly in the UK and USA, but also in New Zealand and Japan (Foliart *et al.* 2001; Payne and Relf 2001; Matsushima *et al.* 2002; Payne 2002; Demmer 2003; Field *et al.* 2005). Although not all hospices provide all the services identified, the following represent the main approaches:

- one-to-one support (befriending, counselling);
- telephone support;
- referral to other agencies;
- memorial, remembrance or anniversary services;
- written information and advice;
- support groups;
- drop-in support.

A variety of personnel are involved in delivering such bereavement services, although in the UK the largest group is nurses (Field *et al.* 2004). Other personnel involved include religious workers, social workers, doctors, psychologists, administrative and clerical staff, therapists and psychiatrists. This underlines the importance of a co-ordinated, multidisciplinary approach, with professionals, volunteers and lay people working together (Bouton 1996). However, small numbers of people tend to be involved in bereavement services; typically two or three paid members of staff are assisted by 11 or 12 volunteers, most working part-time (Field *et al.* 2004).

Internationally, volunteers play a major role in bereavement support services and tend to be involved in the majority of services (Payne *et al.* 1999; Foliart et al. 2001; Payne 2001; Matsushima et al. 2002; Payne 2002; Field *et al.* 2004). Volunteers can help normalise the grief process (Relf 2006) and are also viewed as a cost-effective means of supporting the bereaved (Payne 2002; Field *et al.* 2004). However, some concerns have been raised about whether the cost-effectiveness of volunteers could potentially be exploited, particularly as most volunteers are women (Payne 2002; Field *et al.* 2004) and many are over 60 years of age.

Training of both health and social care professionals and volunteers involved in bereavement care varies, as does the duration of programmes. In both the UK and USA the majority of staff receive specialist bereavement training (Demmer 2003; Field *et al.* 2004). However, in the UK this is more likely to be provided if individuals are involved in services provided by an in-patient unit (Field *et al.* 2004). Such training within palliative care settings is rarely transferred to other health and social care settings and yet deaths in hospices represent only about 5 per cent of all deaths. This promotes the view that those who work in palliative care are 'experts' in bereavement care. It is certainly the case that bereavement care is given greater priority in palliative care and, given this, the model developed could be transferred to all health and social care settings.

However, cultural and ethnic diversity does not appear to be well addressed in the provision of follow-up bereavement services. For example, there appear to be few volunteers in hospices from ethnic minority backgrounds (Payne and Relf 2001; Payne 2002). Spruyt (1999) has specifically highlighted a lack of bereavement support for Bangladeshi carers. This ethnic group commonly uses children as interpreters and it is suggested that bereaved children of this and other ethnic minorities may be at particular risk of complicated grief.

Inevitably, even within palliative care, time constraints and lack of staff have been identified as barriers to providing bereavement care (Demmer 2003; Field *et al.* 2004). The number of staff involved in bereavement services has declined since 1986 (Field *et al.* 2004). These authors argue that increasing demands on specialist palliative care community nurses impact negatively on bereavement support work, which was continually deferred because of other priorities. Time and staffing constraints highlight the need to ensure that bereavement services are targeted at those most at risk of developing mental or physical health problems. Assessment tools exist, such as that described above; however, in the UK, fewer than 50 per cent of hospices have been found to use a formal risk assessment tool (Field *et al.* 2004) although, as Stephen and colleagues (2009) highlight, assessment may be undertaken through informal methods, such as discussion at multidisciplinary meetings.

Little information exists about the evidence base for hospice bereavement services or their impact on bereavement outcome. However, in-depth case studies of five hospices in England revealed that most bereaved people were satisfied with the support they received (Field *et al.* 2004). This report also found the successful delivery of support groups problematic, as it frequently becomes difficult for new members to join. Irrespective of type of follow-up support, formal processes for enabling the bereaved to feed back on the services they receive are recommended so that provision can be adapted (Field *et al.* 2004). However, facilitated support groups have been described as resource intensive and may not be cost-effective (Field *et al.* 2004). Although some may disagree with the economic arguments, NICE (2004) also highlights the need for evaluative research to determine the cost-effectiveness of bereavement support services.

A recurring theme in the literature is the presumption that 'something should be done' for people who are bereaved, and it is not always clear whose needs are being met. Kaunonen and colleagues (2000a) describe setting up a system to phone family members after the death of a relative on an oncology ward in Finland. No evidence of effectiveness in terms of enhanced bereavement outcomes is apparent. However, in their review of the role of bereavement support groups in oncology services, Lorenz (1998) states that not providing support has medical and emotional implications for surviving family members.

Although there is general agreement on the need for assessment of individuals and families in the bereavement period, particularly to identify those at most risk, there is a lack of consensus on how this should be carried out, by whom and at what time. You may offer follow-up services in your own area of practice and there is evidence that it is usually well received by the bereaved and can offer opportunity to ask questions about the death as well as provide support. In addition, it is normally the case that only a small number of the bereaved will take up the offer of follow-up support.

NICE (2004) recommends that a three-component model of bereavement support should be implemented in all cancer networks in England and Wales (Table 5.3). This could be equally applied to all settings.

Table 5.3 A three-component model of bereavement support (NICE 2004)

Component 1	Component 2	Component 3
Recognises that grief is normal following the death of a loved one and most support will be provided by family and friends. All bereaved individuals should be offered information about the bereavement experience and how to access different forms of support regardless of place of death or services accessed before death. Health care professionals involved in end of life care should assess the coping abilities, available support and needs of individuals and families in preparation for bereavement	Offers more formal opportunities to reflect on the bereavement experience and may involve volunteers in preference to health care professionals. Processes should be in place to ensure those with complicated grief reactions are referred to the appropriate professionals	Is for the small number of people who will require specialist bereavement support, including mental health services and psychological support, including specialist counselling services. For those at risk of prolonged or complicated grief and provision for meeting the specialist needs of bereaved children and young people

Conclusion

Bereavement care and support is an integral part of palliative care, although many practitioners only glimpse the impact that loss has on the bereaved. The provision of services for the bereaved and the development of understanding and knowledge to support practice is also probably greater in palliative care services than elsewhere. However, this has the effect of viewing palliative care practitioners as 'experts' on bereavement and bereavement care, which can prevent development of services in, for example, acute and community-based settings, where the majority of people will die.

This chapter has highlighted the importance of assessment, albeit there is no specific way of assessing the risk of bereavement becoming complicated or pathological. It is also acknowledged that this is more likely to be carried out in specialist palliative care contexts. Those whose grief may be complicated by the loss and whose bereavement becomes problematic can be identified and referred to specialist practitioners. The chapter has also highlighted the need to anticipate likely grief reactions, assess appropriately as part of the supportive care provided to individuals and families, and be aware of the individual and cultural differences that impinge on the provision of supportive care.

Finally, the approaches and knowledge and understanding developed in palliative care settings need to be transferred to all health and social care settings to address the inequity of provision for the bereaved.

References

Addington-Hall JM and Higginson IJ (2001) *Palliative care for non cancer patients*. Oxford: Oxford University Press.

Arber A and Gallagher A (2003) Breaking bad news revisited: the push for negotiated disclosure and changing practice implications. *International Journal of Palliative Nursing* 9(4): 166–172.

Baile WF, Buckman R, Lenzi R, Glober G, Beale EA and Kudelka AP (2000) SPIKES – a six step protocol for delivering bad news: application to the patient with cancer. *Oncologist* 5(4): 302–311.

Beardsmore S and Fitzmaurice N (2002) Palliative care in paediatric oncology. *European Journal of Cancer* 38: 1990–1997.

Bouton BL (1996) The interdisciplinary bereavement team: defining and directing appropriate bereavement care. In: Infield DL and Penner NR (eds) *Bereavement: client adaptation and hospice services*. Binghampton, NY: Haworth Press.

Charmaz K (1980) *The social reality of death*. Reading, MS: Addison-Wesley.

Clark D and Seymour J (1999) *Reflections on palliative care*. Buckingham: Open University Press.

Clark D, Hockley J and Ahmedzai S (1997) *New themes in palliative care*. Buckingham: Open University Press.

Clukey L (2008) Anticipatory mourning: processes of expected loss in palliative care. *International Journal of Palliative Nursing* 14(7): 316–325.

Cobb M (2001) *The dying soul: spiritual care at the end of life*. Buckingham: Open University Press.

Copp G (1999) *Facing impending death*. London: Nursing Times Books.

Costello J (1990) Dying at home. *Nursing Times* 86(8): 49–52.

Costello J (1996) The emotional cost of palliative care. *European Journal of Palliative Care* 3(4): 171–174.

Costello J (1999) Anticipatory grief: coping with the impending death of a partner. *International Journal of Palliative Nursing* 5(5): 223–231.

Costello J (2004) *Nursing the dying patient: caring in different contexts*. London: Palgrave.

Costello J (2009) *Caring for someone with a long term illness*. Manchester: Manchester University Press.

DeCinque NL, Monterosso L, Dadd G, Sidhu R, Macpherson R and Aoun S (2006) Bereavement support for families following the death of a child from cancer: experience of bereaved parents. *Journal of Psychosocial Oncology* 24(2): 65–83.

Demmer C (2003) A national survery of hospice bereavement services. *OMEGA: Journal of Death and Dying* 47(4): 327–341.

Department of Health (2008) *End of life care strategy: promoting high quality care for all adults at the end of life*. London: Department of Health.

Dickenson D, Johnson M and Katz JS (2000) *Death, dying and bereavement*. London: Open University Press in association with Sage.

Doka K (ed.) (2002) *Disenfranchised grief: new directions, challenges and strategies for practice*. Champaign IL: Research Press.

Evans AJ (1994) Anticipatory grief: a theoretical challenge. *Palliative Medicine* 8: 159–165.

Field D, Reid D, Payne S and Relf M (2004) Survey of UK hospice and specialist palliative care adult bereavement services. *International Journal of Palliative Nursing* 10(12): 569.

Field NP, Gao B and Paderna L (2005) Continuing bonds in bereavement: an attachment theory based perspective. *Death Studies* 29(4): 277–299.

Foliart DE, Clausen M, Siljestrom C (2001) Bereavement practices among California hospices: results of a statewide survey. *Death Studies* 25(5): 461–467.

Glackin M and Higgins A (2008) The grief experience of same sex couples within an Irish context. *International Journal of Palliative Nursing* 14(6): 297–302.

Glick IO, Weiss RS and Parkes CM (eds) (1974) *The first year of bereavement*. New York: John Wiley.

Huber R and Gibson JW (1990) New evidence for anticipatory grief. *Hospice Journal* 6(1): 49–67.

Kaunonen M, Päivi Å-K, Paunonen M and Erjanti H (2000) Death in the Finnish family: experiences of spousal bereavement. *International Journal of Nursing Practice* 6: 127–134.

Klein S and Alexander DA (2003) Good grief: a medical challenge. *Trauma* 5: 261–271.

Leader D (2008) *Mourning, melancholia and depression*. London: Hamish Hamilton.

Lindemann E (1944) Symptomatology and management of acute grief. *American Journal of Psychiatry* 101: 155–160.

Lorenz L (1998) Selecting and implementing support groups for bereaved adults. *Cancer Practice* 6(3): 161–166.

Mallon B (2008) *Dying death and grief: working with adult bereavement*. London: Sage.

Martin TL and Doka KJ (2000) *Men don't cry women do*. Washington, DC: Taylor & Francis.

Matsushima T, Akabayashi A and Nishitateno K (2002) The current status of bereavement follow-up in hospice and palliative care in Japan. *Palliative Medicine* 16(2): 151–158.

Moos LN (1995) An integrative model of grief. *Death Studies* 19: 337–364.

Mount B, Hanks G and McGoldrick L (2006) The principles of palliative care. In: Fallon M and Hanks G (eds) *ABC of palliative care*, 2nd edn. London: Blackwell and BMJ Books.

National Institute for Clinical Excellence (2004) *Guidance on improving supportive and palliative care for adults with cancer*. London: NICE.

Parkes CM (1974) The effects of bereavement on physical and mental health: a study of the case records of widows. *British Medical Journal* 2: 274.

Parkes CM (1990) Risk factors in bereavement: implications for the prevention and treatment of pathologic grief. *Psychiatric Annals* 20(6): 308–313.

Parkes CM and Weiss RS (1983) Recovery from bereavement. *Psychiatry* 33: 44–467.

Parkes CM, Stevenson-Hinde J and Marris P (eds) (1995) *Attachment across the life cycle*. London: Routledge.

Payne S (2001) The role of volunteers in hospice bereavement support in New Zealand. *Palliative Medicine* 15(2): 107–115.

Payne S and Relf M (2001) The assessment of need for bereavement follow up in palliative care and hospice care. In: Field D, Clark D, Corner J and Davis C (eds) *Researching palliative care*. Buckingham: Open University Press.

Payne S, Horn S and Relf M (1999) *Loss and bereavement*. Buckingham: Open University Press.

Payne S, Seymour J and Ingleton C (2008) *Palliative care nursing: principles and evidence for practice*. Buckingham: Open University Press.

Prigerson, HG, Shear MK, Jacobs SC, Kasl SV, Maciejewski PK, Silverman GK, Narayan M and Bremner J (2000) Grief and its relationship to PTSD. In: Davidson J, Nutt D and Zohar J (eds) *Post-traumatic stress disorder: diagnosis, management and treatment*. New York: Martin Dunitz.

Rando TA (ed.) (1986) *Anticipatory grief and loss*. Lexington, MA: Research Press.

Rando TA (2000) *Clinical dimensions of anticipatory mourning: theory and practice of working with the dying, their loved ones and caregivers*. Champaign, IL: Research Press.

Relf M (2006) Bereavement. In: Fallon M and Hanks G (eds) *ABC of palliative care*, 2nd edn. London: Blackwell and BMJ Books.

Sandman L (2005) *A good death*. Buckingham: Open University Press.

Schoenberg B, Carr AC, Kutscher AH, Peretz D and Goldberg IK (eds) (1974) *Anticipatory grief*. New York: Columbia University Press.

Scottish Partnership Agency for Palliative and Cancer Care (1998) *Palliative care in community hospitals: report of a working party of the Scottish Partnership Agency for Palliative and Cancer Care*. Edinburgh: SPACC.

Seymour J (2001) *Critical moments in intensive care*. Buckingham: Open University Press.

Sheldon F (1997) *Psychosocial palliative care*. Cheltenham: Stanley Thornes.

Spruyt O (1999) Community-based palliative care for Bangladeshi patients in east London: Accounts of bereaved carers. *Palliative Medicine* 13(2): 119–129.

Stephen AI, Wimpenny P, Unwin RF, Dempster P, Macduff C, Wilcock SE and Brown A (2009) Bereavement and bereavement care in health and social care: provision and practice in Scotland. *Death Studies* 33(3): 239–261.

Strauss A (1984) *Chronic illness and the quality of life*. St Louis: Mosby.

Sweeting HN and Gilhooley MLM (1991) Anticipatory grief: a review. *Social Science and Medicine* 30: 1073–1080.

Tadman M and Roberts D (2006) *Oxford handbook of cancer nursing*. Oxford: Oxford University Press.

Teel CS (1991) Chronic sorrow: analysis of the concept. *Journal of Advanced Nursing* 16: 1311–1319.

Walter T (1999) *On bereavement: the culture of grief*. Buckingham: Open University Press.

Watson M, Lucas C, Hoy A and Back I (2005) *Oxford handbook of palliative care*. Oxford: Oxford University Press.

Wee B and Hughes N (2007) Learning and teaching palliative care. In: Wee B and Hughes N (eds) *Education in palliative care: building a culture of learning*. Oxford: Oxford University Press.

Wimpenny P , Unwin R, Dempster P, Grundy M, Work F, Brown A and Wilcock S (2007). A literature review on bereavement and bereavement care: developing evidence based practice in Scotland. *Bereavement Care* 26(1): 7–10.

Woodhouse J (2004) A personal reflection on sitting at the bedside of a dying loved one: the vigil. *International Journal of Palliative Nursing* 10(11): 537–541.

6 Mental health, trauma and bereavement

David Alexander and Susan Klein

Key messages

This chapter will concern itself with mental health issues relating to traumatic deaths, and will address the following key messages:

- Grief is not an illness; most people cope without professional help.
- Attitudes and reactions to death have changed and these may now influence the manner in which we grieve and mourn.
- Risk factors for complicated grief have been identified.
- There are some common components of complicated grief and post-traumatic stress disorder (PTSD). PTSD may interfere with grieving in particular ways.
- Traumatic death, violent death and multiple loss are commonly associated with adverse grief reactions.
- The lack of a body or body part can hinder grieving.
- The resilience of individuals in the face of trauma and adversity can be significant and can be enhanced by health and social care professionals.

Introduction

This chapter addresses the association with trauma, mental health and bereavement. It is acknowledged that what follows can be only generalisations since the reactions of the bereaved will depend on many factors, including the personal meaning of the death as well as the socio-cultural context in which it occurred. There are therefore no simple formulaic approaches to traumatic death for either the bereaved or the caregiver.

Death arrives in many guises: it can be the end point of a prolonged physical illness; it may be sudden but not wholly unexpected in individuals with some known physical vulnerability (e.g. cardiovascular disease), but it may arrive suddenly and unexpectedly because of a number of traumatic events. ('Traumatic events' are those which do or threaten to overwhelm the ability of an individual, family or even community to cope with their consequences.) Globally there is no shortage of contemporary circumstances which are traumatic. Some massive events may be of natural origin (e.g. earthquakes) or due to human malevolence (e.g. the terrorist attacks on the World Trade Center and the Pentagon), and their effects reverberate locally, nationally and even internationally. Others may have a more local focus, and may include domestic, industrial and traffic incidents, acts of criminality (e.g. murder) or self-harm (e.g. suicide).

Such events are capable of creating very powerful and even contradictory emotions for which the bereaved (and, indeed, their helpers) have little or no time to prepare. Sensitivities surrounding such tragedies also pose challenges to researchers; rarely is there an opportunity for developing elegant research protocols, and there is the omnipresent concern to avoid retraumatising the traumatically bereaved through vigorous research enquiry (Klein and Alexander 2007). Nonetheless, research evidence is beginning to emerge and, reassuringly, it has been shown that sensitively conducted trauma research may even represent a constructive step towards adjustment for those who have suffered during a traumatic experience (Dyregrov 2004).

A 'case history' is also presented to highlight some of these issues. To guarantee complete anonymity, this is a compound vignette containing features relating to several patients treated by the first author.

Attitudes and reactions to death

Although we may wish sometimes to deny the reality of death (particularly on the grounds of advances in contemporary medicine which themselves encourage the belief that death can be fought off), we also show a fascination with death. Confirmation of this can be found in the widespread interest in traumatic events, depicted in the media, including disasters and gory stories – factual and fictional.

Because most deaths now occur in institutions, few people have personally witnessed a dead body or a dying person (Gorer 1965). In Victorian times, most deaths occurred at home, and coffins were traditionally left open for viewing by the mourners. More commonly now, if viewing of the deceased does take place, it does so in funeral parlours, although some UK rural and fishing communities adhere to more traditional practices. There has also been a move in our society towards more abbreviated and sanitised mourning rituals and practices, with a more secular tone, unlike those which prevail in other cultures and religions, which may extend for days. It is also noticeable that, in the UK, younger individuals are less likely to wear black clothing following the death, even at funerals, and the black veiled widow is a rarity. This change in our behaviour is likely to influence (although we do not know in what way) how we mourn the dead (Littlewood 1992), by addressing the 'tasks' facing us (Worden 2003) and/or by coming to terms emotionally with the reality of the death (Kastenbaum 2008). The consensual view is that mourning rituals facilitate grieving and, when there are multiple losses after major catastrophes, they may facilitate community support (Alexander 2001).

Complicated grief

Hereafter, the term 'complicated grief' will be used to embrace reported synonyms and related syndromes, such as 'pathological grief', 'abnormal grief', 'morbid grief', 'chronic grief' and 'absent grief' (Middleton *et al.* 1996) and 'traumatic grief' (Zisook and Shear 2009). To avoid confusion, it is also important to bear in mind that, with few exceptions, psychiatric disorders are not categorical; they are dimensional or on continua. In other words, there is no clearly defined, empirically based cut-off between that which is 'normal' and that which is 'abnormal'. This is true in the case of the two primary systems currently in use: the ICD-10 International Classification of Mental and Behavioural Disorders (World Health Organization 1992) and the *Diagnostic and Statistical Manual* (4th edn) (DSM-IV; American Psychiatric Association 1994).

More specifically, with regard to bereavement reactions, the normal/abnormal distinction is a difficult one to make, and there are competing views. However, most authorities (e.g. Klein and Alexander 2003) would regard the following four criteria as grounds for distinguishing between the two states:

* severity of symptoms/reactions;
* duration of symptoms/reactions;
* delayed onset of symptoms/reactions;
* level of dysfunction (e.g. at home and/or at work).

Neither the ICD-10 nor the DSM-IV contains a specific diagnostic category of 'complicated grief', although the term is widely used by clinicians and researchers. Indeed, there has been much support for the formal recognition of such a term (Jacobs 1999; Prigerson *et al.* 2000; Lichtenthal *et al.* 2004; Bonanno *et al.* 2007; Simon *et al.* 2007), including the proposal for the inclusion of a complicated grief syndrome in DSM-V (Zhang *et al.* 2006).

'Grief reactions' do surface in the ICD-10 within the category of 'Adjustment Disorders' (F43.2), and within the (rarely used) diagnosis of 'Other enduring personality changes after bereavement' (F62.8). In DSM-IV, bereavement appears as a clinical issue in recognition of the fact that some individuals will experience such severe grief reactions that they should be regarded as suffering from a Major Depressive Episode. According to Hensley (2006), about 7 per cent of the bereaved are likely to be classified as suffering from this condition. Others claim that complicated grief is a subset of clinically significant grief reactions which has its own specific phenomenology, with different features from bereavement-related depression, anxiety and PTSD (e.g. Boelen *et al.* 2008). Bereavement can also be found in the DSM-IV TR as a V code diagnosis (V62.82) in recognition of the fact that certain individuals display symptoms not considered to be normal (e.g. guilt, suicidal thoughts, worthlessness, and hallucinations).

Forstmeier and Maercker (2007) have further investigated complicated grief by comparing two different methods of classifying it. They have proposed two main categories of distinctive symptoms. The first is 'separation distress' (e.g. the preoccupation with thoughts of the deceased), and the second is 'traumatic distress' (e.g. shock and disbelief). Not surprisingly, they confirm that much more research is required to explore different methods of classifying and defining features of grieving which may be identified as being 'complicated', because they are qualitatively and/or quantitatively different. What we must not do, however, is to regard all grief as an illness or assert that professionals must be available to help all bereaved persons. Also, we should not make the mistake of thinking that there is some 'correct' formula for successful grieving; individuals, families and communities should be free to follow those practices and rituals which have been found to be helpful to them in the past (also see Chapter 1).

At risk factors of complicated grief

Although most individuals cope with bereavement without adverse long-term effects and without professional help, certain factors can lead to a complicated grief reaction. The accurate detection of individuals at risk is important (Hawton 2007). Within the general adult population, it has been suggested in surveys that somewhere between 8 per cent and 9 per cent of individuals experience significant problems in grieving (Byrne and Raphael 1994; Middleton *et al.* 1996). Complicated grief is more common among younger individuals (Jacobs 1999), although the elderly, for obvious reasons, are more likely to experience the death of friends and loved ones. As a consequence, they are more likely to experience what has been called 'bereavement overload' (Kastenbaum 1969). Zisook and DeVaul (1983) suggest women are more likely than men to display 'abnormal grief', particularly when it is associated with numbness, denial and depressive symptoms. Grief has also been strongly associated with a miscellany of psychological and physical pathologies, including myocardial infarction ('death from a broken heart'), alcohol misuse, depression, anxiety, arthritis and rheumatic conditions. The underlying mechanisms have not been fully established, but the compromised integrity of the immune system is a likely contender (Klein and Alexander 2003).

Parkes and Weiss (1983) have set out an Index of Bereavement to help us to identify those at greater risk of adverse reactions. Similar guidance is provided by Parkes (1985) in an excellent review article. These factors may be categorised according to the following four sets of features:

Features of the death

- Sudden, untimely and unexpected.
- Death of a child or spouse (in contemporary Western society, all children's deaths are 'untimely').
- A painful, horrifying and/or mutilating death.
- (Perceived as) mismanaged (e.g. by hospital and emergency care personnel).
- Missing body (discussed later).

Features of the bereaved

- Insecure, anxious and poor self-esteem.
- Previous psychiatric history (helpers should not be squeamish about asking about this).

- Excessively angry and guilty (in relation to the death).
- Physical disability/illness.
- Previous unresolved losses (they may have an additive effect and compromise coping with the most recent loss).
- Unable to express emotions (this does not mean individuals must be coerced into expressing feelings in the more conventional fashion; there are subcultural and personality factors to be respected).
- Concurrent problems of living (in assessing the bereaved, it is important to establish with what else they are coping).

Features of the relationship

- Highly dependent on the deceased.
- An ambivalent relationship (that is to say, one characterised by intense 'love/hate' feelings) (the death may occur at a bad time in the relationship, inducing guilt in the remaining survivor – 'If only we hadn't . . .').

Features of the bereaved's circumstances

- Unsupportive or unavailable family.
- Lack of social, religious and other supports.
- Low socio-economic status. (This is probably because people in this stratum may have more problems of living and ill health, and because of their inability to access the appropriate social and other support systems.)

Trauma, PTSD and grief

Typical reactions to trauma have been widely described (e.g. Hodgkinson and Stewart 2001; Gibson 2006; Benedek 2007; Alexander and Klein 2009a). Largely in response to the longer-term and unexpected effects of the Vietnam War among veterans following demobilisation, the American Psychiatric Association introduced into the third edition of the DSM (American Psychiatric Association 1980) a new diagnosis, that of PTSD. (Although 'new' in one sense, it had many recognisable antecedents, including 'nostalgia', 'shell-shock' and 'combat stress', mainly deriving from military observations of combat troops over centuries; Alexander and Klein 2008).

There has been an extended debate about the relationship between grief and PTSD. Prigerson and colleagues (2000) offer a helpful review of this debate. The diagnosis of PTSD can be difficult, partly because the ICD-10 and the DSM-IV use different criteria, particularly with regard to what kind of events are sufficiently disturbing to constitute a 'trauma' (Klein and Alexander 2007). On the other hand, each taxonomy is sufficiently flexible to accommodate certain deaths as 'traumatic'. For example, the death of an elderly grandparent, who has died quietly in sleep, following an extended illness, would not be considered by most practitioners to be 'traumatic', although it is accepted that it could undoubtedly be distressing. On the other hand, to suffer the sudden and unexpected death of a child when a drunk driver slews off the road and crashes into the child's pram could only be described as 'traumatic' by medical, legal, and lay personnel. Again, however, it has to be conceded that defining what is traumatic and what is not does require a matter of judgement; there never could be any clearly defined cut-off point, universally accepted.

What is important, from the point of view of this chapter, is that both classification schemes recognise three core symptoms (although overall the DSM-IV requires the identification of more symptoms for the diagnosis of PTSD to be made). The symptoms in common are as follows.

- The re-experiencing of the trauma (e.g. through unbidden memories, flash-backs, and nightmares).
- Avoidance of reminders of the event (e.g. this might include avoiding the scene of the event and/or any other reminders of the event – including people associated with it).
- Hyperarousal (commonly revealed by irritability, sleep loss, and an exaggerated acoustic startle response). This symptom is also often accompanied by hypervigilance whereby the survivors have an exaggerated sense of risk, not only for themselves but sometimes for other loved ones, including their children.

Post-traumatic symptoms may interfere with grieving (Hodgkinson and Stewart 2001) in at least four particular ways. These are:

1 through the constant re-experiencing of traumatic images and memories of the death scene;
2 becoming totally preoccupied with aspects of the death (including the – real or feared – contribution to it of the bereaved);
3 constantly avoiding reminders of the death and the deceased, thereby not allowing the bereaved opportunities to become desensitised and to adjust to the death;[1] and
4 post-traumatic numbness, which may cause the bereaved to become distanced from individuals and circumstances that could be supportive and facilitate grieving.

Grief reactions in relation to traumatic death

Complicated grief and PTSD are not co-extensive even after traumatic deaths. However, if the bereaved bore witness to the traumatic death, then they could have, as comorbid conditions, complicated grief and PTSD. Kaltman and Bonanno (2003) have explored the relationship between traumatic events and bereavement with sudden and violent deaths. Generally, the suddenness of the death does not prove to be a particularly influential feature, but the violence associated with the death certainly does. Most evidence suggests that man-made traumas, such as terrorist incidents, are more difficult for survivors to come to terms with than are natural events such as tsunami and earthquakes (Klein and Alexander 2009). Of particular research interest has therefore been those deaths which may include a dimension of violence (e.g. certain types of suicide and murder) and those which have involved multiple loss due to a disaster.

Violent deaths

Although the definition of what constitutes a 'violent' death is open to some debate, it is generally recognised that violent deaths are commonly associated with adverse grief reactions (Kaltman and Bonanno 2003; Asaro and Clements 2005). Violent deaths may not necessarily result from acts of deliberate malevolence. For example, certain motor vehicle accidents may themselves be violent (Lehman *et al.* 1987).

Suicide

Fortunately, suicide is relatively uncommon. Even if it is not always easy to define an act as 'suicide' to the satisfaction of a Coroner's Court (in England) or a Fatal Accident Inquiry (in Scotland) (Callander and Eagles 2009), what evidence there is points to suicide as a high risk factor for complicated grief (e.g. Bailley *et al.* 1999; de Groot *et al.* 2007). Some (e.g. Lindqvist *et al.* 2008) have suggested that teenage suicide (which is becoming more common, particularly among young males) can be a particularly devastating experience for a family, who struggle with their guilt and with their attempts to find a meaningful explanation. A particularly informative study was conducted by Miyabayashi and Yasuda (2007) in which those bereaved by suicide, accidents, and acute and chronic illness were compared. After controlling statistically for factors such as the age of the bereaved, the age of the deceased and the time since the death, suicide was found to be the most emotionally damaging kind of loss for the bereaved; however, physical symptoms such as insomnia and anxiety did not differentiate between the group bereaved by suicide and those bereaved by other losses. Moreover, Voracek (2008) observed an increased level of suicides among spouses bereaved by suicide, although he admits it is unclear what underlies this association – assortative mating has been proposed as a possibility.

Social stigma has long been associated with suicide. In the eighteenth century, the property and goods of the dead were forfeited to the Crown; their bodies were commonly mutilated and they were given no honourable burial. It is argued by Cvinar (2005) and others that this stigma against suicides, albeit now more covert, continues to prevail, and this factor may compromise the process of grieving. The surveys by Alexander and colleagues (2000) and Dewar and colleagues (2000) represent persuasive testimony that even mental health professionals whose patients commit suicide may legitimately be included among the ranks of the bereaved.

Murder

One reaction among the bereaved, commonly associated with murder, is anger; an emotion which may be directed at the perpetrator, the victim (for getting into a vulnerable position) and the authorities (especially the police) who 'failed' to protect the individual. There may also be guilt experienced by the bereaved for not taking more steps themselves to protect the victim. The legal proceedings unintentionally, but particularly because of the adversarial climate in which they are conducted and their complexity (Alexander *et al.* 2006), may also evoke anger among the bereaved. The attributions of blame (especially if they are directed at the victim) may be particularly painful to the bereaved.

Sudden and/or unexpected deaths in the UK are likely to require examination of the body to obtain a fuller understanding of the cause of death. Inevitably, this occasions a further delay in the funeral arrangements, and may inspire anxiety, uncertainty and suspicions which complicate grieving.

However, murders sell newspapers and viewing time on television. Thus, families of victims (as well as those of the perpetrators) become the target for the popular media, which may display few concerns about unearthing (or even inventing) sensationalist headlines and 'stories'. Parkes (1993) laid bare, in a follow-up of 17 individuals bereaved by murder, the pressures both public and intra-familial to which the bereaved are exposed. Those who had witnessed the death or had found the body described themselves as being haunted by disturbing images, and others were equally troubled by what they feared might have happened to their loved one. Emotionally, cases of murder are made particularly complex by the fact that most murders are committed by family members and not by strangers. This can cause disturbed dynamics within the family. Also, the return of the perpetrator to the area in which the family live, and in which the killing may have taken place, can be very difficult for the bereaved to cope with.

Multiple loss

As a number of authorities have indicated (e.g. Ursano *et al.* 2007), the experience of multiple loss is a common feature of disasters. There are many forms of these and with a number of causes; some are natural (e.g. earthquakes) whereas others are man-made (sometimes they are technological accidents and on other occasions they are due to acts of human malevolence, including terrorism). The key features of such events, however, are that they are usually sudden and that their effects are widespread, paralysing and devastating in terms of loss of life, facilities and resources.

Epidemiological surveys (e.g. Norris *et al.* 2002; Sundnes and Birnbaum 2003; Neria 2008) confirm that disasters are common events and that their effects can be catastrophic, including in terms of their death toll, which may often be incalculable, generating a host of bereaved. Following such major incidents, the authorities ought to be alert to their secondary effects (Gist and Lubin 1989). These have more recently been described as the 'ripple effect' (e.g. Strous and

Kotler 2004); a metaphor that refers to the fact that there may be a succession of 'victims' following the initial incident, just as there is a series of waves following a stone dropping in the water. First responders can be adversely affected by the nature of very unpleasant duties (Alexander and Klein 2009b), but it should also be remembered that they are often not only 'secondary victims', owing to the nature of their disaster work, but they may also be 'primary victims' because they too may have suffered the personal loss of their loved ones, homes and/or possessions. This was most obvious to the authors after the Sri Lankan tsunami and the Pakistan/Kashmir earthquake. A particularly moving case involved a Pakistani surgeon who had to continue operating in a tent knowing that his own son lay dead in the street outside.

Bereavement after major catastrophe may also be made all the more difficult to cope with because of the scale of the incident. It may have exposed the bereaved to many scenes of dying and injured individuals; communities and whole families may have been wiped out (their sources of support); other losses may have been extensive, including those of the communications systems and public health and welfare facilities. In addition, there may be a continuing threat of further calamity, as was the case in Pakistan when the 2005 earthquake was followed by a succession of aftershocks (PACTT 2008).

After a disaster, although many individuals may be well-meaning, there is often an uninvited influx of aid workers, counsellors and other 'helpers'. Their arrival can be extremely unhelpful, as the bereaved become the victims of 'over-care'. Similarly, this convergent phenomenon involves the media, who are always hungry for a 'good story'. Although, in one sense, the bereaved may appear to volunteer to be interviewed by the media, it is the authors' experience that many have later regretted revealing their deeper feelings in public so prematurely after a tragedy. One has to ask to what extent, in the immediate aftermath of a tragedy, the bereaved can give genuinely informed consent.

Another feature of major disasters is that they tend to have a long tail. In the 'honeymoon phase' (Raphael 1986), there may be plenty of competent and accessible help, but after a few weeks these helpers move on (sometimes to another tragedy), and the bereaved are often left in a trough in which little help is available. Society can be remarkably intolerant and have unrealistic expectations of people and their ability to recover from a tragic loss. For the survivors, however, it is commonly only after a few months that the real significance of the loss becomes evident, and that is often the time when legal proceedings are initiated, revitalising the predatory interest of the media. Moreover, after about 6 months, it is the common expectation that the family should have 'got over it'. Two to four years is a more realistic period, depending on the nature of the death and the relationship between the bereaved and the deceased.

Missing bodies and 'ambiguous loss'

Boss (2006) introduced the useful concept of 'ambiguous loss', reflecting the fact that a body, or even a body part, can facilitate grieving. Many years ago, in the aforementioned review, Parkes (1985) identified the lack of a body as a poor prognostic indicator for the bereaved. Without a body, denial and wishful thinking may unhelpfully persist. Alexander (1991) noted that, after the Piper Alpha oil platform disaster, some families (who had no bodies returned) lived in the vain hope that their loved ones had been picked up by some foreign sea vessel and would soon be returned to them. The availability of a body provides the bereaved with the opportunity to say 'goodbye', 'I am sorry', 'I love you' and so on. Relatedly, the physical reality of a body (through its appearance, touch and smell) helps to release emotions, which otherwise can be 'frozen'. Also, a body, or even a body part, allows families and colleagues to initiate mourning rituals and practices which, as has been argued above, further facilitate grieving and mourning. It is noteworthy that kamikaze pilots commonly left symbolic nail and hair cuttings before departing on their missions of self-destruction.

The importance of body retrieval is widely recognised by the authorities, and is reflected in the extreme efforts the authorities make to retrieve human remains after major catastrophes, although this can be a very difficult and distasteful task (Alexander and Wells 1991). Identification through DNA analyses and odontology has increased the likelihood of identification. For the military, 'Missing in Action' is a not uncommon but certainly a very unwelcome outcome after combat. Modern weaponry is so powerful that bodies can be completely atomised: there is nothing to be retrieved. In an effort to at least partially provide some closure for families and colleagues, most countries set up a tomb to 'The Unknown Warrior' (Alexander and Klein 2008).

There are other kinds of 'ambiguous loss'. These include the loss of personal identity through dementia and strokes, 'permanent vegetative states' and other major medical conditions. In such cases, the families are in a difficult position because they are faced with a 'psychological death' in the absence of a definitive physical one. Special attention needs to be paid to children's reactions to different kinds of loss (Goldman 2001), and family-focused grief therapy may be required (Kissane and Bloch 2002).

The viewing of human remains

The importance of retrieving a body or body parts raises the delicate and complex question whether or not the bereaved should be allowed to view what has been found. There are two legitimate but antithetical opinions among professionals. Some authorities claim that certain sights (and smells) are too horrific for the bereaved and would leave them with enduring and too disturbing memories of a loved one. Others argue, on the other hand, that the reality of what is to be seen or what smelled is frequently much less awful than the bereaved fear. This dilemma has been discussed in detail elsewhere (e.g. Joseph *et al.* 1997; Alexander and Klein 2000).

Although one must not be too prescriptive about this, as there is insufficient evidence, what little evidence exists suggests that most individuals report that the viewing of human remains is a valuable step in coming to terms with a death. However, care must be taken to conduct this circumstance sensitively and professionally. Families must be allowed to reach an *informed* decision. They should be:

- given sufficient information as to what they will see, smell or feel (if they touch the body) (resuscitation marks should be explained);
- offered some privacy before and after the viewing;
- offered to be accompanied by a member of staff who is competent to answer any questions which might arise about the state of the remains (some families prefer staff not to be present during the visit, but an informed professional should certainly be available after the viewing); and
- reassured that there is no 'right' or 'wrong' decision; it has to be a free one, and none of the family should feel that he/she ought to view the remains.

One cannot escape the risk that, even after competent professional preparation and post-viewing support, some individuals may find the experience deeply disturbing. Even in such cases, however, it is important to bear in mind that viewing the remains does offer some important advantages. These include:

- dispelling myths and rumour as to how the deceased will look, smell and feel;
- enabling 'goodbyes' and the like to be expressed; and
- defusing denial, and false hopes and expectations.

It is crucial that respect be shown towards the human remains, particularly when there may be religious and cultural sensitivities and mores regarding death and dead bodies. This is a crucial issue after major catastrophes involving victims of different faiths and cultures.

Resilience and recovery

So far the focus has been on the adverse effects of bereavement, suffering and loss. It is essential, however, that we remember the resilience of the human spirit.

As Linley and Joseph (2004) have emphasised, positive adaptation to psychological trauma has a long and well-documented heritage. They assert that adaptation is not just about a homeostatic return to the pre-loss level of adjustment (although the value of that should not be underestimated). However, some individuals reach a higher level of achievement, sometimes referred to as 'post-traumatic growth' (Tedeschi *et al.* 1998). Individuals, families and communities may come through adversity the stronger, having revised their life priorities, strengthened relationships and acquired a stronger view of their future.

A review by Bonanno (2004) confirms three important principles relating to resilience such that:

1 It is more than mere recovery.
2 It is more common than previously acknowledged.

3   There are probably several pathways to resilience, including through training, previous experience and even genetics. (It should be noted, however, that to describe somebody as 'resilient' does not mean that they have not suffered, e.g. through bereavement.)

Williams (2008) has identified certain personal skills, beliefs and attitudes associated with resilience:

Personal skills
- Capacity to receive social support
- Good cognitive skills
- Good communication skills
- Active problem-solving skills
- Flexibility – the ability to adapt to change
- Ability to cope with stress.

Personal beliefs and attitudes
- Self-efficacy (general expectation of competence)
- Self-esteem
- Hope
- Sense of purpose
- Religion or having a sense of belonging
- Positive emotion and humour
- Belief that stress can have a strengthening effect
- Acceptance of negative feelings.

Resilience has been conceptualised in a variety of ways, including as a disposition that promotes positive outcomes (e.g. adaptation) in the face of challenging or stressful circumstances. Dispositional resilience (Bartone 2007) derives from the term 'hardiness', which was originally coined by Kobasa (1979) to explain why certain individuals, often similar in so many ways (including their training and background), cope quite differently when exposed to extreme and/or serial adversities. Research by Alexander and Klein (2001) and Paton (2005) have confirmed how variable can be the coping abilities of even experienced paramedics and other emergency service personnel. According to its advocates, 'hardiness' comprises three primary components: (i) 'commitment' (the capacity to view potentially stressful events as meaningful and understandable); (ii) 'control' (the capacity to see oneself in control of life events and circumstances); and (iii) 'challenge' (the capacity to see adversities not just as barriers and impedimenta but as challenges and opportunities for achievement). Viewing tragic and traumatic events, including bereavement, through a more constructive prism, is also known as 'salutogenesis' (Antonovsky 1991). Again, it is important to note that being possessed of such positive attitudes and traits does not mean that there has been no pain and suffering; these remain just as real as is the case for other persons.

Resilient individuals may indeed display transient signs of complicated grief, or of some other pathology, and they are equally capable of displaying the full gamut of so-called 'normal grief reactions'. However, they seem able to transcend these reactions in the longer term.

Help for the bereaved

It is worth repeating that most people do not suffer a mental illness after bereavement: relatively few people will suffer from complicated grief or some bereavement-related psychopathology. This does not imply, however, that professionals have no role to play in facilitating the adjustment of a bereaved person following traumatic death. In a recent review, Scott (2007) has described how emergency care personnel have the opportunity to assist with regard to, for example, the practical aspects of pronouncing the death, explaining the cause of death and conducting the deceased's last offices, as well as providing support and information – including that in the fashion of leaflets, such as *What to do after a death in England and Wales* (Department for Work and Pensions 2009) and *Help is at hand: a resource for people bereaved by suicide and other sudden, traumatic death* (Department of Health 2010). Providing this level of care does, however, require adequate training and preparation, as dealing with emotionally distressed relatives can be threatening (Scott 2007). There are also steps which the bereaved can take to help themselves. The Sudden Trauma Information Service Helpline (http://www.stish.org/) advises that individuals, following trauma, should:

- keep up their usual daily routines;
- talk (when they feel able to do so) to those whom they trust;
- find time for relaxation;
- eat regular meals;
- use physical exercise;
- be aware that certain drugs and potions may interfere with sleep (e.g. caffeine-containing drinks);
- develop positive sleep habits; and
- avoid excessive use of alcohol (it should be remembered that alcohol is a 'depressant' drug and more commonly disturbs sleep, particularly in the later stages of the sleep cycle).

Following major incidents, Psychological First Aid (Raphael 1986) is widely favoured by experts in the field. It is not in itself a formal treatment; however, it contains a series of recommended interventions which will promote individual as well as community resilience. It is strongly associated with Maslow's 'Hierarchy of Needs', which is a well-established model of human priorities and motivations (Maslow 1954). Most importantly, it places physical needs as the top priority rather than psychological ones. With regard to the bereaved, first ensure they have sources of food, shelter and safety, before engaging with their sense of loss.

Ørner and Schnyder (2003) have provided a detailed list of the elements of Psychological First Aid, but below are some of its key elements:

- attention to basic needs (e.g. food, shelter, security and communication);
- early interventions (e.g. reducing physiological arousal, mobilising support for those in greatest need, keeping families together, providing clear and accurate information);
- needs assessment and screening (e.g. assessing each individual's personal needs and identifying what is required);
- monitoring the rescue and recovery environment (e.g. identifying additional threats and stressors, ensuring services are being provided, and monitoring media coverage and the spreading of rumours);
- outreach and information dissemination (e.g. ensuring the effective use of community facilities and public information programmes).
- technical assistance, consultation and training (e.g. supporting family recovery, encouraging cohesion and resilience, and safeguarding community infrastructures);
- foster resilience, coping and recovery (e.g. encouraging social interaction at family, group and community levels, and providing psycho-education in relation to stress responses etc.);
- assessing different levels of immediate need (e.g. 'triage', i.e. identifying those who may require more professional help);
- treatment (e.g. treating those who require active medical/psychiatric care by means of either pharmacotherapy or psychotherapy).

Throughout this list, it will be seen that there is an emphasis on mobilising individual, family and community resources. Professional helpers should not 'take over' a tragedy. Most individuals will gain most help, support and encouragement from their family, colleagues and others already known to them rather than from a group of (albeit well-intended) strangers who have descended (usually uninvited) upon the scene. It is important to be aware, however, that after major trauma, such as tsunamis and earthquakes, whole families and communities may have been wiped out.

With regard to those who have genuine psychopathologies, such as complicated grief, what treatment is provided should be, whenever possible, evidence-based (Hawton 2007).

Case history

A 34-year-old married man, Donald, suffered the death of his wife when he went to get help after their car broke down in a blizzard. Unfortunately, whilst he was away, the driving snow blocked the exhaust outlet. (He had left the engine running to keep her warm.) When he returned with a mechanic, he found his wife dead. It was established at her post-mortem that she had died of carbon monoxide poisoning.

Donald had the painful task of breaking the bad news to their 5-year-old son and 7-year-old daughter, who subsequently blamed him for their mother's death. For weeks, Donald's friends and colleagues described his behaviour as through he were 'in a dream'; he never spoke about his wife's death and spoke as though she were still alive. Subsequently Donald began to drink heavily, showed no interest in his children, took up an 'extreme sport' (for which he was physically unsuited), bought a very expensive sports car (out of his wife's insurance) and was twice charged with speeding and 'careless driving'. Despite suffering the loss of his driving licence, Donald continued to drive. On one occasion, he crashed his car. He suffered serious chest and facial injuries as he had not been wearing a seatbelt. From being, prior to his wife's demise, a quiet, introspective and introverted man he became, according to his colleagues and friends, 'loud-mouthed', disinhibited in social settings (particularly those in which young women were present) and 'cocky'. When drunk, he became tearful and maudlin, and expressed profound guilt over his wife's death. (Such guilt he never expressed when sober.)

Physically, his health suffered; he became very thin, with poor appetite and suffered headaches and insomnia (early-morning wakening). His blood pressure (systolic and diastolic) was raised. Several of his family reported his showing signs of poor personal hygiene.

Psychologically, Donald denied being depressed, but his parents described him as having extended spells of low mood, showing signs of having been crying, and displaying poor memory and concentration. They were also concerned about his apparent lack of concern for his children's welfare, frequently requiring his parents to 'baby sit' whilst he went out socialising. (He claimed his evenings out were 'business meetings'.)

These changes began after about 2 months following the death of his wife, and worsened over a 3-year period. He then struck up a new relationship with a much younger woman, whom his parents described as 'totally unsuitable' for him, and was the antithesis of his wife in terms of her looks, manner and behaviour.

Commentary

This was not a 'normal' grief reaction. Donald was clinically depressed but tried to mask it. He displayed extended denial of the reality of his wife's death (partly revealed by his not talking about it and creating a totally atypical lifestyle). Guilt leaked out only when he had too much alcohol. There were moreover signs of self-destructive behaviour (e.g. alcohol abuse, taking risks when driving and 'extreme' sporting activity). Other signs causing concern were self-neglect (e.g. food intake and personal hygiene), lack of concern for the children, impaired cognitive functions and chronic insomnia.

In accordance with the National Institute for Health and Clinical Excellence clinical guideline 90 (NICE 2009) on the treatment and management of depression in adults, Donald was successfully treated with a combined regimen of an antidepressant (an SSRI) and cognitive behavioural therapy (CBT) over a period of 5 months. He has resumed a more appropriate lifestyle, particularly with regard to his children.

Conclusion

Adjusting to the death of a loved one through trauma is unquestionably a psychological challenge for the bereaved. It is reassuring, however, that so many individuals do not develop a psychiatric illness, and it is important we do not 'medicalise' normal reactions. Resilience is the human norm in the face of adversity. However, we must remember three points.

First, we can augment that resilience by providing a level of support and information for the bereaved, even although it is accepted that we must continue to seek a stronger evidence base for what is most helpful, for whom and when.

Second, we need to be ever alert to the risk of compromising that resilience by failing to recognise and respond appropriately to the needs of the bereaved. This chapter has confirmed that there are some guidelines to help us to identify those individuals who may have most difficulty in adjusting to a traumatic loss.

Finally, we must not forget that the nature and level of the impact of the loss may be such that the person's difficulty in coping may legitimately be described as a psychiatric condition which requires to be treated with skill, care and evidence-based practice.

Note

1   The association between avoidance and adjustment is complex. Boelen and colleagues (2006) showed that 'anxious' avoidance (as opposed to avoidance driven by depression) may facilitate adjustment because the individuals, by deflecting themselves from a preoccupation with the loss, are able to redirect their energies to positive aspects of living.

References

Alexander DA (1991) Psychiatric intervention after the Piper Alpha disaster. *Journal of the Royal Society of Medicine* 84(1): 8–11.

Alexander DA (2001) Nairobi terrorist bombing: the personal experience of a mental health adviser. *International Journal of Emergency Mental Health* 3(4): 249–257.

Alexander DA and Klein S (2000) Bad news is bad news: let's not make it worse. *Trauma* 2(1): 11–18.

Alexander DA and Klein S (2001) Ambulance personnel and critical incidents: the impact of accident and emergency work on mental health and emotional well-being. *British Journal of Psychiatry* 178(1): 76–81.

Alexander DA and Klein S (2008) Combat-related disorders: a persistent chimera. *Trauma* 154(2): 96–101.

Alexander DA and Klein S (2009a) Psychological reactions to trauma. In: Greaves I, Porter K and Garner J (eds) *Trauma care manual*, 2nd edn. London: Hodder Arnold.

Alexander DA and Klein S (2009b) First responders: a review of stress reactions, at risk and vulnerability, and resilience factors. *Prehospital and Disaster Medicine* 24(2): 87–94.

Alexander DA and Wells A (1991) Reactions of police officers to body-handling after a major disaster: a before-and-after comparison. *British Journal of Psychiatry* 159(4): 547–555.

Alexander DA, Klein S, Gray NM, Dewar IG and Eagles JM (2000) Suicide by patients: a questionnaire study of its effects on consultant psychiatrists in Scotland. *British Medical Journal* 320(7249): 1571–1574.

Alexander DA, Badial R and Klein S (2006) Personal injury compensation: no claim without pain? *Psychiatric Bulletin* 30(10): 373–375.

American Psychiatric Association (1980) *Diagnostic and statistical manual of mental disorders*, 3rd edn. Washington, DC: American Psychiatric Association.

American Psychiatric Association (1994) *Diagnostic and statistical manual of mental disorders*, 4th edn. Washington, DC: American Psychiatric Association.

Antonovsky A (1991) The structural sources of salutogenic strengths. In: Cooper CL and Payne R (eds) *Personality and stress: individual differences in the stress process*. Chichester: Wiley.

Asaro MR and Clements PT (2005) Homicide bereavement: a family affair. *Journal of Forensic Nursing* 1(3): 101–5, 128.

Bailley SE, Kral MJ and Dunham K (1999) Survivors of suicide do grieve differently: empirical support for a commonsense proposition. *Suicide and Life-Threatening Behavior* 29(3): 256–271.

Bartone PT (2007) Test–retest reliability of the dispositional resilience scale-15: a brief hardiness scale. *Psychological Reports* 101(3): 943–944.

Benedek DM (2007) Acute stress disorder and post-traumatic stress disorder in the disaster environment. In: Ursano RJ, Fullerton CS, Weisaeth L and Raphael B (eds) *Textbook of disaster psychiatry*. Cambridge: Cambridge University Press.

Boelen DA, van den Bout J and van den Hout MA (2006) Negative cognitions and avoidance in emotional problems after bereavement: a prospective study. *Behaviour Research and Therapy* 44(11): 1657–1672.

Boelen DA, van den Hout MA and van den Bout J (2008) The factor structure of post-traumatic stress disorder symptoms among bereaved individuals: a confirmatory factor analysis study. *Journal of Anxiety Disorders* 22(8): 1377–1383.

Bonanno GA (2004) Loss, trauma and human resilience: have we underestimated the human capacity to thrive after extremely aversive events? *American Psychologist* 59(1): 20–28.

Bonanno GA, Neria Y, Mancini A, Coifman, KG, Litz B and Insel B (2007) Is there more to complicated grief than depression and posttraumatic stress disorder? A test of incremental validity. *Journal of Abnormal Psychology* 116(2): 342–351.

Boss P (2006) *Loss, trauma, and resilience: therapeutic work with ambiguous loss*. London: Norton and Co.

Byrne GJA and Raphael B (1994) The psychological symptoms of conjugal bereavement in elderly men over the first 13 months. *Psychological Medicine* 24(2): 411–421.

Callender JS and Eagles JM (2009) Coping with suicide: a perspective from Scotland. *Advances in Psychiatric Treatment* 15(1): 17–22.

Cvinar JG (2005) Do suicide survivors suffer social stigma: a review of the literature. *Perspectives in Psychiatric Care* 41(1): 14–21.

de Groot M, de Keijser J, Neeleman J, Kerkhof A, Nolen W and Burger H (2007) Cognitive-behaviour therapy to prevent complicated grief among relatives and spouses bereaved by suicide: cluster randomised controlled trial. *British Medical Journal* 334(7601): 994–996.

Department for Work and Pensions (2009) *What to do after a death in England and Wales.* DWP1027. London: Department for Work and Pensions. Available at: http://www.dwp.gov.uk/docs/dwp1027.pdf (accessed 24 May 2010).

Department of Health (2010) *Help is at hand: a resource for people bereaved by suicide and other sudden, traumatic death.* London: Department of Health. Available at http://www.dh.gov.uk/en/Publicationsandstatistics/Publications/PublicationsPolicyAndGuidance/DH_115629 (accessed 24 May 2010).

Dewar I, Eagles JM, Klein S, Gray N. and Alexander DA (2000) Psychiatric trainees' experience of and reactions to patient suicide. *Psychiatric Bulletin* 24(1): 20–23.

Dyregrov K (2004) Bereaved parents' experience of research participation. *Social Science and Medicine* 58(2): 391–400.

Forstmeier S and Maercker A (2007) Comparison of two diagnostic systems for complicated grief. *Journal of Affective Disorders* 99(1–3): 203–211.

Gibson M (2006) *Order from chaos*, 3rd edn (revised). Bristol: Policy Press.

Gist R and Lubin B (1989) *Psychosocial aspects of disaster.* New York: Wiley.

Goldman L (2001) *Breaking the silence: a guide to helping children with complicated grief: suicide, homicide, AIDS, violence and abuse.* Bristol, PA: Taylor and Francis.

Gorer G (1965) *Death, grief and mourning in contemporary Britain.* London: Cresset.

Hawton K (2007) Complicated grief after bereavement: psychological interventions may be effective. *British Medical Journal* 334(7601): 962–963.

Hensley PL (2006) Treatment of bereavement-related depression and traumatic grief. *Journal of Affective Disorders* 92(1): 117–124.

Hodgkinson PE and Stewart M (2001) *Coping with catastrophe: a handbook of post-disaster psychosocial aftercare.* New York: Routledge.

Jacobs S (1999) *Traumatic grief: diagnosis, treatment and prevention.* London: Brunner/Mazel.

Joseph S, Williams R and Yule W (1997) *Understanding post-traumatic stress.* Chichester: John Wiley.

Kaltman S and Bonanno GA (2003) Trauma and bereavement: examining the impact of sudden and violent deaths. *Journal of Anxiety Disorders* 17(2): 131–147.

Kastenbaum R (1969) Death and bereavement in later life. In: Kutcher A (ed.) *Death and bereavement.* Springfield, IL: Charles C Thomas.

Kastenbaum R (2008) Grieving in contemporary society. In: Stroebe MS, Hansson RO, Schut H and Stroebe W (eds) *Handbook of bereavement research and practice: advances in theory and intervention.* Washington, DC: American Psychological Association.

Kissane DW and Bloch S. (2002) *Family focused grief therapy.* Buckingham: Open University Press.

Klein S and Alexander DA (2003) Good grief: a medical challenge. *Trauma* 5(4): 261–271.

Klein S and Alexander DA (2007) Post-disaster research issues. In: Niaz U (ed.) *Pakistan 2005: earthquake: the day the mountains moved.* Karachi: SAMA Editorial and Publishing Services.

Klein S and Alexander DA (2009) Epidemiology and presentation of post-traumatic disorders. *Psychiatry* 8(8): 282–287.

Kobasa SC (1979) Stressful life events, personality and health: an inquiry into hardiness. *Journal of Personality and Social Psychology* 37(1): 1–11.

Lehman DR, Wortman CB and Williams AF (1987) Long-term effects of losing a spouse or child in a motor vehicle crash. *Journal of Personality and Social Psychology* 52(1): 218–231.

Lichtenthal WG, Cruess DG and Prigerson HG (2004) A case for establishing complicated grief as a distinct mental disorder in DSM V. *Clinical Psychology Review* 24(6): 637–662.

Lindqvist P, Johansson L and Karlsson U (2008) In the aftermath of teenage suicide: a qualitative study of the psychosocial consequences for the surviving family members. *BMC Psychiatry* 21(8): 26.

Linley PA and Joseph S (2004) Positive change following trauma and adversity: a review. *Journal of Traumatic Stress* 17(1): 11–21.

Littlewood J (1992) *Aspects of grief: bereavement in adult life*. London: Tavistock/Routledge.

Maslow A (1954) *Motivation*. New York: Harper and Row.

Middleton W, Burnett P, Raphael B and Martinek N (1996) The bereavement response: a cluster analysis. *British Journal of Psychiatry* 169(2): 167–171.

Miyabayashi S and Yasuda J (2007) Effects of loss from suicide: accidents, acute illness and chronic illness on bereaved spouses and parents in Japan: their general health, depressive mood, and grief reaction. *Psychiatry and Clinical Neurosciences* 61(5): 502–508.

Neria Y, Nandi A and Galea S (2008) Post-traumatic stress disorder following disasters: a systematic review. *Psychological Medicine* 38(4): 467–480.

NICE (2009) *Depression: the treatment and management of depression in adults*. National Clinical Practice Guideline 90. Available at: http://guidance.nice.org.uk/CG90 (accessed 24 May 2010).

Norris FH, Friedman MJ, Watson PJ, Byrne CM, Diaz E and Kaniasty K (2002) 60,000 disaster victims speak: part I. An empirical review of the empirical literature, 1981–2001. *Psychiatry* 65(3): 207–239.

Ørner RJ and Schnyder V (2003) Progress towards reconstructing early intervention after trauma: principles of evidence based practice. In: Ørner RJ and Schnyder V (eds) *Reconstructing early intervention after trauma*. Oxford: Oxford University Press.

PACTT (2008) The psychological and psychosocial impact of the Pakistan Kashmir earthquake after 8 months: a preliminary evaluation by PACTT. *International Psychiatry* 5(2): 43–46.

Parkes CM (1985) Bereavement. *British Journal of Psychiatry* 146: 11–17.

Parkes CM (1993) Psychiatric problems following bereavement by murder or manslaughter. *British Journal of Psychiatry* 162(1): 49–54.

Parkes CM and Weiss RS (1983) *Recovery from bereavement*. New York: Basic Books.

Paton D (2005) Posttraumatic growth in protective services professionals: individual, cognitive and organisational influences. *Traumatology* 11(4): 335–346.

Prigerson HG, Shear MK, Jacobs SC, Kasl SV, Maciejewski PK, Silverman GK, Narayan M and Bremner J (2000) Grief and its relationship to PTSD. In: Davidson J, Nutt D and Zohar J (eds) *Post-traumatic stress disorder: diagnosis, management and treatment*. New York: Martin Dunitz.

Raphael B (1986) *When disaster strikes*. London: Hutchinson.

Scott T (2007) Sudden traumatic death: caring for the bereaved. *Trauma* 9(2): 103–109.

Simon NM, Shear KM, Thompson EH, Zalta AK, Perlman C, Reynolds CF, Frank E, Melhern NM and Silowash R (2007) The prevalence and correlates of psychiatric comorbidity in individuals with complicated grief. *Comprehensive Psychiatry* 48(5): 395–399.

Strous RD and Kotler M (2004) The ripple effect of the toll of terror. *Israel Medical Association Journal* 6: 425–426.

Sundnes KO and Birnbaum ML (2003) Health disaster management guidelines for evaluation and research in the Utstein style. Vol 1: Conceptual framework of disasters. *Prehospital and Disaster Medicine* 17 (Suppl. 3): 1–177.

Tedeschi RG, Park CL and Calhoun LG (1998) *Posttraumatic growth: positive changes in the aftermath of crisis*. Mahwah, NJ: Erlbaum.

Ursano RJ, Fullerton CS, Weisaeth L and Raphael B (2007) Individual and community responses to disasters. In: Ursano RJ, Fullerton CS, Weisaeth L and Raphael B (eds) *Textbook of disaster psychiatry.* Cambridge: Cambridge University Press.

Voracek M (2008) Cross-national social ecology of intelligence and suicide prevalence: integration, refinement, and update of studies. *Perceptual & Motor Skills* 106(2): 550–556.

Williams RJ (2008) Resilience and risk in children and young people. In: Jackson C, Hill K and Lavis P (eds) *Child and adolescent mental health: a handbook.* Brighton: Pavilion.

Worden JW (2003) *Grief counselling and grief therapy*, 3rd edn. Hove: Brunner-Routledge.

World Health Organization (1992) *The ICD-10 classification of mental and behavioural disorders: clinical descriptions and diagnostic guidelines.* Geneva: WHO.

Zhang B, El-Jawahri A and Prigerson HG (2006) Update on bereavement research: evidence-based guidelines for the diagnosis and treatment of complicated bereavement. *Journal of Palliative Medicine* 9(2): 1188–1203.

Zisook S and DeVaul RA (1983) Grief, unresolved grief, and depression. *Psychosomatic* 24(3): 247–256.

Zisook S and Shear K (2009) Grief and bereavement: what psychiatrists need to know. *World Psychiatry* 8(2): 67–74.

7 Bereavement and primary care

Sally Lawton and Ken Lawton

Key messages

- Grief is a normal healthy process for the majority of people.
- The journey through grief is unpredictable and it is important that community practitioners can determine the need for appropriate intervention so that the medicalisation of grief is avoided.
- Bereavement does not occur in isolation, but is subject to the influencing factors of family, the community, professionals and society.
- Death occurs within the context of a personal, local community of which health care professionals are a part.

Introduction

The purpose of this chapter is to examine the evidence and critically discuss responses to bereavement within the primary care setting. The key message is that death, bereavement and grieving are normal life events and that the medicalisation of grief should be avoided. Bereavement does not occur in isolation, but is subject to a greater or lesser degree by the influencing factors of family, the community, professionals and society.

Although it is recognised that there is morbidity and mortality associated with bereavement for a small proportion of individuals, most people will not require any professional intervention to manage grief (Stroebe *et al.* 2007). Primary care practitioners may become involved only in complex situations, but can help the bereaved by acknowledging that a death has occurred.

In order to understand the different responses to bereavement, we propose the following simple diagram that aims to capture the various influencing factors on the way individuals and social groups respond to death and the links between them (Figure 7.1). This is not a hierarchical diagram, but aims to show how inter-linked individuals are both to their close family and friends as well as to the local community and wider society. We think this is helpful because, although the experience of bereavement is an intensely personal experience (Silverman 2007), a death occurs within the context of a personal, local community of which health care professionals are a part. Throughout the chapter, authentic examples are taken from clinical practice.

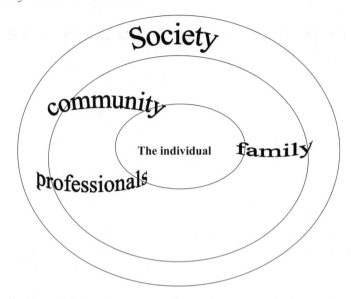

Figure 7.1 Influencing factors on the response to death.

The individual: the story of the interface between private and public grief

The central element of Figure 7.1 is the individual responses made toward death. All bereavement affects individuals in a unique way. This will be dependent on the relationship between the mourner and the deceased, the context of the death and previous experiences of loss. The processes of bereavement depend on circumstances, such as whether the death is sudden, unexpected or the result of a long illness. There is evidence by Steeves (2002) that a death can have a great effect on daily life. The findings indicated that the experiences of the bereaved blurred between initial numbness, waves of emotion and loneliness. Although the rhythm of the bereavement varied among individuals, all 15 respondents reported the impact of the death on normal daily life. For example, they described how their sleep was disturbed and how difficult they found mealtimes.

Reimers (2001) notes that bereavement has both internal and external elements to it: the internal feelings associated with a loss, and external action. This means that the person may put on a public 'brave face' to the outside world while feeling completely bereft when alone, as shown in the following example. This was Kirsty's experience. She was considered to be coping well by neighbours, friends and work colleagues 2 months following the death of her husband. She was frightened to go out apart from going to work in case she cried in front of anyone. Whilst at work, she managed to put on a very brave face as long as she did not enter into conversation about herself. She described her anxiety as thinking that she was going mad. She worried that she would upset other people if she cried in front of them.

The loneliness associated with bereavement may manifest itself within a person's own environment as well as having an impact on their social functioning. Zisook (2005) observes that loneliness may be the most enduring expression of grief. David was widowed after 40 years of marriage. His wife died following a short, unexpected illness and he described how this sense of loneliness was heightened whenever he returned to their house. Bowman has eloquently described this sense of loneliness as 'the constant presence of absence' (Bowman 2006, personal communication).

Individuals may use strategies such as resilience, denial or extreme emotional feelings to help them cope with their grief. Whether this is a process of recovery or of adaptation continues to tax theorists, but there seems to be some process of transformation (Paletti 2008). Furthermore, there is certainly a change of circumstances that will never be restored.

What comfort measures do people seek and find helpful? Our combined clinical experience has encountered a range of different comfort measures that individuals use. Examples may include spending time with family and friends, engaging in a variety of activities, giving back by becoming involved in voluntary work, withdrawal from a normal routine, reflection to try to find some meaning in the death and working out strategies to cope with more poignant events such as birthdays, festivals, anniversaries or holidays.

One source of support for the bereaved might be their religious affiliation. A systematic review was undertaken (Becker *et al.* 2007) to investigate whether a person's spiritual or religious beliefs influenced their ability to cope with bereavement. Thirty-two studies were reviewed and 22 identified positive links between religious belief and bereavement. The study sample tended to focus on white female Protestants. Furthermore, many studies failed to distinguish religious belief from spirituality. Therefore, the results were inconclusive. It may be that a person gains great comfort from their faith or spiritual beliefs because the beliefs give them a framework to understand why something has happened. It also provides a recognised framework for a funeral.

The facility to 'tell the story of their loss' appears to be an important element in dealing with bereavement. However, Silverman (2007) observes that 'personal experience does not always seem to coincide with popular theories of grief' (p.168). This mismatch may lead to conflict between the public understanding of grief and personal experience. It is this link between individual experience, the person's local community and wider society that we move on to now.

The local community: family, local community and professional responses

In relation to Figure 7.1 the second element is concerned with the people who are close to the individual. Those most intimate to the bereaved person may be their family or close friends and neighbours. These people can play an important role in the life of the bereaved and, as Machin (2007) notes, a person's ability to cope with a loss can be influenced by the family that surrounds them and the cultural mores that they follow. This is of particular relevance if a bereaved person then has to face other people's losses when they are experiencing grief themselves.

However, not all family members will react in the same way to a death. For example, whereas some feel completely bereft, others may feel a sense of relief or guilt at the death. An example of this is the dedicated daughter who felt guilt for placing a parent in care that overshadowed her grief when the parent subsequently died. In addition, as the illustration of Morag shows, family support may be difficult.

> During a lengthy illness, Morag was completely absorbed in caring for her husband to the extent that the grown-up children felt left out and frustrated. Following her husband's death, she became increasingly dependent on her family. Initially they were keen to support her; however, they were going through their own grieving process for their dad. This resulted in great anxiety and feelings of overwhelming responsibility and intrusion into their lives.

Local community

The experience of bereavement is lived out within the context of a person's own sense of community, with many people coping with this painful but normal life experience without the need for any formalised bereavement care. This sense of 'own community' was discussed by Walter (1994) when he commented on the frequency of *sharing death* in settled communities in contrast to the privacy of death in suburban communities, where people rely on their own family or professional services.

There is a connection between the people who are directly affected by the death and people from the local community. This is manifested in the reactions of others to death based on what they say or don't say, or how they react.

An example of the connection between the private and public elements of bereavement occurs at the funeral. Pennebaker and colleagues (2001) identify this as social sharing, observing that this is often a time when a family hears about the qualities of the person who has died and their impact on others.

Reimers (2001) observes that when people are labelled as being bereaved, others respond differently to them. This was made very clear in a recent radio broadcast when Barbara Want, the widow of the BBC journalist Nick Clarke, investigated people in her own community who did not speak to her following Nick's death (British Broadcasting Corporation 2008). Barbara wanted to know why people found it so hard to speak to her and described how aware she was of the averted eyes of acquaintances when she went by and the pain this caused. Her investigation suggested that because people do not know what to say, they remain silent. Walter (1994) labels this as *mutual avoidance*. Alternatively, family members may act in the role of gatekeeper in an attempt to protect the bereaved person. This may include making decisions about who has access to the bereaved person or protecting them from callers.

A different response of the local community was reported in a study exploring how teachers respond to bereaved children (Lowton and Higginson 2003). The results confirmed that the influence of culture, local communities and families were important elements of the teachers' interactions with bereaved children. A surprising finding was the mature way that other secondary-age pupils reacted to their bereaved classmates with shows of impeccable behaviour such as politeness, wearing uniform and 'doing what they thought was expected' (p. 734).

Professional responses

For practitioners working in primary care, the key issue in bereavement care is recognising who might be vulnerable to a complicated grief reaction (see Chapter 6 for further description and discussion of complicated grief). A person who is experiencing a traumatic or complicated grief reaction may be at risk of suicidal ideation. This is particular to men over 75 according to Szanto and colleagues (2002). However, there is the challenge in determining what is meant by the term 'complicated' grief as opposed to 'normal' grief. A study undertaken by Prigerson and colleagues (1995) sought to identify the symptoms that would define complicated grief. The results, based on a follow-up series of inventory completion with widowed elderly individuals over an 18-month period following the death of a spouse, suggested that symptoms such as yearning, searching, disbelief and a sense of being stunned about the death were indicative of complicated grief as well as the mourner being preoccupied with the person who had died, excessive crying and an inability to accept the death.

In addition, participants reported loss of sleep, low mood, feelings of low self-esteem and a decline in overall functioning. The authors suggested that, taken together, these symptoms were different from clinical depression. Furthermore, a prospective cohort study undertaken in Scotland on married couples found that bereaved spouses have a higher risk of dying than non-bereaved spouses and that this risk does not lessen over time (Hart *et al.* 2007).

The physical and mental health consequences of bereavement are well documented and GPs are frequently the first formal contact with the health service when problems arise (Birtwistle and Kendrick 2001). Such problems may include an exacerbation of an existing chronic condition. An Australian study of bereaved elderly men indicated that the unexpected nature of a death, even in the presence of a long-term illness, seemed to cause a more severe bereavement reaction than other factors such as income or education (Byrne and Raphael 1994). GPs may be at the forefront of assessing patients who have bereavement-related problems and deciding what the best course of action, if any, for that person is.

In order to understand the views of bereaved patients, a study was undertaken in a single general practice to find out what people expected in the way of bereavement care (Main 2000). The findings highlight the appreciation felt when a death is acknowledged. The majority of the sample felt that bereavement support was an important aspect of the GP's role. Some comments related to specific aspects of care, such as those who would have appreciated contact from the surgery to discuss aspects of the death. Certain practical steps, such as ensuring bereaved patients could be readily identified within the system, were considered in the surgery to make staff aware of people who were recently bereaved so that they could be more sensitive to their needs. One approach that this group of bereaved patients would have welcomed was a letter of sympathy from the practice, or a 'tag' in the notes, with fewer feeling a visit was actually necessary. Some of the respondents who had seen a GP following the bereavement felt unable to raise the issue because the GP did not mention it either.

The differing reasons why people die will have an influence on how well the patient and family has been known to the GP and other members of the care team.

The relationship with the GP

The relationship between the GP and the family prior to death was a key finding reported by Saunderson and Ridsdale (1999). The study highlighted that where prior strong relationships existed before death, it was more likely that contact would be made after death by the GP. This included strong relationships between individual family members. What was clear was the need for professionals to *reach out to the bereaved person,* but not necessarily in their capacity as a GP. The decision about professionals attending funerals is also affected by the individual circumstances, context of the death and relationships between the family and professionals. It may help to provide some closure for the health care professional.

However, in the event of an unexpected death, the pattern between GP and individual was not clear; much depended on the circumstances. Peters and Lewin (1994) studied the relationship between GPs and the intensive care unit within one local health authority. The GPs survey generated a 59 per cent response rate ($n = 67$) with the findings suggesting that 50 per cent of GPs were informed of the death in intensive care by a relative, rather than directly from the unit.

GPs' beliefs and attitudes to death and bereavement play a part here. Saunderson and Ridsdale (1999) found that GPs may have feelings of guilt about the death of patients, and require support to manage their own and their patient's bereavement. Some doctors expressed their lack of confidence and training in tackling bereavement. In particular, 23 of the 25 doctors interviewed felt that their undergraduate training had left them ill-equipped to deal with death and bereavement.

Wiles and colleagues (2002) explored the factors that influenced GP referrals to a bereavement counselling service. They uncovered the views of GPs regarding what constitutes abnormal bereavement. The indicators included such factors as the nature of the death, level of social support and the reaction to the death. Participants also made a judgement based upon who they thought might benefit most from counselling. However, this may have excluded other individuals who did not fit into their *notional* criteria, emphasising the importance of clinical judgement.

Different counselling strategies are known to exist in the community and Payne and colleagues (2002) interviewed counsellors to uncover their approaches for counselling the bereaved in general practice. Most counsellors saw their work within the broader agenda of being concerned with loss and relationship management. Strategies used included telling the 'story' of loss, active listening, establishing a supportive relationship and enabling the person to deal with unfinished business.

The role of community nurses

The role of the district nurse was explored by Birtwistle and colleagues (2002) through surveying a sample of 522 nurses. Ninety-five per cent of the respondents believed that they should visit bereaved relatives and carers of patients they had nursed (19 per cent thought they should visit even if it was not their patient). Although they felt they should be involved, there was evidence that this involvement lacked structure and rationale and it was suggested that there were implications for training and support. A study undertaken by Lyttle (2001) investigated the perspectives of both district nurses visiting bereaved relatives as well as the individuals being visited. One of the key findings was the importance of having known the family prior to the death.

Davidson (2001) wrote about the potential role of the health visitor in offering bereavement services to the clients who suddenly find themselves bereaved – a service she argued was necessary. However, in the light of evidence highlighted in this chapter, the establishment of contact prior to death is a major challenge for primary care staff in relation to unexpected death.

Community Macmillan nurses

Community Macmillan nurses are clinical nurse specialists in palliative care who address the holistic needs of patients affected by cancer or other life-threatening illness. They support the family and the patient at any stage in their illness to death and bereavement. Therefore, a link is made with the family prior to the death.

There is little evidence of the amount of time Macmillan nurses spend supporting the bereaved. An activity analysis performed by Newbury and colleagues (2008) examined their clinical activity. The study revealed a variation between individual Macmillan nurses, but showed that bereavement is a small yet significant part of their caseload. This correlates with a German study (Weber and Grohmann 2004) identifying how palliative care nurses spend their time, revealing that 8 per cent of caseload time is spent on bereavement counselling.

The same study shows that these nurses spent 27 per cent of their time supporting relatives through the patient's illness, therefore it is realistic to expect that these nurses are well placed to identify which relatives are more likely to suffer a complicated bereavement.

One approach to assist primary care teams is the Gold Standards Framework (n.d.), 'a systematic evidence based approach to optimise the care for patients nearing end of life in the community'. This can be applied to any patient with an advanced illness. The GSF highlights the necessity for carer support and considers that Primary Care Teams ideally should plan for bereavement support. The GSF suggest a practice bereavement protocol. However, such a framework will not account for those suddenly bereaved.

The reactions of health care professionals to death may be similar to those of the local community. In particular, the way a person is informed about a sudden, unexpected death may have an impact on the subsequent grief reaction (Wright 1999). There may be different attitudes towards death in primary and secondary care. Within the setting of an accident and emergency department, for example, unhelpful strategies include failing to communicate effectively, making inappropriate comments or being evasive about the use of the word 'death'. Furthermore, if the health care professional blocks emotional expression by the person being told, it may well adversely affect the grief reaction (Harwood-Nuss 2005).

Brysiewicz's (2008) study explored the lived experiences of family members whose relative died suddenly or unexpectedly. Its relevance to primary care related to how the reaction of staff made a profound impact on the relatives, both positive and negative. From a positive perspective, it was the little things that staff did that made a difference, even the acknowledgement that the person was bereaved. From a negative point of view, the coldness of the staff they encountered gave the impression of a lack of emotional involvement in their work, which negatively affected the bereaved relative. This was Susan's impression when her grandfather died in hospital after sustaining a severe injury in a fall. Although she was saddened by his death, she was horrified by the lack of humanity she perceived in the staff who were meant to be looking after him. This included their lack of personal care and poor communication.

Wright (1999) comments that the support work that is undertaken with bereaved relatives in an emergency department helps family members to begin the normal process of grieving. This suggests that a lack of sensitivity towards relatives at the time of death may be a trigger for a complicated grief reaction.

Society

The outer element of the diagram is concerned with the broader reactions of society to death and bereavement and it is acknowledged that our perspective is based within the UK.

When death is unexpected, and often when a young person dies, society responds in a demonstrative way. It is relatively common in contemporary society to see public expressions of loss through rituals such as roadside shrines where flowers are placed at the scene of an accident, although these have also created some controversy. Tragic events are often presented as headlines in newspapers and regularly feature on television news.

Reimers (2001) argues that the media has an important role in representing 'normal' grief and that bereavement, grief and mourning are dependent on cultural norms including a set of acceptable mourning behaviours. Reimers argues that the problem here is that the bereaved can be stigmatised both by the death and by the unacceptable way in which mourning takes place. This demonstrates the inter-linking between the three elements of the diagram in that there may be a clash between individual reactions to grief and what appears to be 'normal' to the local community and society.

An example of this is in the clearing out of the dead person's wardrobe. If it is done too soon, then it is judged to be too hasty and a sign of disrespect for the dead person. However, if a person chooses not to clear out the clothes, then this might not be 'normal' either! One way of finding comfort that we have observed in clinical practice may be keeping some element of clothing close by. Margaret reported keeping a jumper belonging to her father on a bedside shelf for a couple of years after he died. Occasionally, she would clutch it as though it had some connection to him. As time passed, she realised that she no longer needed to do this and donated the jumper to a charity shop.

A bereaved person reminds others of their own mortality and this is a cause of unease within the community. However, Reimers argues that bereavement should be socially constructed to enable it to be less constraining. Silverman (2007) argues that one of the difficulties in the professionalisation of grief is the disempowerment of the individual's own responses to the loss. Because of this reminder of mortality, it has been proposed that modern Western society is death denying and that the subject of death is a taboo subject (Devlin-Friend 2006). Lendrum and Syme (1992) outline the changes in Western society's attitudes to dying and bereavement from a historical perspective. They propose that in earlier times, death was much more a part of everyday life, with people having a more focused awareness of their own mortality. In contrast, today, death has been largely removed from daily life, with approximately 60 per cent of people dying in hospital settings. Many years ago, the deceased would be cared for within the home. In modern times, the mechanics of dealing with the dead has been professionalised by funeral directors.

Mount (1976) highlighted the explosion of technology and information within medicine and the false assumption that good care equates with aggressive intervention and treatment. Although this was written over 30 years ago, our experience suggests that it remains relevant today. Could it be argued, therefore, that the process of denying death has been driven by healthcare itself in that death could be seen as a failure, rather than the natural conclusion to life?

However, the view that society is death denying is not universally accepted. Zimmerman and Rodin (2004) observe that death is frequently reported, challenging the death denial argument, but noting that people find it difficult to discuss. Perhaps it is the power of the emotions that may be triggered by a death that prevent people from talking about it. This is not a new human experience. The poet and writer Ted Bowman (1994) refers to grief being like a companion throughout our lives, but suggests that we have devised ways of trying to ignore it.

Art, literature and music have explored bereavement, grief and loss over many centuries. Reading poems, listening to music and looking at art can touch the senses profoundly and bring comfort in knowing what other people have experienced. An early example of the depth of emotion is a short poem expressing the sadness of losing a dear friend written in the sixteenth century called 'A remembrance of my friend Mr Thomas Morley' (Downie 1994). More recently, collections of secular and spiritual writing have been collated, with an example by Emerson (2004) that focuses on celebrating life, the emotions that occur following a death, and finding peace.

Individuals, local communities and society need further understanding of the wide range of manifestations of grief and the recognition of an abnormal grief reaction. One way that information about loss can be obtained is through the Internet. How do the new technologies support the bereaved? A search on the Internet about grief and bereavement yields over a million hits. There are information-giving sites, interactive sites to share experiences from the safety and anonymity of your own cyber-space, or details of groups and organisations offering face-to-face support. This reflects the ability for people to gather information about all aspects of grief and bereavement that can be tailored to reflect the particular type of loss.

Face-to-face support may provide comfort and be helpful, when hearing about other people's experiences. However, bereavement support groups were not universally welcomed by participants in a study that compared the reasons why people opt to join or choose not to participate in bereavement support groups (Levy and Derby 1992). This American study found that the people who joined a bereavement support group had more symptoms of depression, stress or anger and the people who chose not to join perceived the other group as being less able to help themselves. There may be other personality traits which result in individuals joining groups or not. This shows that bereavement is an individual experience that requires an individual response from staff in primary care settings, albeit this will be framed in a community and societal context.

Conclusion

In this chapter, we have reviewed differing responses to bereavement from the individual through to wider society, using a simple diagram for illustration. Throughout this chapter, we have stressed the individualised nature of grief and bereavement, and agree with the sentiments expressed by Pennebaker and colleagues (2001: 28) that 'during bereavement, people usually work through grief naturally and do not need intervention strategies to help them cope with their grief'.

The chapter has also emphasised that grief is a normal process for the majority of people, but the journey through it is unpredictable. Perhaps it is wise not to try and explain bereavement as a 'one size fits all' approach and accept the individual nature of this experience. There is a need for health care professionals working in primary care to be flexible when caring for a bereaved person. The ability to listen and respond in an individualised way is crucial, as is the ability to recognise abnormal grief. Experience from practice and research indicates the importance of acknowledging the death, whether you are a family member, part of the local community or a health professional.

References

Becker G, Xander C, Blum H, Lutterbach J, Momm F, Gysels M and Higginson I (2007) Do religious or spiritual beliefs influence bereavement? A systematic review. *Palliative Medicine* 21(3): 207–217.

Birtwistle J and Kendrick T (2001) The psychological aspects of bereavement. *International Journal of Psychiatry in Clinical Practice* 7(3): 91–95.

Birtwistle J, Payne S, Smith P and Kendrick T (2002) The role of the district nurse in bereavement support. *Journal of Advanced Nursing* 38(5): 467–478.

Bowman T (1994) *Loss of dreams: a special kind of grief.* St. Paul, MN: Ted Bowman.

British Broadcasting Corporation (2008) 'I don't know what to say'. Broadcast on BBC Radio 4, 12 May.

Brysiewicz P (2008) The lived experience of losing a loved one to a sudden death in KwaZulu-Natal, South Africa. *Journal of Clinical Nursing* 17(2): 224–231.

Byrne G and Raphael B (1994) A longitudinal study of bereavement phenomena in recently widowed elderly men. *Psychological Medicine* 24(2): 411–421.

Davidson A (2001) Bereavement: implications for health visiting practice. *Community Practitioner* 74(5): 182–184.

Devlin-Friend N (2006) Bereavement in primary education: a study of a group of schools. *Bereavement Care* 25(2): 31–32.

Downie R (ed.) (1994) *The healing arts: an Oxford illustrated anthology.* Oxford: Oxford University Press.

Emerson S (ed.) (2004) *In loving memory: a collection for memorial services, funerals and just getting by.* London: Little, Brown.

Gold Standards Framework (n.d.) Available at: http://www.goldstandardsframework.org.uk/GSFInPrimary+Care (accessed 3 September 2008).

Hart C, Hole D, Lawlor D, Smith G and Lever T (2007) Effect of conjugal bereavement on mortality of the bereaved spouse in participants of the Renfrew/Paisley study. *Journal of Epidemiology and Community Health* 61(5): 455–460.

Harwood-Nuss A (2005) Bereavement and grief reactions. In: Wolfson A, Hendey G, Hendry P and Linden C (eds) *Clinical practice of emergency medicine*, 4th edn. London: Lippincott, Williams and Wilkins.

Lendrum S and Syme G (1992) *Gift of tears: a practical approach to loss and bereavement counselling.* London: Routledge.

Levy L and Derby J (1992) Bereavement support groups: who joins; who does not; and why. *American Journal of Community Psychology* 20(5): 649–662.

Lowton K and Higginson I (2003) Managing bereavement in the classroom: a conspiracy of silence? *Death Studies* 27(8): 717–741.

Lyttle P (2001) Bereavement visiting: older people's and nurses' experiences. *British Journal of Community Nursing* 6(12): 629–632.

Machin L (2007) Resilience and bereavement, part 1. In: Monroe B and Oliviere D (eds) *Resilience in palliative care.* Oxford: Oxford University Press.

Main J (2000) Improving management of bereavement in general practice based on a survey of recently bereaved subjects in a single general practice. *British Journal of General Practice* 50(460): 863–866.

Mount B (1976) We're a 'death-denying' society, Montreal surgeon charges. *Canadian Family Physician* 22(1378): 20.

Newberry J, de Leeuw W and Newton C (2008) What do community palliative care nurse specialists do? *International Journal of Palliative Nursing* 14(6): 264–271.

Paletti R (2008) Recovery in context: bereavement, culture and the transformation of the therapeutic self. *Death Studies* 32(1): 17–26.

Payne S, Jarrett N, Wiles R and Field D (2002) Counselling strategies for bereaved people offered in primary care. *Counselling Psychology Quarterly* 15(2): 161–177.

Pennebaker J, Zech E and Rimé B (2001) Disclosing and sharing information. In: Stroebe M, Stroebe W, Hansson R and Schut H (eds) *Handbook of bereavement research: consequences, coping and care*. Washington, DC: American Psychological Association.

Peters H and Lewin D (1994) Bereavement care: relationships between the intensive care unit and the general practitioner. *Intensive and Critical Care Nursing* 10(4): 257–264.

Prigerson H, Frank E, Kasl S, Reynolds C, Anderson B, Zubenko G, Houck P, George C and Kupfer D (1995) Complicated grief and bereavement-related depression as distinct disorders: preliminary empirical validation in elderly bereaved people. *American Journal of Psychiatry* 152(1): 22–30.

Reimers E (2001) Bereavement: a social phenomenon? *European Journal of Palliative Care* 8(6): 242–244.

Saunderson E and Ridsdale L (1999) General practitioners' beliefs and attitudes about how to respond to death and bereavement: qualitative study. *British Medical Journal* 319(7205): 293–296.

Silverman P (2007) Resilience and bereavement, part 2. In: Monroe B and Oliviere D (eds) *Resilience in palliative care*. Oxford: Oxford University Press.

Steeves R (2002) The rhythms of bereavement. *Family and Community Health* 25(1): 1–10.

Stroebe M, Schut H and Stroebe W (2007) Health outcomes of bereavement. *Lancet* 12(1): 1960–1973.

Szanto K, Gildengers A, Mulsant B, Brown G, Alexopoulos G and Reynolds C (2002) Identification of suicidal ideation and prevention of suicidal behaviour in the elderly. *Drugs and Aging* 19(1): 11–24.

Walter T (1994) *The revival of death*. London: Routledge.

Weber M and Grohmann L (2004) Time expenditure in patient-related care provided by specialist palliative care nurses in a community hospice service. *Palliative Medicine* 18(8): 719–726.

Wiles R, Jarrett N, Payne S and Field D (2002) Referrals for bereavement counselling in primary care: a qualitative study. *Patient Education and Counselling* 48(1): 79–85.

Wright B (1999) Responding to autonomy and disempowerment at the time of a sudden death. *Accident and Emergency Nursing* 7(3): 154–157.

Zimmerman C and Rodin G (2004) The denial of death thesis: sociological critique and implications for palliative care. *Palliative Medicine* 18(2): 121–128.

Zisook S (2005) Death, dying and bereavement. In: Sadock B, Sadock V (eds) *Kaplan and Sadock's comprehensive textbook of psychiatry*, 8th edn. Baltimore: Lippincott, Williams and Wilkins.

8 Acute care and bereavement

Peter Wimpenny

Key messages

- Although there is no evidence of the effectiveness of follow-up from acute care/hospital settings, it would appear to offer an opportunity for relatives to seek answers to questions surrounding the death and also for health care professionals to receive feedback on the provision of care at the time of death.
- The choice of witnessing resuscitation has been identified as potentially helpful and not detrimental to bereavement and should be available. In addition, enabling and accompanying relatives to view the body is also helpful.
- There is a need to ensure appropriate physical resources, irrespective of hospital setting but particularly in areas where resuscitation and acute/unexpected deaths may occur.
- The provision of all forms of information and services should be identified as important, appropriate and of high quality.
- Hospitals may benefit from having an individual 'in charge' of bereavement services in conjunction with national guidance.
- A palliative care approach might be considered for all areas of an acute hospital to ensure consistency of care for the dying and bereaved.
- Health care professionals identify the need for education and support. Different professional groups may have different needs in respect of this provision.

Introduction

This chapter sets out to review the range of evidence that relates to bereavement in acute care settings, particularly in units such as accident and emergency (A&E) departments, intensive therapy units (ITUs) and coronary care units (CCUs). It would appear that it is within such settings that bereavement has most significance as the environments are often clinical and unfamiliar to relatives (Fauri *et al.* 2000). Death is often sudden and unexpected (Edlich and Kübler-Ross 1991) and the resultant grief more pronounced (Parkes 1972). Thus, death in acute hospital-based settings has the potential to have a greater impact on the bereavement process for relatives and others close to the deceased. It can also be extremely challenging for staff to provide 'good quality' bereavement care.

Additionally, it must be recognised that the majority of deaths will occur in hospital and, for acute units such as ICU, this may be in the region of 17 per cent of admissions (ICNARC 2011), which increases to 25 per cent when ultimate hospital mortality is considered and 34 per cent when considering only non-surgical cases. These figures correspond with earlier estimates of deaths in UK ICUs of 11–31 per cent of admissions (Rowan *et al.* 1993) and are in line with other countries; for instance around 20 per cent in the USA (Angus *et al.* 2004). Therefore, the likelihood of dealing with death and needing to provide bereavement care in acute care settings is high.

Most practitioners, however, find bereavement a challenging part of their practice. It may be useful to begin by thinking about or reflecting on your own experiences and understanding of bereavement and bereavement care if you work in an acute care setting. For example, how have you approached those who are bereaved or are likely to be bereaved and how do you know this is 'best practice'? Questions that are important to ask at the outset may be 'where does bereavement care begin in acute care and where does it end?'

Bereavement care in acute care/hospital settings may traditionally have been associated with the period of time at the point of and just after the death, until relatives and friends leave the ward or unit. However, it is important to consider the period before death, if the opportunity exists, and also the period beyond death, which can be equally influential on the bereavement journey for the individuals concerned. Of course, the period of time around the death is also important and the issues related to how to break bad news and communicate with relatives and others are vital in the provision of end of life care (Coombs and Long 2008; ICU Liverpool Pathway n.d.). End of life care is an important subject in its own right and includes many factors related to care of the patient as well as those who may be bereaved. This chapter will not dwell on the end of life care related to the patient but will seek to illuminate evidence for best practice for the bereaved. You should also read Chapter 5 on end of life aspects of bereavement care.

Background

It has been suggested that bereavement care in acute hospital settings has been neglected, as the focus is on interventions to promote repair and rehabilitation (Kissane 2000). Although you may disagree with Kissane's perspective, there is a lack of rigorous research studies to identify actions and interventions for the bereaved in acute care, which may be an indication that it has been neglected, particularly in relation to the on-going journey for the bereaved.

However, there are some general aspects of bereavement care identified as helpful in acute care settings which you could consider. Kent and McDowell's (2004) literature review of bereavement in acute care settings highlights aspects of care which can enhance the care of the bereaved. Their review identified that whenever possible relatives should:

- not be informed by phone of death unless they have far to travel;
- be allocated one nurse, which is often identified as helpful by the bereaved family;
- be provided with an appropriate room which has identified facilities, such as a phone.

It goes on to suggest that relatives should not necessarily be excluded from resuscitation [a view identified in a range of evidence; Resuscitation Council (UK) 1996; Royal College of Nursing 2002; Hadders 2007] and if they wish to be present they should be accompanied by a nurse to explain what is happening. However, as Axelsson and colleagues (2005) point out, from a review of evidence in this area, there is a need for policy agreement, training, preparation of staff and supervision. These views are echoed by Walker (2007) in a review of evidence on A&E staff opinions in which the risks associated with relatives' presence were seen as greater than the benefits. It is not something to enter into without planning.

Kent and McDowell (2004) also indicate that the manner in which the death is communicated is more important than the professional identity of the person undertaking the role, which casts doubt on the view that it should be the 'most senior intensive care doctor' (Granger and Shelly 2002). Having a multiprofessional approach can allow the bereaved to gain a better understanding of the circumstances surrounding the death, with nurses and medical staff undertaking different roles in this situation (Coombs and Long 2008). Answering questions, listening, sitting with and showing emotion are identified as assisting this process. Furthermore, Kent and McDowell (2004) suggest that viewing the body is important in the facilitation of the grief process (a point supported by, for example, Haas 2003) but that this should be encouraged, rather than forced on relatives. Involvement in last offices is also identified as possibly helpful in accepting and adjusting to the death, as is appropriate packaging (bag or box) to convey the deceased's clothing, with an explanation for any damaged or soiled clothing. There is also a need to accommodate cultural/religious rituals and any specific personal requirements. The above apply to many hospital areas where people die and are by no means easy to achieve, but often are not discussed or we assume they will happen and therefore rarely question the approach taken in the ward or unit.

In addition it is suggested that some form of follow up should occur, with a recommended time of 1–2 weeks after the death, when a handwritten note or telephone call is appropriate and can be welcomed by families. This may demonstrate concern for those whose bereavement is sudden or unexpected (Walsh *et al.* 2008). Such follow-up is often part of the type of bereavement service offered in palliative care settings and it may be suggested that the ideals and standards of palliative care could be transferred to the general acute hospital setting (Street *et al.* 2004). This is echoed in a UK context by Rogers and colleagues (2000), who identify dissatisfaction with dying in hospital and advocates the use of palliative care approaches/standards across all settings. (These are discussed more fully in Chapter 5.) Follow up allows the bereaved to ask questions of the clinicians that may, if not answered, be detrimental to a 'natural or healthy' bereavement.

In order for bereavement care to be enhanced, it is suggested that specific plan-ning and increased education for staff is required. This is particularly so as it is an area of practice about which hospitals usually receive most complaints and in which the UK health service ombudsman gets most involved (for example 54 per cent of complaints in England and Wales were related to death, dying and bereavement in 2007). Striving for best practice can be helpful to health and social care practitioners, the bereaved and the health care organisation you work in. This is clearly demonstrated by Walsh and colleagues (2008), whose model of bereavement care (Beaumont model; see Figure 8.1) provides a useful structure to the development and provision of services, rather than ad hoc provision.

Often hospital staff do not see the consequences of their involvement with the bereaved as the bereavement journey continues well beyond the hospital. If they were made aware, it has been suggested, improved outcomes could result (Wright 1996; Brysiewicz 2006). Good bereavement care can help to facilitate optimal bereavement experiences or identify those who may be at risk of complicated grief and reduce the dissatisfaction with bereavement care that motivates complaints.

> Do you believe that good bereavement care is offered in your own area? You might want to consider if you know how care for the bereaved occurs. Do other staff talk about this and how could it be enhanced?

There is also a more general acute care perspective that can be added to the discussion. If we continue the issue of follow-up, Ellison and Ptacek (2002)

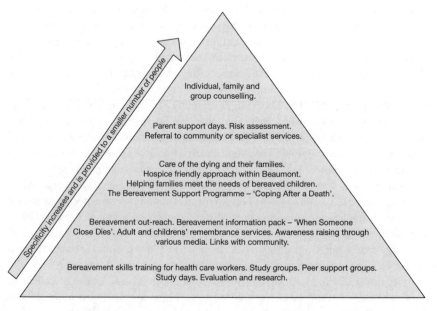

Figure 8.1 A model for bereavement support in an acute hospital (adapted from Walsh *et al.* 2008).

indicated that medical staff working in hospital-based services perceived that the bereaved should have follow up through an institutionally generated mailing service and programme, rather than personal involvement of physicians. Ferris and colleagues' (1998) study reported similar findings in junior medical staff, in that although they were usually involved in a number of deaths, it was often only at the time of death and not much beyond. In addition, although they had some concerns about death and bereavement care, they considered themselves competent for future practice in this area. Although they considered they had learned most of their knowledge in this area 'on the job', over half recognised a need for further training. This raises some possible differences in perspective between medical and other healthcare staff. You may find that differences exist within your own area of practice but may rarely be discussed. Unless there is an understanding of roles at such a critical period, for the bereaved, then care may not be optimal.

However, within the medical profession there appears to be a need to address the subject more fully. The 'neglect' may have been created by a perception that professional distance and objectivity were key parameters for successful practice. Redinbaugh and colleagues (2003) identify that junior doctors have the greatest need for emotional support following death (greatest in females and related to the time they had provided care to the patient), but consultants rarely provide such support. Role modelling from consultants, it is suggested, may lead to less stress and burnout in junior medical staff. However, consultants also report a lack of available help in discussing issues related to death and bereavement. This is supported by Delvecchio Good and colleagues (2004), who, in a study of narrative experiences of death in a variety of doctors, found that all levels have issues when dealing with death. Such issues are perhaps not unusual but when doctors may be identified as the ones to 'break bad news' (Lloyd Richards and Rees 1996), it can place an increased burden on them. Providing multidisciplinary workshops (as well as bereavement services) (Fauri *et al.* 2000) may provide greater opportunity to identify stressors and consider the roles of the team more fully in bereavement care. Edlich and Kübler-Ross (1992) endorse the need for 'systematic educational training programs' in addition to death education being a greater part of medical curricula generally, although at present it is likely that limited attention is paid to this.

There is a range of other evidence, identified particularly with specific acute care settings, that highlights additional factors which may impact on the way in which bereavement and bereavement care is managed. These may add to the general aspects already highlighted.

The provision of bereavement care in A&E departments

Dealing with death and bereavement in A&E is particularly challenging as the deaths are usually sudden, there is limited opportunity to develop a relationship with the bereaved and the distress experienced can be significant (Wright 1993). Nurses in A&E identify dealing with death and bereavement as the most difficult aspect of caring for families (Hallgrimsdottir 2004), although this may not be the case for doctors, as they have reported less emotional involvement (Redinbaugh *et al.* 2003).

In 1995 the Royal College of Nursing and the British Association of A&E Medicine (RCN/BAAEM) developed guidelines for bereavement care based on a review of death, dying and bereavement in A&E departments in England and Wales. It could be argued that these have already improved standards of care although no evidence exists to support this. However, when the guidelines were being developed, although there were examples of good policy and practice, there were considerable shortfalls in allocation of staff to bereaved relatives and to telephone responses related to a death. Only a minority of the bereaved were asked about organ donation (which has been noted as helping with bereavement in some cases; Wellesley *et al.* 1997; Cleiren and Van Zoelen 2002) and it appears that relatives were often excluded from resuscitation and last offices within the department (something that is changing as both practitioners and relatives question such exclusion). Follow-up support to the bereaved was often limited and information given to relatives often more related to post-death tasks. Although such tasks are important, for example registering the death, these are often dealt with in a more procedural manner.

The review (RCN/BAAEM 1995) identified that facilities were often not private and were variable in providing essential fixtures and fittings such as a telephone. Formal training was not available in half of the A&E units surveyed and where it was available often did not include issues related to organ donation and spiritual/cultural issues. In addition staff support was not always available beyond debriefing sessions. Medical staff are more likely to inform relatives of death, whereas nurses appeared to be more likely to be involved in the care of bereaved. The guidelines are still relevant and useful if you are considering your own approaches and facilities for bereavement and bereavement care and the extent to which your present position complies with them.

You may also consider the value of having a multidisciplinary protocol, an educational programme and an information pamphlet for the bereaved, as these have been identified as advantageous in A&E (Adamowski *et al.* 1993). Providing education for staff, as Adamowski and colleagues (1993) and Tye (1996) have also identified, is essential in meeting the needs of staff in A&E departments. When did you, or the department, last undertake professional development related to bereavement?

Lopez Soccoro and colleagues (2001) remind us that bereavement support should also be considered for staff in this area. Their study, carried out in Spain, highlights the lack of education in how to break news and support for relatives when viewing bodies and illustrates the global difficulties. The use of reflection and sharing as a means of coping is the main approach encouraged. This theme is also identified by Wakefield (2000) and Fauri and colleagues (2000), who consider that nurses may harbour disenfranchised grief (Doka 1999) and need some means of expressing their feelings and reflecting on experiences. Disenfranchised grief is when there is no recognition of your right to grieve, a perspective that may often be made worse by those in senior positions who fail to acknowledge its existence.

> Do you feel you understand the bereavement process? If not just go back and review Chapter 1. Are you aware of the guidelines available (RCN/BAEM)? Is there opportunity to express feelings about death and reflect on practice in your department? Importantly, does practice vary depending on who is on duty – that is, is care consistent for both patients, relatives and staff in respect of bereavement?

Another issue is whether relatives should be allowed to witness resuscitation and how this might affect bereavement care. Robinson and colleagues (1998), in a controlled pilot study in A&E, found a trend towards lower symptoms of grief and intrusive imagery and post-traumatic avoidance if relatives witnessed the resuscitation process. There was no evidence of detrimental effects up to 9 months later. Merlevede and colleagues (2004) similarly, but in a Belgian setting, also identify the value of allowing relatives to be present during resuscitation and being accompanied to see the body if desired. This would suggest that this is an area for further development in A&E units, although not without arousing strong feelings (Wright 2004). Considerable debate exists about allowing relatives to witness resuscitation as it can be viewed as an opportunity for staff to be put under the spotlight. However, the evidence points to enhancements for staff as well as relatives in A&E departments, particularly in assisting relatives with their bereavement journey (Axelsson *et al.* 2005).

Challenges to good care in A&E departments

There are often cultural and religious aspects to consider when dealing with bereavement in A&E, particularly as there may be limited opportunity to obtain information and provide culturally competent care. For example, Li and colleagues (2002) ranked the perspectives of bereaved people in respect of helpful actions in a Hong Kong A&E. Giving information after death and during resuscitation, seeing the body and respecting customs and religions were ranked as most helpful. Least helpful were being offered sedation and being discouraged from seeing the body, and being offered a drink was seen as an insult! Although these results obviously need to be interpreted in the light of differences in culture, as Chinese culture has different mourning rituals and responses, it highlights how important the perspective of the bereaved can be to the development of services in A&E. How this is undertaken may be through some type of audit or as part of a follow-up service or through local religious and bereavement groups who may provide advice. Many health care organisations have established guidance on the needs of different faith groups; however, we should be aware that intracultural differences exist and we should avoid stereotyping (Parkes *et al.* 1997).

Consider the following scenario, which may be typical but may help to tie up some of the key issues raised so far.

Agnes's husband Bill (75 years of age) had complained of some chest pain whilst sitting reading his paper. He often had indigestion and so she had fetched some of his antacid mixture and told him that he had perhaps eaten his tea too fast again! He complained again a short time later and was looking a bit 'peaky' but he often took a while to settle down after his antacids, although it did seem worse this time. They were just getting ready for bed when she noticed he was still holding his chest. 'Should I call for a doctor Bill?' 'No, I'll be fine I'm sure.' She wasn't convinced and decided a short time later to ask for advice. An ambulance arrived and Bill was whisked away to hospital. Agnes phoned her son and he arrived to pick up his mum and for them to travel in together to the hospital. When they arrived they were directed to a small room and told that the doctor would be with them shortly. She duly arrived and informed Agnes and her son that Bill had had a cardiac arrest when he arrived at the hospital and had 'not recovered'. 'Do you mean he is dead?' asked Agnes. 'Yes, I am sorry', said the doctor and indicated that the nurse would be in to see the family and give them information about what to do next. She then asked if Agnes or her son had any questions but they could not think of anything to ask.

The nurse arrived and he asked if they wanted to see Bill. Agnes did but his son didn't ('I'd sooner remember dad as he was'). Agnes entered the resuscitation room where Bill was. The staff had put out some flowers and dimmed the lights. They left Agnes alone with Bill. She sat by him and didn't know what to do. After a short while the nurse returned and suggested that Agnes return home with her son and come back the next day to collect Bill's clothes and belongings and the death certificate. He gave Agnes a 'bereavement pack' and pointed out the telephone number to call the next day to check if the death certificate was available. When the death certificate was finally collected it stated that Bill died of an anterior myocardial infarction.

The above scenario misses out a considerable amount of detail but represents the sort of speed of death that can occur in acute care and the extent to which dealing with such rapidity is challenging, particularly in the midst of seeking to 'maintain life'. However, for Agnes and her son their bereavement journey has only just begun and will be on-going.

Which bits of the scenario are significant, why might this be so and is it possible for you to consider what you believe would have assisted Agnes and her son setting out on the bereavement journey?

Providing a follow-up service from A&E has been described as beneficial to staff and relatives (Williams *et al.* 2000), although no evidence of the effectiveness of such a service is available. After having considered the scenario, you may reflect on whether it may have offered the opportunity for Agnes and her son to ask some specific questions, such as 'If we had got Bill to hospital sooner would this have meant he wouldn't have died?' ' Was he conscious when he arrived at the hospital and what did he say?' 'Why did he have a cardiac arrest?' In addition it is also an opportunity to ask Agnes and her son their views on what had helped and what could be improved.

When a follow-up service is offered it is often taken up by only a small number of relatives and so should not be overwhelming for staff. Parris and colleagues (2007) held meetings with 14 per cent of their follow-up contacts, the majority (75 per cent) of whom wanted an explanation of medical terms on the death certificate or post-mortem examination form, 12 per cent to get an explanation of the circumstances and treatment related to the death, 4 per cent advice about medical screening for relatives, 4 per cent reassurance that they could not have prevented the death and 11 per cent 'miscellaneous', which included concerns about treatment and requests for support. Those who provided the service believed it facilitated the bereavement process by providing answers to questions that would have gone unanswered and potentially led to prolongation of the grieving process. It may also be the case that it had other effects such as a reduction in morbidity and mortality in the bereaved and also a reduction in complaints to the service. If Agnes and her son had had such an opportunity they might have had questions related to a number of the areas identified above.

The provision of bereavement care in ITUs

Bereavement care will of course be associated with end of life care. Historically ITUs have focused more on therapy/treatment rather than palliation, but this is changing (Morgan 2008). There is, however, little doubt that the care provided, to both patient and those close to them, will impact on bereavement. What appears to be particularly important in end of life care related to the bereaved is the communication that occurs with relatives and others and also with the health care team (Lautrette *et al.* 2006; Levy and McBride 2006; Truog *et al.* 2008). Such communication may also stretch beyond the death if follow up is considered or issues related to communication before or at the time of death identified.

Cuthbertson and colleagues (2000) sought to establish the value of a follow-up bereavement service from ITUs (follow up is also identified as part of the Intensive Care Society guidelines for bereavement care which were published in 1998). Those followed up identified that relationships and communication with staff were key factors before and at the time of death and that the majority of the bereaved have support from family and friends and few use professional services after the death (a finding that is also reported by Billings and Kolton 1999). They make the practical point that a lack of adequate recording at admission can make follow up problematic, highlighting how accurate assessment and records are important in a variety of ways. The evaluation by Cuthbertson and colleagues (2000) does not establish in what ways the intervention of follow up was effective and there is an implicit assumption that it is of value. Similarly, Tunnicliffe and Briggs (1997) and Williams and colleagues (2003) highlight the perceived value of follow up from perspectives of the bereaved and the staff of the unit, but again evidence of effectiveness is not described.

This raises a key issue: can practice be based on such evidence? There is no doubt that establishing the effectiveness of a follow-up service would be beneficial; however, if this is not forthcoming, what should you do? Of course you could set up your own research, although it is more likely that you will have to make a decision based on existing evidence. This will always be influenced by the context in which you work. For example, if you have a large number of complaints related to death, dying and bereavement then there may be an increasing impetus to review practice and put a follow-up service into place. Alternatively, if your unit has fewer deaths each year, as it is a surgical ITU, you may feel that follow up may not be warranted but an annual memorial service may be more appropriate (Platt 2004).

Granger and colleagues (1995), in a survey of UK ITUs, identified that staff considered they needed more than training to deal with breaking bad news and dealing with bereaved relatives. Other issues they raised were a need to improve facilities for relatives, particularly practical issues such as relatives having an available phone and direct physical access to the deceased in a private setting. Granger and colleagues (1995) also found that the range and type of information available in ITUs and given to relatives suggested duplication of effort and the possibility that the quality of some of this home-produced information may be poor.

Communication and information giving about end of life care giving are issues which need to be addressed in ITUs (Jastremski 1998). A more recent multicentre study (Lautrette *et al.* 2007) sought to compare 'normal' end of life care with an enhanced conference process with relatives. This enhanced process was based on acknowledging emotions, listening, gaining understanding of the patient as a person, eliciting questions from the family and a new bereavement brochure. The results indicated that the enhanced approach could have an impact on the bereavement journey through lower levels of on-going stress, depression and anxiety.

There is also a need to ensure communication between units such as ITUs and primary care practitioners. The latter may be in a better position to conduct follow-up. General practitioners (GPs), for example, indicate they would welcome quicker accurate information on deaths in ITUs so that they could follow up the bereaved relatives, although, in the main, they do not then refer on to other services (Peters and Lewin 1994). However, a visit by the GP, if undertaken, may provide an opportunity for relatives (it would probably only be immediate next of kin, for example spouse, who receive such a visit), to ask questions about the death and to be informed about available services in the community if they need them.

The provision of bereavement care in CCUs

Edwards and Shaw (1998) in a review of literature related to bereavement in CCUs identified issues similar to those in A&E and ITUs. Their review highlights that relatives wished to be present during resuscitation, viewing the body was regarded as a positive factor in facilitating bereavement, and the provision of appropriate private facilities was seen as being important. However, it also questions the need for an allocated nurse, as some relatives may not wish this, and advocated the distribution in England and Wales of a booklet entitled *What to do after a death* and other information on support such as bereavement counselling. It also suggested that clinical staff were not good at breaking bad news and communicating at the time of death, something that seems to be common across all settings. In addition, the lack of available education and support for staff was once again noted. The idea of follow up appears to be viewed with more ambivalence in CCUs and there are questions around whether hospital staff are best placed to undertake it. This may be because of clearer reasons for death, or because the focus of care is geared to issues such as rehabilitation or on-going treatment.

Although information from health care staff has been shown to be valued by relatives in the CCU context (Olsson 1997), it is not clear that staff showing their emotions is helpful. The coping needs of the family when death occurs in a CCU may be difficult to assess, particularly in relation to the degree of support available through family and social networks. The support that may be required from health or social care staff is therefore uncertain at this point, as relationship building within such a short space of time can be challenging. It may be suggested that some form of follow up could seek to address this and again provide feedback on performance.

> Who do you think should undertake follow up? Should it be a hospital responsibility, or each unit/ward, or should it only be undertaken by a practitioner in the community such as a GP or District Nurse?

Policy development

The development of policy on bereavement care by the NHS in England and Wales (Department of Health 2005) drew on perspectives from the bereaved who suggested that the journey from pre-death to bereavement is often affected by poor communication from all staff and between staff internally and to external sources, not being fully involved in the process, staff being unaware of relevant policies, problematic environmental factors, a lack of specialised staff for advice and support, and a need for good-quality information (such areas are also identified by others, for example Warren 2002).

These shortfalls in care have also been highlighted in the USA (Billings and Kolton 1999; Curtis and Engelberg 2006), although it must be noted that the majority of people surveyed registered overall satisfaction with care. The issues of respect, dignity and communication covered the majority of the shortfalls. As Silvey (1990) points out from a small sample of interviews with relatives after a death in hospital, 'All remarked positively about any member of staff who responded to them in a caring or empathetic way. These people and their actions were remembered with clarity and described with great warmth' (p. 17). It might be assumed that such responses could impact positively on the bereavement process.

A follow-up survey of NHS organisations (Trusts) in England and Wales carried out in 2005 by the Department of Health (a repeat of a 2001 survey) indicated that improvements to bereavement care were happening but there were still considerable gaps. The main conclusions were:

- a need for someone to be in charge of bereavement services at Trust level;
- a desire to have national guidelines;
- an urgent need for information packs in a variety of languages, and a need for dedicated rooms; and
- greater consistency in approach through 'training more (if not all) hospital staff in basic bereavement awareness and communication skills' (p. 5).

Twelve areas on which bereavement care should be based were also highlighted:

- respect for the individual;
- equality of provision;
- choice;
- communication;
- information;
- partnership;
- recognising and acknowledging loss;
- environment and facilities;
- staff training and development;
- staff support;
- health and safety; and
- review and audit.

It was also recommended that all NHS organisations in England and Wales should have in place a written policy on death and bereavement which should identify bereavement care pathways (e.g. Gold Standards Framework), be based on consultations with appropriate stakeholders and include awareness of consent to post-mortem (Department of Health 2003). There should be clear responsibility at executive and managerial level, with a senior manager who has appropriate skill and training taking primary responsibility. Identified education and support should be available and utilised.

Similar developments related to bereavement care are being developed in Scotland and Northern Ireland within the UK context where centralised provision of health and social care provide opportunities to develop, co-ordinate and evaluate services to the bereaved in acute care settings.

Conclusion

This chapter has covered a range of issues related to acute care settings, based around the available evidence. It is clear that there are a number of aspects related to the provision of bereavement care that are worthy of consideration, particularly around the time of death and beyond. There is a need for better organisation and co-ordination of service provision, which includes education and communication between services that, at present, appear to be lacking.

It may be argued that development of bereavement care is already something that is being promoted in government circles – this is the case, for example, in many developed countries (Nucleus Group 2004; Department of Health 2005; Walsh *et al.* 2008). In addition there is evidence that developments are happening on the ground where improvements to services for the bereaved are occurring such as employment of bereavement co-ordinators who are able to assess local provision of care to the bereaved; for example, improving the journey to the mortuary or viewing area, which can often be along little-used corridors full of old chairs and beds. The challenge is to see such improvements as part of standard care provision, rather than the exception.

You may want to reflect on your own position.

> What does your acute care setting offer in respect of bereavement care? Do you ever have any contact with bereaved relatives after the death – is this a thank-you card or perhaps a complaint about care? Is this type of feedback the best available? How do you know that your care for the bereaved is always appropriate and how could you determine this? When did you last consider what to do about bereavement in your ward or unit?

References

Adamowski K, Dickinson G, Weitzman B, Roessler C and Carter-Snell C (1993) Sudden unexpected death in the emergency department: caring for the survivors. *Canadian Medical Association Journal* 149(10): 1445–1451.

Angus DC, Barnato AE, Linde-Zwirble WT, Weissfield LA, Watson RS, Rickert T and Rubenfeld GD on behalf of the Robert Wood Johnson Foundation ICU End-of-Life Peer Group (2004) Use of intensive care at the end of life in the United States: an epidemiologic study. *Critical Care Medicine* 32(3): 638–643.

Axelsson AB, Zettergren M and Axelsson C (2005) Good and bad experiences of family presence during acute care and resuscitation: what makes the difference? *European Journal of Cardiovascular Nursing* 4(2): 161–169.

Billings JA and Kolton E (1999) Family satisfaction and bereavement care following death in the hospital. *Journal of Palliative Medicine* 2(1): 33–49.

Brysiewicz P (2006) A model for dealing with sudden death. *Advances in Nursing Science* 29(3): E1–E11.

Cleiren MPHD and Van Zoelen AAJ (2002) Post-mortem organ donation and grief: a study of consent, refusal and well-being in bereavement. *Death Studies* 26(10): 837–849.

Coombs M and Long T (2008) Managing a good death in critical care: can health policy help? *Nursing in Critical Care* 13(4): 208–214.

Curtis JR and Engelberg RA (2006) Measuring success of interventions to improve the quality of end-of-life care in the intensive care unit. *Critical Care Medicine* 34(11): S341–S347.

Cuthbertson SJ, Margetts MA and Streat SJ (2000) Bereavement follow-up after critical illness. *Critical Care Medicine* 28(4): 1196–1201.

Delvecchio Good M-J, Gadmer NM, Matthew L, Redinbaugh E, Ruopp P, Sullivan A, Arnold RM and Block S (2004) Narrative nuances on good and bad deaths: internists' tales from high-technology work places. *Social Science and Medicine* 58(5): 939–953.

Department of Health (2003) *Families and post mortems: a code of practice.* London: HMSO.

Department of Health (2005) *When a patient dies: advice on developing bereavement services in the NHS.* London: HMSO.

Doka KJ (1999) Disenfranchised grief. *Bereavement Care* 18(3): 37–39.

Edlich RF and Kübler-Ross E (1992) On death and dying in the emergency department [Review]. *Journal of Emergency Medicine* 10(2): 225–229.

Edwards L and Shaw DG (1998) Care of the suddenly bereaved in cardiac care units: a review of the literature. *Intensive Critical Care Nursing* 14(3): 144–152.

Ellison NM and Ptacek JT (2002) Physician interactions with families and caregivers after a patient's death: current practices and proposed changes. *Journal of Palliative Medicine* 5(1): 49–55.

Fauri DP, Ettner B and Kovacs PJ (2000) Bereavement services in acute care settings. *Death Studies* 24(1): 51–64.

Ferris TGA, Hallward RL and Billings MD (1998) When the patient dies: a survey of medical housestaff about care after death. *Journal of Palliative Medicine* 1(3): 231–239.

Granger C and Shelly M (2002) Bereavement care. In: Griffiths RD and Jones C (eds) *Intensive aftercare.* Oxford: Butterworth-Heinemann.

Granger CE, George C and Shelly MP (1995) The management of bereavement on intensive care units. *Intensive Care Medicine* 21(5): 429–436.

Haas F (2003) Bereavement care: seeing the body. *Nursing Standard* 17(28): 33–37.

Hadders H (2007) Relatives' presence in connection with cardiopulmonary resuscitation and sudden death at the intensive care unit. *Nursing Inquiry* 14(3): 224–232.

Hallgrimsdottir EM (2004) Caring for families in A&E departments: Scottish and Icelandic nurses' opinions and experiences. *Accident and Emergency Nursing* 12(2): 114–120.

ICNARC (2011) CMP case mix and outcome summary statistics: 1 April 2009 to 31 March 2010. Available at: https://www.icnarc.org/documents/Summary%20statistics%20 rebranded.pdf (accessed 16 June 2011).

ICU Liverpool Care Pathway (LCP) Available at: http://www.mcpcil.org.uk/liverpool-care-pathway/lcp-specialist-icu.htm (accessed 16 June 2011).

Jastremski CA (1998) Caring for the families of those who die in the critical care unit. *Critical Care Medicine* 26(7): 1150–1151.

Kent H and McDowell J (2004) Sudden bereavement in acute care settings. *Nursing Standard* 19(6): 38–42.

Kissane D (2000) Neglect of bereavement care in general hospitals. Editorial. *Medical Journal of Australia* 173 (9): 453.

Lautrette A, Ciroldi M, Ksibi H and Azoulay E (2006) End-of-life family conferences: rooted in the evidence. *Critical Care Medicine* 34(11): S364–S372.

Lautrette A, Darmon M, Megarbane B, Joly LM, Chevret S, Adrie C, Barnoud D, Bleichner G, Bruel C, Choukroun G, Curtis JR, Fieux F, Galliot R, Garrouste-Oregas M, Georges H, Goldgran-Toedano D, Jourdain M, Loubert G, Reignier J, Saidi F, Souweine B, Vincent F, Barnes NK, Pochard F, Schlemmer B and Azoulay E (2007) A communication strategy and brochure for relatives of patients dying in the ICU. *New England Journal of Medicine* 356(5): 469–478.

Levy ML and McBride DL (2006) End-of-life care in the intensive care unit: state of the art in 2006. *Critical Care Medicine* 34(11): S306–S308.

Li SP, Chan CW and Lee DT (2002) Helpfulness of nursing actions to suddenly bereaved family members in an accident and emergency setting in Hong Kong. *Journal of Advanced Nursing* 40(2): 170–180.

Lloyd Richards C and Rees C (1996). Clinical management. Hospital nurses' bereavement support for relatives: study report. *International Journal of Palliative Nursing* 2(2): 106–110.

Lopez Socorro L, Tolson D and Fleming V (2001) Exploring Spanish nurses' lived experience of the care provided for suddenly bereaved families. *Journal of Advanced Nursing* 35(4): 562–570.

Merlevede E, Spooren D, Henderick H, Portzky G, Buylaert W, Jannes C, Calle P, Van Staey M, De Rock C, Smeesters L, Michem N and Van Heeringen K (2004) Perceptions, needs and mourning reactions of bereaved relatives confronted with a sudden unexpected death. *Resuscitation* 61(3): 341–348.

Morgan J (2008) End-of-life care in UK critical care units: a literature review. *Nursing in Critical Care* 13(3): 152–161.

Nucleus Group (2004) *Review of specific grief and bereavement services: final report*, Melbourne: Department of Human Services, Victoria. Available at: http://www.health.vic.gov.au/palliativecare/archive/finalrep_grief.pdf (accessed 16 June 2011).

Olsson M (1997) Social support in bereavement crisis: a study of interaction in crisis situations. *Social Work in Health Care* 25(1): 117–130.

Parkes CM (1972) *Bereavement: studies of grief in adult life*. London: Penguin.

Parkes CM, Laugani P and Young B (1997) *Death and bereavement across cultures*. London: Routledge.

Parris RJ, Schlosenberg J, Stanley C, Maurice S and Clarke SFJ (2007) Emergency department follow-up of bereaved relatives: an audit of one particular service. *Emergency Medicine* 24(5): 339–342.

Peters H and Lewin D (1994) Bereavement care: relationships between the intensive care unit and the general practitioner. *Intensive and Critical Care Nursing* 10(4): 257–264.

Platt J (2004) The planning, organising and delivery of a memorial service in critical care. *Nursing in Critical Care* 9(5): 222–229.

Redinbaugh EM, Sullivan AM, Block SD, Gadmer NM, Lakoma M, Mitchell AM, Seltzer D, Wolford J and Arnold RM (2003) Doctors' emotional reactions to recent death of a patient: cross sectional study of hospital doctors. *British Medical Journal* 327(7408): 185.

Resuscitation Council (UK) (1996) *Should relatives witness resuscitation? A report from a project team of the Resuscitation Council (UK)*. London: Resuscitation Council (UK).

Robinson SM, Mackenzie-Ross S, Campbell Hewson GL, Egleston CV and Prevost AT (1998) Psychological effect of witnessed resuscitation on bereaved relatives. *The Lancet* 352(9128): 614–617.

Rogers A, Karlsen S and Addington-Hall J (2000) All the services were excellent. It was when the human element comes in that things go wrong: dissatisfaction with hospital care in the last year of life. *Journal of Advanced Nursing* 31(4): 768–774.

Rowan KM, Kerr JH, Major E, McPherson K, Short A, Vessey MP (1993) Intensive Care Society's APACHE II study in Britain and Ireland – II: outcome comparisons of intensive care units after adjustment for case mix by the American APACHE II method. *British Medical Journal* 307(6910): 977–981.

Royal College of Nursing (2002) *Witnessing resuscitation: guidance for nursing staff*. London: RCN.

Royal College of Nursing/British Association for Accident and Emergency Medicine (1995) *Bereavement care in A&E departments: report of a working group*. London: RCN.

Silvey S. (1990) Bereavement care in hospitals. *Bereavement Care* 9(2): 17–18.

Street AF, Love AW and Blackford J (2004) Exploring bereavement care in inpatient settings. *Contemporary Nurse* 17(3): 240–250.

Truog RD, Campbell ML, Curtis JR, Haas CE, Luce JM, Rubenfield GD, Rushton CH and Kaufman DC (2008) Recommendations for end-of-life care in the intensive care unit: a consensus statement by the American Academy of Critical Care Medicine. *Critical Care Medicine* 36(3): 953–963.

Tunnicliffe R and Briggs D (1997) Introducing a bereavement support programme in ICU. *Nursing Standard* 11(47): 38–40.

Tye CC (1996) Sudden bereavement in accident and emergency: the development and evaluation of a short educational course for qualified nurses. *Accident and Emergency Nursing* 4(2): 88–93.

Wakefield A (2000) Nurses' responses to death and dying: a need for relentless self-care. *International Journal of Palliative Nursing* 6(5): 245–251.

Walker W (2007) Accident and emergency staff opinion on the effects of family presence during adult resuscitation: critical literature review. *Journal of Advanced Nursing* 61(4): 348–362.

Walsh T, Foreman M, Curry P, O'Driscoll S and McCormack M (2008) Bereavement support in an acute hospital: an Irish model. *Death Studies* 32(8): 768–786.

Warren NA (2002) Critical care family members' satisfaction with bereavement experiences. *Critical Care Nursing Quarterly* 25(2): 54–60.

Wellesley A, Glucksman E and Crouch R (1997) Organ donation in the accident and emergency department: a study of relatives' views. *Journal of Accident and Emergency Medicine* 14(1): 24–25.

Williams AG, O'Brien DL, Laughton KJ and Jelinek GA (2000) Improving services to bereaved relatives in the emergency department: making healthcare more human. *Medical Journal of Australia* 173(9): 480–483.

Williams R, Harris S, Randall L, Nichols R and Brown S (2003) A bereavement after-care service for intensive care relatives and staff: the story so far. *Nursing in Critical Care* 8(3): 109–115.

Wright B (1993) *Caring in crisis: a handbook of intervention skills*. Edinburgh: Churchill Livingstone.

Wright B (1996) *Sudden death: a research base for practice*, 2nd edn. London: Churchill Livingstone.

Wright B (2004) Difficulties around family presence during resuscitation [Editorial]. *Accident and Emergency Nursing* 12(2): 65–66.

9 Children's deaths and bereavement

Brother Francis

Key messages

- Where an illness is life-limiting, bereavement care should start at diagnosis.
- Families may have more than one life-limited child and so may lose children rather than a child.
- Children die in hospitals, at home and in children's hospices, so families' experiences will be different. However, home is normally the preferred place for the dying child.
- Parents need good information and should be involved in all aspects of their child's care.
- Issues of bereavement need to be integrated into mainstream services and policies for children and young people rather than being isolated specialist services.
- The consequences of the death of a sibling should be considered particularly within the context of the family group and the stage of development of the surviving child.
- We need to take the 'long view' when thinking about support for siblings.
- Strategies in practice may include creating a sacred space for the child and family where they can express their 'soul pain'.

Introduction

> My attempts to prepare Andrew's sister were totally insufficient. It should have started earlier and with professional help. The prospect of my own loss was so great I could not sufficiently appreciate my daughter's loss.
>
> (Darnill and Gamage 2006)

I write this chapter as a practitioner who has spent most of his professional life working with children and with parents of dying children. The writing is driven by my personal experience and from a 'deep place' within me, and I hope will be of some use to the reader as you work with families who are going to lose or who have lost a child.

This chapter considers the needs of dying children by examining the evidence and ways in which interventions can be meaningful and helpful to the dying child, their parents and siblings. It is illuminated with a number of illustrations from practice as I believe that such evidence can also assist practitioners to enhance the provision of care and make connections with their own clinical work.

Background

Children die every year from a range of causes. However, the majority will still die in hospital despite concerns about choice in the place of death. The Association for Children's Palliative Care (ACT 2003a) and Craft and Killen (2007) suggest these concerns are due to a lack of support and services in the community, for example for care at home. Home may be considered the preferred place for a child to die, although children's hospice care may offer an intermediate and acceptable alternative (ACT 2003b; CLIC Sargent 2009)

Best care related to bereavement and children's death may be interpreted as holistic or family-centred concepts, which paediatric clinicians and carers appear committed to (Thompson 1985; Casey 1988; Palmer 1993; Darbyshire 1994). However, they may also be the first to admit, like other groups of clinicians, that they find this dimension of care difficult to address with children, particularly those from many different cultural and religious backgrounds who may be dying (Winkelstein 1989). In addition they can be faced with many different priorities in their work and not necessarily know what is best care or how to deliver it. This is reflected in a Delphi study by Steele and colleagues (2008) which sought to identify research priorities in paediatric palliative care, one of which was: what are the bereavement needs of families in paediatric palliative care? Such identification of establishing needs through research suggests a desire to enhance care through the use of available evidence.

In the late 1960s and into the 1970s, for example, when a child diagnosed with cancer faced a high probability of death, psychosocial researchers focused on how much the child knew about his or her impending death and how best to communicate with and support that child. They found that children with cancer often reach an understanding of what death means for them at an earlier age than their peers and earlier than their level of development would suggest. Dying children, even those who are very young (under the age of 5) and whose understanding is still not fully developed, may express their knowledge and emotions about death in various ways, both verbal and non-verbal (Waechter 1971; Spinetta 1974; Bluebond-Langner 1978).

My clinical experience suggests that the more information and support we can offer all the family before their child dies and at the time of death, the less we will need to do for them after the death in the way of support. This theme will be developed further as the chapter progresses. I think the key is to help them prepare and not complicate their journey, so they are left free to grieve after the death. As professionals we perhaps need to learn the art of 'walking alongside' the families we have the privilege of working with and learn to stay with the pain and sit with the mystery of death as there will be no easy answers. Although theories, models and research may have some usefulness to developing our understanding, they also have limitations. A bereaved parent recently wrote on a palliative care website:

> Excuse me, but all of this seems to be rather a lot of unnecessary complicated tosh. When your child is seriously ill and terminally ill; everything then depends on quality and time. The energy you have to care for your child and the professionalism and communicating qualities of the experts and carers around you . . . the relationships you develop are crucial, as are the sensitivities of those working with your child to you. Stress as such is not dependant on being a carer, but due to loss of control and hope. Hope comes from being there for your child in even the smallest ways . . . through everything, don't rely on models ask real people.
>
> (From a parent on Paedpal Care mailing group, which is run by ACT)

The aim of good bereavement care is to enable siblings and parents to be left with what can only be described as a 'good enough' memory of the life, dying, death and after care of their child or in some cases children or their parents. It is also about leaving staff with a 'good enough' memory of the encounter. How this can be achieved, I suggest, is through a combination of knowledge, clinical supervision that helps us make sense of our experience and understanding.

Parents' responses to the death of a child

> Becoming a bereaved parent is like joining a club that no one wants to belong to.
>
> (Tonkin 2008: 4)

Rolls and Payne (2007) found parents had difficulty in maintaining their parenting role as they struggled with their own bereavement and the disruption in their circumstances. The loss of a child is considered intense and overwhelming and, as Rando (1986) and Klass (1996) state, for parents the death of a child contains dimensions not seen in other losses, including a sense of failure in their parental role. This includes the 'protector role', and a sense of loss of self because of the investment of their hopes for the future embodied in their children. Grief for parents is now often considered an on-going experience that has no fixed end point but which normally changes over time as adaptation occurs (Davies 2004). This has clear implications for any interventions that bereaved parents are offered and when and how they are offered.

Janzen and colleagues (2003–2004) illustrate parents' experiences and their advice to those professionals who might be in the front line to provide such services, for instance police, nurses, doctors, coroners, social workers/crisis counsellors, funeral directors and clergy.

They divide advice into three areas:

- instrumental assistance (e.g. providing access, allowing time, respecting decisions);
- provision of information (e.g. details of death, what to expect and do, rituals and memorials);
- compassion and empathy (e.g. give control, actively listen, be present, respect for the child's body, respect their faith).

One parent in the study by Janzen and colleagues (2003–2004: 161) stated:

> It is amazing what an impact the actions/reactions of others can have during this traumatic and very vulnerable time. I remember very clearly the things that were said and done which were comforting. I remember just as clearly, in fact, perhaps more clearly, the things that were said and done which were hurtful and upsetting.

The quote from the grieving parent illustrates the impact of professionals around the time of death and afterwards and the need for consideration of what is said and how it is said. Often health and social care professionals will highlight a need for better training and education to develop communication skills in sensitive topics, such as death and bereavement. What should I say? is a common response made by professionals, for which I suggest what can you say? In certain circumstances, it may be appropriate to say very little and instead to listen, be still and try to be present with them, utilising non-verbal communication such as eye contact, touch and gestures to offer comfort and support. This may be a more appropriate response than trying to fill the space with words and advice. What we do and say can have a negative impact on grieving parents, so saying very little is perhaps a safer response.

The death of a child is one of the most stressful events for any parent and they can struggle to move out of the loss phase [see Chapter 1, Stroebe and Schut's model (1999)], which will hinder their long-term restoration and could lead to complicated grief. So how we care for them before their child dies, at the time of death and beyond are key factors in their long-term survival and their adjustment to life without their child (Surkan *et al.* 2006; Riley *et al.* 2007).

Before death and at the time of death, parents need to maintain some sense of control. Moulton (1997) found that parents who had control found some 'peace and serenity'. Conversely, those that had no control over the situation felt guilty (a finding also supported by Surkan *et al.* 2006 and by Rolls and Payne 2007 in the context of their parenting role). My experience suggests that positive outcomes in situations such as this are about enabling the parents to make choices available to them so they can plan for the death of their child. In addition, as Craft and Killen (2007) identified in their independent review of services, families require bereavement support for siblings.

A useful qualitative research paper by Davies (2005), 'Mothers' stories of loss: their need to be with their dying child and their child's body after death', is a study from which we can reflect on and consider what we offer. The study highlighted the need of mothers to have time, space and privacy with their dying child and, I think more importantly, time with their child after the death. Nothing can turn the clock back at this stage but how we engage and work with them can help or hinder their bereavement journey. Surkan and colleagues' (2006) findings indicate that families who reported that their child's care was suboptimal frequently cited feelings of guilt in their bereavement, as compared with families who felt that they and their child were well cared for.

I have not yet met a parent who has not known at a deep level that their child is dying. However, their surface behaviour or what they present to the outside world may be seen as denial (Kübler-Ross 1985). In fact, what they are doing is 'coping' or 'getting through the day in one piece'; it is called 'maintaining their hope'. If we misread this, we may well intervene in the wrong way. They need their hope as this gets them through the day and helps them 'hold it together' for the rest of the family, and they need us to support them in this. This is not some form of collusion; it is understanding how they cope and what they need at that time. If we fail to understand how a family works, what roles they have and how they process information, we may well miss important information and again intervene in a way that can be unhelpful and subsequently affect our relationship with the parents, which in turn will affect the care given to the child or sibling (see also Chapter 3 about families and bereavement).

The above point was well illustrated to me when a well-meaning medical consultant and a community nurse felt a mother did not fully understand how ill her child was and they saw it as their job to tell her. They took the mother into a side room, late one Friday afternoon, and told her that her child was very ill and could die very soon, maybe even over that weekend. The mother left the room very angry with the two professionals and took her child home, never to return.

These professionals did not fully understand how the mother and child talked with each other, nor how the mother liked to transmit messages to her child. What the professionals did not know was that the mother and child had both spoken about it and had made plans together. The mother wanted to be given 'bad news' at a time when she was away from her child and that she had the time and space after to process the information and think about how she would tell her child. This she normally did at bedtime when they would both lie on the bed and talk about such things. Following the meeting, she had to come out of one room and go straight into the next room where her child was. She had no space or time to compose herself before facing her child and her child could see that she was upset and wanted to know why. Planning meetings after this event had to take place in a GP's office, as the mother would not attend the hospital.

The child died at home some weeks later in bed with her mother. Another sad aspect of this story was that shortly after, the mother had another child who became unwell and she could not bring herself to return to the hospital but had to go to a hospital in another town.

It is also the case that we need to be aware that there is evidence that parental grief reactions will be different (Dyregov 1990). The differences can continue beyond the child's death. For example the father may go back and get lost in work and the mother may be left at home with her grief. It is a common mistake in situations like this to become judgemental about fathers who appear to be escaping when in practice they are in a very painful place, and are using work as a coping strategy when all they want to do is run away.

Childhood/sibling bereavement

Although this chapter is focused on children's deaths, it is also important not to forget that surviving children will also be affected. The wider issue of anticipatory grief, when the dying person and the family may be grieving simultaneously before death, is covered by Costello in Chapter 5. Moreover, data from empirical studies relating to childhood bereavement in health and social care contexts are reviewed more fully in Chapter 2. However, there is a clear need to develop good evidence in paediatric care and bereavement support for the dying child, their parents, siblings and grandparents as well as the child's school or college community. On the one hand there is a tension around conducting ethical research with this group and on the other there is now emerging evidence that this can be undertaken if it is done sensitively and that parents view this in a positive light (Hynson *et al.* 2006). Parents often want to know that their child may make a difference to the way care is delivered in the future and therefore will readily agree to participate in research.

There are often short- and long-term bereavement consequences for children that are reported (Silverman and Worden 1992). These will be influenced by the type of bereavement experienced. For example, a 6-year-old sibling may not fully understand the meaning of their brother or sister's death before they become a young adult (Ribbens-McCarthy and Jessop 2005). It is at the latter stage that they may need the support and input. The loss of a sibling will be different from that of a parent. There are also differences between boys and girls and between the loss of a mother and of a father (Black 1998; Kalter *et al.* 2003; Sandler *et al.* 2003).

Some of the literature on childhood bereavement looks at the 'meaningfulness' of care (Davies *et al.* 2006). This is very important in giving the remaining child(ren) and their family the opportunity to express grief at the time of death, which can be referred to at a later date with the child. For example, a parent can remind the child by saying, 'do you remember we did this at the time' and so on (Corr 1999; Ribbens-McCarthy and Jessop 2005).

Rolls and Payne (2007), in their study of children and young people's experience of UK childhood bereavement services, identified that children expressed:

- difficulties in managing and expressing their feelings;
- isolation;
- problems at school;
- fear for their surviving parent.

Although in this context the fear of losing a surviving parent is not the focus, the impact of a child's death on the parents can mean that they are often 'disabled' and the surviving child(ren) may have concerns for both parents (see also Chapter 2) which they may struggle to meet.

When a sibling loses a brother or sister, they are saying goodbye to one of the longest-lasting relationships that they may ever have (Davies 1999). This may well bring about a change in the surviving child, which may be their way of getting some attention from their bereaved parents. The age of the sibling may well be significant with regards to their 'acting out' behaviour or need for support. For example, adolescents may deny and suppress their emotions (Mearns 2000).

The role of the surviving child may change, as may the relationships within the family, so these should be considered when dealing with sibling loss (see also Chapters 2 and 3). More aggressive behaviour in the surviving child(ren) has been identified, particularly in younger children, and has been interpreted as a cry for attention (McCown and Davies 1995). Similar analysis carried out by Birenbaum (2000) highlights the need for better assessment of children to establish the problems associated with the death of a sibling. Potts and colleagues (1999) demonstrate the value of a 'Treasure Weekend' as one means by which bereaved siblings can express their grief, remember their sister or brother and potentially move on.

An earlier literature review on sibling loss by Huntzinger (1995) has two recurrent threads: one that is focused on the relationship between the siblings and the consequences of the loss and a second focusing on the loss of 'attention' because of the parents' own grief reactions (McCown and Davies 1995; Potts *et al.* 1999). Robinson and Mahon (1997) highlight (although this is related more to adult siblings) that specific changes occur relating to self-perception and changes in world views, which will be governed by the context surrounding the child, the stage of their development, the family system and the nature of the death.

In my clinical work, siblings are one of the most important groups of people to work with. With our understanding of pain and symptom management, we know we can care for the dying child and manage their symptomatology. However, working with siblings is not so well understood and at times it can be hard to access them, for one reason or other. As Rolls and Payne (2007) have highlighted, they can feel isolated, they have difficulties in expressing their feelings and they can be confused about what they are feeling. It may be that they feel guilty or angry. They can have problems at home and at school. They may not be able to speak with their parents, as they see that they are upset. They deserve just as much of our (health and social care professionals') time and attention.

Helping children express grief

Helping children address their feelings can be difficult for health and social care professionals, but children of all ages can express their inner worlds and all that goes to make up that world through play, music, art, image work and dream work (D'Antonio 1984). In this way they can remain in control, and choose to reveal as much or as little as they can cope with (Bach 1990). Children often express themselves more naturally and spontaneously through art than through words. Even when the child draws a picture which symbolically represents thoughts and feelings that might be too painful to express verbally, he is still able to maintain his ego strength; his art work, therefore, may be used as an indication of his thoughts and emotions.

They may just need us to give them the time and the space. The painting by an 8-year-old sibling (Figure 9.1) depicts the death of a brother from a brain tumour. The brother of the dying child was asked to paint a picture of his 'perfect world'. He was asked this before his brother had died and when his brother was very much taking all the attention in the family home. In the picture you cannot see his dying brother, only his younger sister and baby brother. He is standing right in the middle of the picture, which in reality is the centre of the family. His mother and father are holding hands and smiling for the first time in a long time. The sun is shining and the world looks calm, something home never was for him. The only way to get an attention was to shout, something the baby learnt very quickly.

So where is his dying brother in all of this? If we look closer at the picture we can see that his dying brother is in the picture, but has been painted as a ghostlike figure and put behind the tree; take a look at the trunk and how the brush strokes have been applied (Figure 9.2).

The case studies and qualitative research reviewed and presented by Ribbens-McCarthy and Jessop (2005) highlight how significant bereavement is in young people's lives and how it can affect them well into the future. Social relationships, including increasing risk and vulnerability caused by the death of a sibling and social isolation, coupled with lack of opportunity to talk are major themes from

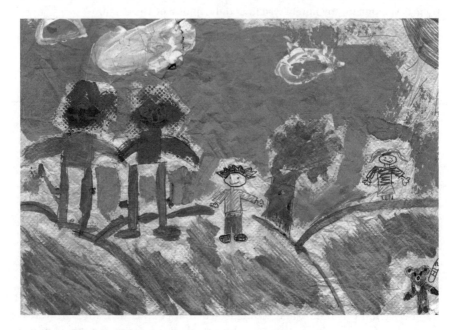

Figure 9.1 My Perfect World or Death and the Child.

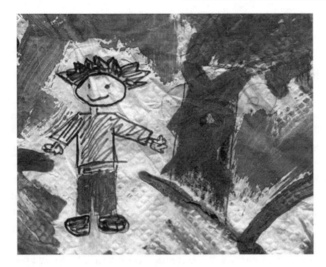

Figure 9.2 Detail from *My Perfect World or Death and the Child.*

the voices of young people. Black (1998) clearly indicates that bereaved children benefit from involvement and discussion and not exclusion and denial. These themes are echoed in the available research where there is evidence of short- and long-term consequences, particularly when personal, social and material resources are low and other stressors are high. Approximately 17 per cent of bereaved children will show significant behavioural problems beyond about 4 months after the death (Silverman and Worden 1992).

Family relationships

The roles and dynamics within the family will change following the death of a child (McCown and Davies 1995). A few years ago I was working with a family of four: mum, dad and two children. After the death of one of the children, the family dynamic changed with the parents supporting each other and having more time for their own relationship, which had been 'put on hold' in some way during the years their child had been ill. The remaining child could see that mum and dad needed time, but she felt lost. It was like a double bereavement for her: she had lost her brother and now it looked as if she was losing her parents. She had also played a key part in the care of her sibling and now she was alone. However, in this situation, with the work that had gone on before the child had died, the parents could see this happening and we were all able to discuss what was going on and put in place space for the sibling.

We need to say a word here about grandparents and their experience of loss at this time. Reed (2000) talks about the 'double pain of bereaved grandparents', by which they suffer the loss of their grandchild and also the pain of their own child's loss. Rothman (1999) illustrates the role of the grandchild for the grandparent, which is around ensuring eternity in some way for the grandparent. The implication for practice has to be around making sure the feelings of grandparents are raised, acknowledged and addressed.

Approaches to care

In the light of experience over many years and emerging evidence the Association of Children's Palliative Care (ACT 2007) developed a care pathway for dying children. This pathway recognises that preparation and adaptation to bereavement for parents and others starts at diagnosis, which is when care and support also commence.

The ACT pathway is an example of a comprehensive care pathway for children with palliative care needs. It is designed to facilitate the individual needs of the child or young person and their family. It starts from diagnosis or recognition that this child will die, through to death and beyond. This approach enables families to make choices and plan for the care and death of their child in the place of their choice. Choice is a big theme in this work. Helping and supporting parents and children make choices at this time may well help them in years to come.

ACT is the only organisation working nationally to achieve the best quality of life and standard of care for all children and young people with life-threatening or life-limiting conditions and their families.

ACT's mission is to influence and promote excellence and equity in the provision of care and support for children and young people with life-threatening or life-limiting conditions and their families by:

* campaigning for improved provision of children's palliative care services;
* working with professionals to support the delivery of the best care possible;
* informing and empowering families to have a voice in the development of the services that affect them.

ACT has adopted a care pathway approach to care for dying children and young people including neonates. More importantly they have produced a family companion to go with the pathway. The significant aspects of the ACT pathway are those that start with the recognition by the family that the end of life is near. (The professionals may have known for some time that death will be the outcome, but it is more helpful to work at the pace of the child and family.) This of course may never be put into words and so picking up on body language and what is not being said is very important and a skill that we need to enhance or develop.

The aim of the last stage of the pathway is to make an assessment of the end of life needs and wishes of the child and family. From this assessment, an end of life care plan can be created with the family.

The pathway subdivides into three sections (Table 9.1) and highlights some of the issues that need to be considered and addressed in relation to for the family/ carer, the child/young person and the wider context of care, which has been described as the environment.

If professionals follow the key components in Table 9.1, family choice is given priority, thus improving the likelihood of the family being left with a 'good enough memory' of the death of their child. Using the table the family are able to grieve and regrets such as 'did we do all that we could have?' may still be present but are minimised.

The child's understanding of death

When working with children it can be helpful for practitioners to have a working knowledge of the child's understanding of illness and death. This is also useful when working with parents, to help them understand just what their child might be thinking and what information they may need at that time and how to impart that information (Kübler-Ross 1985). It can be easy for practitioners and parents to underestimate a child's understanding of loss, to the detriment of the child and their care.

Goldman and Christie (1993) found that only 19 per cent of families of children dying from malignant diseases mutually acknowledged what was going on, and 23 per cent of children felt they knew what was happening but chose not to discuss it. Staff in the study tended to overestimate how often discussions took place about the impending death of the child. However, Bluebond-Langner (1974) demonstrated that children very rarely talk openly about what is happening to them, because of taboos from parents or carers. If they did talk, it tended to be in highly symbolic ways. She states that the child:

> goes through what can often be a long and painful process to discover what it all means. In this process he assimilates, integrates, and synthesises a great deal of information from a variety of sources. With his arrival at each new stage comes a greater understanding of the disease and its prognosis. This leaves him with a great deal to cope with, and it is part of his anticipatory grief process.
>
> (pp. 171–181)

Table 9.1 End of life and bereavement planning (from ACT 2007 with permission)

Family/carers	Child/young person	Environment
Practical support	Pain/symptom control	Place of death
Sibling involvement	Quality of life	Ambience
Emotional support	Friends	Place after death
Spiritual issues	Emotional support	
Cultural/religious issues	Spiritual issues	
Funeral planning	Cultural/religious issues	
Organ donation	Funeral planning	
Grandparents	Organ donation	
	Resuscitation plan	
	Special wishes/visits	
	Memory box	

A child may go from knowing that they are unwell and will get better to knowing that they are very ill and will not get better. In my experience, this is regardless
of their age or stage of development, and children with chronic illness can sadly
deteriorate clinically at an accelerated pace (Bluebond-Langner 1978).

A young teenager girl dying from cancer wrote the following poem. She finds
herself unable to talk about either her disease or her dying to the person she loves
most, her mother, or to the people who care for her: her dad and the doctor. All
three of them had silenced her by their own fears and anxieties. The poem is a
very powerful expression of what I have come to understand as 'soul pain'. This is
a term I use to describe the undescribable; it is a type of deep/internal pain, with
components of spiritual pain and suffering, that children can experience. Soul
pain has very little to do with what you can see or measure happening in a child's
body; it is what is happening in their inner world. Being with a dying child, or a
parent whose child is going to die or has died, is often more important than any
other intervention you might undertake as a practitioner. This poem, along with
many more, was found after her death and they chart her journey from diagnosis
to near death.

Searching for Me

Disillusioned
Discouraged
Despair writ
On his face
The doctor
Holds my hand
Not my attention
He retreats
The moment
I catch his glance
He hurriedly
Looks away.
Neither he, nor my daddy
Can fool me, no way
It's poor Mom
Who is lost to the world
And relies heavily on God
Little does she realise
I don't even have
A lean chance.
I pity her
And sorry be
For none is there
To share
Her loneliness

Her pain, and
longing, for
only I know
how she cares.
She'll go about
her life, as any
normal human being
only it will be her form
her soul will be searching
for me.
    (Badruddin 1982)

Another child, in less poetic terms but with equal clarity, is reported as saying when asked, 'What would make your life easier?': 'If there was someone to look after my mum and dad and brothers and sisters when I die so that they aren't sad' (Department of Health 2008: 9).

Dying and bereavement in hospital

Children dying in hospital and their families can face real challenges when it comes to this part of their journey (Craft and Killen 2007; Department of Health 2008). Some children who die in hospital may well die a 'toxic death' (i.e. while receiving active treatment) while undergoing 'life-saving' treatments or when families and professionals are unable to say 'enough is enough'. Children who die a 'toxic death' will nearly always die in a paediatric intensive care unit (PICU) or high-dependency unit (HDU) setting. Cook and colleagues (2002) and Stack (2003) highlight that these deaths will be more distressing to deal with and may well leave staff and parents feeling vulnerable. Some children will die in A&E departments having been admitted following a trauma or acute illness. In such cases, the families have no time to prepare themselves or the child and siblings for this kind of death, which then leaves them in a strange place and maybe with some very mixed feelings, which may 'complicate' their grief for years to come (Nusbaumer and Russell 2003; Bucaro *et al.* 2005). Professionals in these areas may encounter similar feelings of lack of preparation and challenges in dealing with the bereaved.

Families need to know what their choices are and how they may plan for the death of their child. The quality of the time they have together is sometimes more important than the length of time; in hospital this can get lost. A parent made the comment: 'Sometimes, being the very best parent does not mean fighting to cure, but fighting to do the best you can for your child's quality of life' (Craft and Killen 2007: 10). Another parent pointed out that: 'The goal is to add life to the child's years, not simply years to the child's life' (Craft and Killen 2007: 14).

There is limited robust evidence related to care of children dying in hospital but this should not equate to no action. Some evidence is related to services offered after a child has died: the contentious issue of organ retention and the consequences for bereaved parents (Sque *et al.* 2004) or bereavement services in hospitals (Jennings 2002). Lipton and Coleman (2002) also suggest that providing staff with guidance on assessing the needs of families of critically ill children can be beneficial in the long term. However, Nusbaumer and Russell (2003) suggest that objective evidence of the benefits from this is poor. This again has implications for the kind of services offered or those that need to be developed. What appears clear is that there is a need to foster engagement of staff with the child and family that goes beyond the functional care often provided.

McCallum and colleagues (2000), in a retrospective study of terminal care provided to 236 dying infants and children, examined communication, decision making and symptom management. In the analysis they found that decision making regarding end of life issues in this population was deferred until very close to the time of death, and only after no remaining curative therapy was available. They also found that children are rarely told that they are dying. This leaves some unanswered questions: did the staff not tell the child because they already knew that they were dying? Or were staff unable to discuss this with children and their families directly because they felt they did not have the skills or the emotional space to do so?

An on-going theme here is therefore of choice and communication or lack of choice and poor communication when it comes to end of life care and bereavement. The indications from the evidence and clinical practice are that parents and children who have more say over how and where their child dies seem to manage their bereavement journey more naturally and so do better in the long term (Davies *et al.* 2006; Craft and Killen 2007).

Education and support for staff around these issues are also key factors in most of the literature (Costello and Trinder-Brook 2000), but sadly these aspects are not seen as a high priority and are often under-resourced. Many clinical staff are offered supervision as a matter of course and yet the way clinical staff behave around the death of a child will impact on the family in both the short and the long term (Meert *et al.* 2001). Particularly, children who die in acute settings and their families need to be cared for by staff who not only can provide appropriate technical care, but can also offer the principles of good palliative and bereavement care when required (Liben and Lissauer 2006).

Dying and bereavement at home: the role of ritual

The family home seems to be the preferred place of choice and care for parents and children, as it offers children more dignity around their death and after care (DoH 2008). However, it may not always be possible or appropriate to achieve this, particularly in acute situations. With some end of life care situations, if home is not an option then children's hospices may also offer a 'half-way' house and sometimes parents may want to go to a children's hospice, even if it is only for a few hours, as it can still offer some control and dignity after the child's death (Brook *et al.* 2006). In such situations, the family and the hospice can utilise appropriate rituals such as using candles, music, prayers and other artefacts that provide comfort.

Ritual plays an important role at the end of life, the purpose of which can be overlooked by our society. In some cases, people do not seem to fully understand the importance of ritual in taking people forward on their journey or through a painful life experience. It may be argued that a sense of ritual has vanished from our modern world following the reduction in institutionalised religion and the denial that goes on around death, and more so when that is the death of a child (Clark 1993).

Ritual plays a key psychological role in helping those who struggle with their life story and who suffer dislocation. Ritual can help them get in touch with that part of their inner world or even soul. What we call it seems unimportant; what is important that we acknowledge that we have an inner world which is an essential part of each of us, the world within the world we ignore at our peril (Fisher and Francis 1999).

In practice, when it became clear that Gabriel, a young boy, was going to die, I encouraged his parents to start to think about what they needed to happen when their son passed away. At this stage I also made the point that it was very important to involve his sister and use some of the language and imagery she was used to or may have heard at school, as this would speak to her.

He died in the early hours of the morning with his parents at home and in the morning they called to inform me (their community nurse). They said they had lots to do during the day and asked me to come back at the end of the day and do a blessing with them. I went back at the end of the day; both sets of grandparents had arrived and we had a quiet informal service in his bed room. I think someone said at the time it was just like 'putting him to bed'.

His sister lit a candle in his room, which stayed alight until the day of his funeral. It felt like a sacred time, but also a time set aside for mourning and making the inner journey and a letting go. All sorts of things were going on at different levels for different members of the family – the point is there was the space to do this work.

Five years later the family and close friends returned to his graveside and remembered 'the boy', and his sister, now 12 years old, wrote and read the following poem, which she dedicated to her brother Gabriel:

A Memoir

In memory of Gabriel (28 October 1998 to 18 December 2004)
Auburn hair still shining,
Even from the life that was once lost,
There are memories.
Brown eyes bright and alert,
So deep you could get lost in them,
A vivid replica of dad's.
His face still looking up at me,
Imprinted in my memory,
As strong as the day he died.
Still five to me,

From the journey that has not been forgotten,
His life,
All I remember is everything,
that is remembered,
that will be forever,
remembered in his name.
He was . . .
as innocent as a child should be
as playful as he could be
as naïve as a child always is
He was . . .
as strong as our hopes
as loving as everything
as giving as time
He was . . .
all he should have been, nothing more, nothing less
He was . . .
all he will be in our thoughts
He is . . .
all he was and will be, forever in our hearts.
Love Maya x

(Maya Knox MaCaulay 2007)

This, I believe, is a good example of the value of rituals for the bereaved and how they can become significant moments that allow us to 'move on' but not forget. Follow up of the bereaved can also assist in providing opportunity for rituals, such as memorial services which may be held on a regular basis. Parents value such services as opportunity for some 'closure', and in addition they appreciate the efforts of staff who attend the funeral and who telephone or visit after the death (Macdonald *et al.* 2005).

Follow up can also be helpful to the bereaved as it allows them to ask questions about the death of the child and also to feed back on the performance of staff, which may assist in improving bereavement care provision.

Helpful interventions

Dame Cicely Saunders once suggested that those of us who have spent time in the company of someone with a terminal illness will have learned from this that we are always challenged to know more and to help more effectively, but, above all, to listen. Sometimes there will be no answers to give to those in apparently desperate situations and we find ourselves with nothing to offer but silent attention.

Currier and colleagues (2007), in a review of bereavement interventions with children, pointed out that there is limited support for the effectiveness of interventions in respect of adjustment to loss. Knowing what we mean by 'helpful interventions' at these times is the key for clinical work. What may seem like a helpful intervention such as the presence of a chaplain may have little meaning for the family. Such an intervention can be very helpful, but has little meaning to a family who are atheists. What can we do as health and social care professionals? The answer is, paradoxically, both clear and complicated. In reality there is very little we can do that will make this situation 'better' or go away. However, I think there is a great deal we can do to help children and parents during this time; by the way we are with them and who we are for them during this stage of their painful journey.

I have come to see over the years that suffering or what may well be called 'soul pain' is not a question that demands an answer; it is not a problem that demands a solution; it is a mystery that demands a presence. Being present is an active and demanding way of being with our client group. We can find this hard as we are trained to make things better and always have to be doing something. Attending the child, as well as watching and waiting with a family – sometimes referred to as 'being there' – is far more important than, for example, doing something or bringing presents.

An attending practitioner is someone who is present to the moment, believing that this moment is the moment. To wait with openness and trust is an enormously radical attitude towards life and our work, and more so in these times of great stress on resources and staff. It beckons us to become good listeners and not necessarily doers. Listening is about:

- Focusing on the whole patient. Hearing is not listening. *Hearing* refers to the sounds that you hear.
- Paying attention not only to the story, but to *how it is told*, the use of language, voice and body language.
- For me, more about listening for what is *not being said* or what I call the 'gaps in the story'.

This again is about being present to the child and parents. However, what they need most of all is for us to be present to them and to give them our full attention so they can do the work they need to do before they move on to the next stage of their journey.

Over 10 years ago Michael Kearney defined soul pain for us in his powerful book *Mortally Wounded*. He said: 'Soul pain is the experience of an individual who has become disconnected and alienated from the deepest and most fundamental aspects of him or herself' (Kearney 1996: 60).

Soul pain is a pain no health or social care professional can treat or cure with medication.

How can I evidence this statement? You may well ask. Well, I can't. Evidence is hard to come by in this area, but we do have clinical experience from which we can draw some conclusions and some guidance on how to work with parents and children who are grieving.

We have to create a safe and secure place or what I would call a 'sacred space', where the child or family can express their inner suffering and know that it is all right to do so, that they will be heard and taken seriously.

Sacred space is unique and will mean different things to different people. The uniqueness comes from the meaning and the value that the individual allots to that sacred space. It is a place of safety – emotional and physical. In the context of this chapter it refers to a place a child can go emotionally or physically to get some 'dedicated' or 'devoted' time exclusively for them; a space away from all the 'trauma' that may be going on in their world. It is a space between worlds (inner and outer worlds) where a sense of self can be restored, where an individual can make sense of new experiences and can refresh their energy.

When life feels blurred or confused we need this sacred space to focus on ourselves and restore perspective. If children are supported to spend time in their sacred space, it makes them more available for what may be happening at home or in hospital.

Preparing and holding the space is what we do when I offer 'expert' and effective care and symptom management, or when we create a warm and friendly environment for the families we work with, where we can help open up blocked channels of communication, and as we work with distressed families, who can find no meaning in their child's illness, suffering or death and cannot make sense of the puzzle of life. (A child in physical pain will not be able to undertake this work.)

If we can find a creative way of responding to the challenge of grief, it may open up a path to the very heart of living, even in the shadow of death.

Conclusion

In conclusion, I have no doubt that parents maintain a bond with their dead children. As one mum put it on the eighth anniversary of the death of her son:

> I'm fine thanks, going home again this weekend as Patrick would have been 13 on Monday 16th. I am having a tree planted at the cemetery for him, still cannot believe that it is almost 8 years since he died. I am sure you hear this a lot from other people but the pain and the loss never goes away, you just learn to live with it. Everything is a constant reminder, his cousins growing up, a song, a book . . . I feel that he is just beside me all the time.

The emotional bond is influenced by how we deal with parents, children and others before, at the time of and after the death. The key aim of this chapter has been to highlight a range of written evidence but also to combine this with less tangible evidence from experience in practice. Both should improve the quality of the outcomes and experiences for children, young people and their families and in so doing leave them with what can only be described as a 'good enough memory'.

Grief and bereavement are natural processes and most people will find their way through the maze, but others will need help and support and may even need professional help. They may need a 'menu' of services to be offered at different times. This needs to be built into care strategies. The evidence suggests there needs to be universal provision of bereavement support for the whole family and the wider community. In the case of siblings, they may need support at different key stages.

This chapter has acknowledged that all children grieve, although this may be in a different way from adults and may not always be fully understood. Those working with grieving children and bereaved families need to be trained and supported if we are to accompany children and families on this journey: a journey they had very little choice about taking and from which they would have stayed at home if they could.

References

ACT (Association of Children's Palliative Care) (2003a) *A guide to the development of children's palliative care services*, 2nd edn. Bristol: ACT.

ACT (2003b) *Voices for change: current perception of services for children with palliative care needs and their families*. Bristol: ACT.

ACT (2007) *Integrated multi-agency care pathways for children with life-threatening and life-limiting conditions*, 2nd edn. Bristol: ACT.

Bach S (1990) *Life paints its own span: on the significance of spontaneous pictures by severely ill children.* Einsiedeln, Switzerland: Daimon Verlag.

Badruddin K (1982) *Poems of Gitanjali*. London: Oriel Press.

Birenbaum LK (2000) Assessing children's and teenagers' bereavement when a sibling dies from cancer: a secondary analysis. *Child Care Health and Development* 26(5): 381–400.

Black D (1998) The dying child. *British Medical Journal* 316(7141): 1376–1378.

Bluebond-Langner M (1974) I know, do you? In: Schoenberg B. (ed.) *Anticipatory grief.* New York: Columbia University Press.

Bluebond-Langner M (1978) *The private worlds of dying children.* Princeton, NJ: Princeton University Press.

Brook L, Vickers J, and Barber M (2006) Place of care. In: Goldman, A. Hain R and Liben S (eds) *Oxford textbook of palliative care for children*. Oxford: Oxford University Press.

Bucaro P, Asher L and Curry D (2005) One children's hospital's compassionate plan for parents & families. *Journal of Emergency Nursing* 31(3): 305–308.

Casey A (1988) A partnership with child and family. *Senior Nurse* 8(4): 8–9.

Clark D (1993) *The sociology of death*. London: Blackwell.

CLIC Sargent (2009) More than my illness: delivering quality care for children with cancer. Available at: www.clicsargent.org.uk (accessed 16 June 2011).

Cook P, White DK and Ross-Russell RI (2002) Bereavement support following sudden and unexpected death: guidelines for care. *Archives of Disease in Childhood* 87(1): 36–38.

Corr CA (corresponding author) (1999) Children, adolescents, and death: myths, realities, and challenges. A statement from the Work Group on Palliative Care for Children of the International Work Group on Death, Dying, and Bereavement. *Death Studies* 23(5): 443–463.

Costello J and Trinder-Brook A (2000) Children's nurses' experiences of caring for dying children in hospital. *Paediatric Nursing* 12(6): 28–31.

Craft A and Killen S (2007) *Palliative care services for children and young people in England: an independent review for the Secretary of State for Health*. London: Department of Health.

Currier JM, Holland J and Neiymeyer R (2007) The effectiveness of bereavement interventions with children: a meta-analytic review of controlled outcome research. *Journal of Clinical Child and Adolescent Psychology* 36(2): 253–259.

D'Antonio IJ (1984) Therapeutic use of play in hospitals. *Nursing Clinics of North America* 19(2): 351–359.

Darbyshire P (1994) *Living with a sick child in hospital*. London: Chapman & Hall.

Darnill S and Gamage B (2006) The patient's journey: palliative care – a parent's view. *British Medical Journal* 332(7556): 1494–1495.

Davies B (1999) *Shadows in the sun: the experience of sibling bereavement in childhood*. Philadelphia: Brunner Mazel.

Davies B, Attig T and Towne M (2006) Bereavement. In: Goldman A, Hain R and Liben S (eds) *Oxford textbook of palliative care for children*. Oxford: Oxford University Press.

Davies R (2004) New understandings of parental grief: literature review. *Journal of Advanced Nursing* 46(5): 506–513.

Davies R (2005) Mothers' stories of loss: their need to be with their dying children and their child's body after death. *Journal of Child Health Care* 9(4): 288–300.

Department of Health (DOH) (2008) *Better care: better lives*. London: DoH.

Dyregrov A (1990) Parental reactions to the loss of an infant child: a review. *Scandinavian Journal of Psychology* 31(4): 266–280.

Fisher M and Francis B (1999) Soul pain and therapeutic use of ritual. *Psychodynamic Practice* 5(1): 53–72.

Goldman A and Christie D (1993) Children with cancer talk about their own death with their families. *Pediatric Hematology & Oncology* 10(3): 223–231.

Huntzinger NW (1995) A selective review and discussion of the literature on early sibling loss. *Depression and Stress* 1: 133–163.

Hynson J, Aroni R, Bauld C and Sawyer SM (2006) Research with bereaved parents: a question of how, not why. *Palliative Medicine* 20(8): 805–811.

Janzen L, Cadell S and Westhues A (2003–2004) From death notification through the funeral: bereaved parents' experiences and their advice to professionals. *Omega* 48(2): 149–164.

Jennings P (2002) Should paediatric units have bereavement support posts? *Archives of Disease in Childhood* 87(1): 40–42.

Kalter N, Lohnes KL, Chasin J, Cain AC, Dunning S and Rowan J (2003) The adjustment of parentally bereaved children. I: Factors associated with short-term adjustment. *Omega* 46(1): 15–34.

Kearney M (1996) *Mortally wounded: stories of soul pain, death and healing*. Dublin: Marino Books.

Klass D (1996) The deceased child in the psychic and social worlds of bereaved parents during the resolution of grief. In: Klass D, Silverman P and Nickman S (eds) *Continuing bonds: new understanding of grief*. Washington, DC: Taylor & Francis.

Kübler-Ross E (1985) *On children and death*. New York: Collier.

Liben S and Lissauer T (2006) Intensive care units. In: Goldman A, Hain R and Liben S (eds) *Oxford textbook of palliative care for children*. Oxford: Oxford University Press.

Macdonald ME, Liben S, Carnevale A, Rennick JE, Wolf SL, Meloche D and Cohen SR (2005) Parental perspectives on hospital staff members' acts of kindness and commemoration after a child's death. *Pediatrics* 116(4): 884–890.

McCallum DE, Byrne P and Bruera E (2000) How children die in hospital. *Journal of Pain and Symptom Management* 20(6): 417–423.

McCown DE and Davies B (1995) Patterns of grief in young children following the death of a sibling. *Death Studies* 19(1): 41–53.

Mearns J (2000) The impact of loss on adolescents: developing appropriate support. *International Journal of Palliative Medicine* 6(1): 12–17.

Meert KL, Thurston CS and Thomas R (2001) Parental coping and bereavement outcome after the death of a child in the pediatric intensive care unit. *Pediatric Critical Care Medicine* 2(4): 324–328.

Moulton M (1997) Maternal responses to the life and death of a child with a developmental disability: a story of hope. *Death Studies* 21(5): 443–476.

Nusbaumer A and Russell R (2003) Bereavement support following sudden and unexpected death in children. *Current Paediatrics* 13(7): 555–559.

Palmer SJ (1993) Care of the sick child by parents: a meaningful role. *Journal of Advanced Nursing* 18(2): 185–191.

Potts S, Farrell M and O'Toole J (1999) Treasure weekend: supporting bereaved siblings. *Palliative Medicine* 13(1): 51–56.

Rando TA (1986) Parental bereavement: an exception to the general conceptualisations of mourning. In: Rando TA (ed.) *Parental loss of a child.* Champaign, IL: Research Press.

Reed ML (2000) *Grandparents cry twice.* Amityville, NY: Baywood.

Ribbens-McCarthy J and Jessop J (2005) *Young people, bereavement and loss.* London: National Children's Bureau.

Robinson L and Mahon MM (1997) Sibling bereavement: a concept analysis. *Death Studies* 21(5): 477–499.

Rolls L and Payne S (2007) Children and young people's experience of UK childhood bereavement services. *Mortality* 12(3): 281–303.

Rothman JC (1999) *The bereaved parent's survival guide.* New York: Continuum.

Sandler IN, Ayers TS, Wolchik SA, Tein JY, Kwok OM, Haine RA, Twoheyjacobs J, Suter J, Lin K, Padgettjones S, Weyer JL, Cole E and Kriege G (2003) The family bereavement program: efficacy evaluation of a theory-based prevention program for parentally bereaved children and adolescents. *Journal of Consulting and Clinical Psychology* 71(3): 587–600.

Silverman P and Worden J (1992) Children's reactions in the early months after the death of a parent. *American Journal of Orthopsychiatry* 62(1): 93–104.

Spinetta JJ (1974) The dying child's awareness of death: a review. *Psychological Bulletin* 81: 841–845.

Sque M, Long T and Payne S (2004) *From understanding to implementation: meeting the needs of families and individuals affected by post mortem organ retention.* Executive summary of the Final Report for the Department of Health and the Retained Organs Commission. Available at: http://eprints.soton.ac.uk/9781/1/finalexectutivesummary.pdf (accessed 16 June 2011).

Stack CG (2003) Bereavement in paediatric intensive care. *Pediatric Anesthesia* 13(8): 651–654.

Steele R, Bosma H, Johnston MF, Cadell S, Davies B, Siden H and Straatman L (2008) Research priorities in pediatric palliative care: a Delphi study. *Journal of Palliative Care* 24(4): 229–239.

Stroebe M and Schut H (1999) The dual process model of coping with bereavement: rationale and description. *Death Studies* 23(3): 197–224.

Surkan P, Kreicbergs U, Valdimarsdottir U, Nyberg U, Onelov E and Dickman P (2006) Perceptions of inadequate health care and feelings of guilt in parents after the death of a child to a malignancy: a population-based long-term follow-up. *Journal of Palliative Medicine* 9(2): 317–331.

Thompson J (1985) Family centred care. *Nursing Mirror* 160: 25–28.

Tonkin L (2008) *Coping with the impossible in our own words.* Bristol: CLIC Sargent.

Waechter EH (1971) Children's awareness of fatal illness. *American Journal Nursing* 71(6): 1168–1172.

Winkelstein ML (1989) Spirituality and death of the child. In: Carson VB (ed.) *Spiritual dimensions of nursing practice.* St Louis: WB Saunders.

10 Perinatal bereavement

Elaine Dick and Peter Wimpenny

Key messages

- There are psychological effects of miscarriage and other perinatal death that suggest follow-up care should be available and offered to all women, partners and families. It should contain both informational and emotional support.
- Assessment is helpful to identify those at known greater risk of developing depression, anxiety and complicated grief.
- The approach to dealing with mothers, parents and families at the time of death is challenging and should be based on individual needs (involving cultural and spiritual dimensions) with validation/memory-based interventions available. It should also take place, wherever possible, in a specialist early pregnancy assessment or pregnancy loss unit.
- Multiprofessional education programmes (for all members of the team including pathologists, radiographers, nurses, all levels of medical doctors, psychologists, midwives, health visitors and funeral directors) that are evidence informed may be useful in developing greater understanding about dealing with perinatal death in primary and secondary care.
- Services for perinatal loss should utilise available guidance for dealing with perinatal death at all stages and take account of cultural, generational and sex-based differences for care.

Introduction

The purpose of this chapter is to highlight issues arising from the review of evidence relating to perinatal death in a range of contexts; however, the chapter also takes a pragmatic, practitioner-based focus on a range of issues including the psychological effects of miscarriage and the need for bereavement follow-up care so that women, partners and families can receive informational and emotional support. Moreover, as in other chapters in this book, we take the view that assessment of the impact of the death of a baby may be helpful to identify those at known greater risk of developing depression, anxiety and complicated grief. We also consider it important to consider the context in which bereavement support may be given and to utilise a range of resources including multiprofessional education programmes.

Thankfully, for the majority of people in the UK the death of a baby is a rare event. This is largely as a result of advances in medical science, including attendance at antenatal clinics, and improved standards of living, together with progress in health care generally. In comparison with other areas of bereavement care there is a fair body of evidence exploring, describing and researching perinatal loss. Reasons for this may mirror those relating to the significance of children's deaths: interest in these subject increases as family size diminishes and the loss of a baby becomes increasingly significant. In addition, from the moment of confirmation parents are now led to expect a safe outcome to pregnancy. Perinatal bereavement includes not only the loss of the baby but parents' perceptions of that child and their expectations of their future as a family. We may also question if the level of grief felt by families is greater now because preparation for the child occurs so much earlier than in previous generations. The taboo against having anything prepared until the child is safely born now seems to have gone. Some families have been encountered where the nursery was fully stocked as early as the twentieth week of gestation. There has also been an increase in early-pregnancy ultrasound scans, which might suggest that parents will bond and show attachment at earlier stages of the pregnancy. In addition, the more widespread use of enhanced three- and four-dimensional scans may bring earlier identification with the unborn baby and may influence the bereavement journey.

Historical and contemporary background

The work of Kennell and colleagues (1970) provides a historical marker for much of the evidence that populates the area of writing and research into perinatal bereavement. It may be the case that until this time, loss through miscarriage, perinatal or neonatal death was not recognised as important. Mothers may have been assumed to begin to love and bond with their babies after they had been born and were able to respond to this love. Kennell and colleagues (1970) identified that this process occurred before birth and attachment was not based solely on, for example, seeing and holding the baby. Attachment and loss (Bowlby 1969; Parkes *et al.* 1991) seem to have greater poignancy in perinatal settings as there are a variety of losses that are unique (Mander 2006) and which require understanding if care is to be enhanced.

The types of deaths discussed in this chapter range from conception to the first month after birth (Rybarik 2000) and include early pregnancy loss (miscarriage) and late pregnancy loss (perinatal loss and neonatal death) (Janssen *et al.* 1996). However, not all are legally required to be recorded (Lovell 2001) and as McCreight (2004) and Lovell (2001) note there may still be hospital-based, and within-hospital, differences related to dealing with the outcomes from early loss. We are aware that throughout Scotland there is a move for pregnancy loss to be dealt with in a specialised unit (RCOG 2006), although this may not occur elsewhere. However, many health services will have different admission criteria to specialised units; for example, ectopic pregnancies may be dealt with in the gynaecology ward when in fact this is still a pregnancy loss. You may be aware of differences in your own area and question why this is so.

It has been reported that between 15 and 25 per cent of clinically confirmed pregnancies will end in miscarriage, although other infant deaths will be fewer in number. Thus, issues related to bereavement in miscarriage will be particularly significant as a high number of women, their partners and families will be affected. Within the earlier perinatal period, Cameron and colleagues (2008a) identify that, for those born before 24 weeks (the present UK legal age of viability) approximately 60 per cent will die in the delivery room and a further 30 per cent will die soon after in neonatal intensive care units (NICUs). The level of viability of these extreme preterm infants in NICU terms is always going to be questionable.

In relation to stillbirths (after 24 weeks), Sands (the stillbirth and neonatal deaths charity) indicates that:

- Every day in the UK 17 babies are stillborn or die within their first month of life, almost 6,500 babies dying every year.
- One in every 200 babies born in the UK is stillborn.
- One in every 300 babies born in the UK dies in the first 4 weeks of life.
- In 2006, 10 babies were stillborn every day on average.
- In 2006, on average every day 7 babies died who were aged less than 28 days.
- Stillbirth rates in the UK have remained unchanged for 10 years. The stillbirth rate in 2006 was 5.3 per 1000 live births, the same rate as in 1997. (There was a temporary increase in the stillbirth rate in 2002/3. No clear cause has been identified for this rise.)
- Stillbirths are 10 times more common than cot deaths in the UK.

(Sands website: www.uk-sands.org/information/definitions.html)

Bereavement and perinatal death

A small number of reviews of evidence have been undertaken related to bereavement interventions. This is the only field of bereavement care where Cochrane reviews appear to exist (Chambers and Chan 2005), which in itself highlights the extent to which perinatal death is a distinct area of concern. Unfortunately, the review by Chambers and Chan (2005) highlights the 'difficulty and inadequacy of research in the area of grief support surrounding perinatal death' (p. 3). Although they indicate that no evidence exists to support the effectiveness of interventions in this bereaved group, it is contended that there is a broader range of evidence which can contribute to practice. In a recent review of effectiveness of bereavement interventions in neonatal intensive care, Harvey and colleagues (2008) report a similar lack of rigorous evaluations. It is, however, disconcerting for this deficit to be stated as relating only to evidence-based medicine when the involvement of, for example, midwives, chaplains and neonatal nurses is significant in perinatal bereavement care.

There is a clear indication in reviews and other evidence that a significant percentage of women who experience perinatal bereavement may be at greater risk of developing depression, anxiety and complicated grief (Janssen *et al.* 1996; Janssen 1997; Lasker and Toedter 2000; Toedter *et al.* 2001; Bartellas and Van Aerde 2003; Chambers and Chan 2005). Therefore it appears important to provide some form of assessment and follow up that may assist in identifying and supporting those at risk. As with other areas of bereavement, not everybody needs 'counselling'. Those who will benefit most are those who are at greatest risk (Murray *et al.* 2000).

Frost and Condon (1996) highlight the psychological sequelae of miscarriage and suggest that, from their extensive critical review of a significant number of papers, they are often not recognised by health professionals and may contribute to subsequent depression, anxiety and post-traumatic stress disorder. Despite this, Nikčević (2003) reports that there is no routine follow-up care for women after miscarriage in the UK despite depression rates in the first 6 weeks reported to be between 8 and 48 per cent and anxiety levels of 22–45 per cent up to 6 months. An earlier review, in the USA, by Athey and Spielvogel (2000), reported similar levels of psychiatric morbidity up to 51 per cent and clinically significant levels of depression and anxiety between 22 and 44 per cent. Miscarriage in particular has tended to lack the recognition as a bereavement that other deaths command, and so any accompanying emotional and social support may be absent or diminished (Simmons *et al.* 2006). It still appears to be a 'hidden' subject which may occur before parents have informed anyone and so often they have to face the loss alone. However, there are a number of support groups available for early pregnancy loss, for example the Miscarriage Association and Ectopic Pregnancy Trust.

Prevention of negative psychological impact

There is often no routine follow-up care for women after miscarriage, although recent guidelines from the Royal College of Obstetricians and Gynaecologists (RCOG 2006) suggest that all women should be offered follow up to prevent negative psychological impact. However, an audit of the management of early pregnancy loss (SPCERH 2003) found that 38 per cent of women had not been offered follow-up. Although there is the positive aspect that 62 per cent of women were offered follow up, it is difficult to ascertain how many of the 38 per cent may have subsequently developed depression or complicated grief.

Follow up can cover a range of practices by notifying all relevant health care professionals of perinatal/neonatal loss to help prevent inadvertently adding to parents' distress by cancelling appointments for sessions such as parentcraft, ultrasound, antenatal clinic and records departments. Grieving parents could also be assisted by offering them the opportunity to meet up and discuss the loss with, for example, the community midwife, health visitor or general practitioner (GP).

Descriptive studies identify considerable appreciation and perceived benefit from offering follow up (Turner *et al.* 1991) and additionally attendance is often high (Athey and Spielvogel 2000). However, although there is no evidence of effectiveness of psychological/counselling interventions alone, Nikčević (2003), drawing on other research work, shows that a combination of medical and psychological support can be beneficial. It is interesting to note that one of the randomised controlled trials assessed by Chambers and Chan (2005) (Lilford *et al.* 1994) reports on the beneficial effects of the obstetrician having feedback on performance from a psychoanalytical psychotherapist after joint consultation sessions and the value of a clinical focus as opposed to dedicated psychotherapy. What might this highlight about follow up? Rather than seeking emotional support, parents are perhaps seeking answers to factual questions: Why did it happen? Will it happen again? What can we do to prevent it? Perhaps providing answers to these may help prevent the on-going rumination that may result in increased levels of anxiety and depression.

The following could be considered points for good practice in follow-up:

- Meet with the consultant and the lead midwife who provided care during the pregnancy loss.
- Feed back from all investigations and post-mortem if performed.
- Discuss the couple's physical and emotional well-being.
- Review the care they received in hospital and its 'time lines'. During periods of high emotion with high levels of pain relief, women can find recollection hazy and it is important to give women the opportunity to discuss their care.
- Discuss the implications for future pregnancies and their management.
- Help couples access support groups.

Where follow up should take place should be carefully considered. Some women and their partners may find it difficult to return to the place where the loss occurred. If only ward- or hospital-based follow up is available this may have an impact on take-up.

Furthermore, Lasker and Toedter (2000) comment that outcomes in respect of grieving for parents may be related more to overall satisfaction with the attention given than to specific interventions. Such an intervention, that is 'attention', seems highly achievable and also, as noted by Chambers and Chan (2005), potentially more cost-effective than provision of specialist services. Again we see that what might assist the bereaved is not provision of highly qualified counsellors (although for a minority of cases these are essential) but a more generic need to pay 'attention' to the bereaved. It may also be helpful to consider risk factors, particularly for women; the use of a general health questionnaire may be appropriate to do this (Athey and Spielvogel 2000) or specific indicators of risk, namely (Murray *et al.* 2000):

- lack of perceived social support;
- ambivalent relationship with the baby;
- particular traumatic circumstances surrounding the death;
- other difficult life circumstances;
- difficulty with coping in the past;
- problematic individual characteristics;
- unsatisfactory relationships within the nuclear family.

Ensuring that support is continued beyond the hospital walls is often challenging. Wong (2003) in a well-designed and -reported qualitative study demonstrates clearly the perceived discrepancy between parents' needs and service provision in the community. The health visitor is often identified as the professional in the community who should be key/lead carer, and a formal process for notification should occur, although the extent of linkage between maternity and health visiting services may be geared more towards dealing with live births. Thus, the scope and type of follow up may vary (Friedrichs *et al.* 2000), although this could be through telephone contact, which may quickly identify those at most risk, so that appropriate referrals can be made. Within the locality in which the first author works it is normally the midwife or GP who is the lead professional. Notification of miscarriage or perinatal loss is made to both of these. In the case of pregnancy loss at a gestational age greater than 24 weeks, midwives are still legally required to visit for up to 10 days postnatally.

Consent to post-mortem

As part of any perinatal death, parents are often asked to consent to a post-mortem to determine the nature of death. They are normally shocked, and sensitive handling of such an approach is essential. Parents may perceive the benefits of such an examination as assisting in improving understanding of the reason for the death (Rankin *et al.* 2002). Parents also request that medical terminology and concepts should be fully explained and an opportunity to ask questions at a later date should be built in (Rankin *et al.* 2002). This may form part of the medical support identified by Nikčević (2003). Considering who is best placed to provide information about the death and how this is communicated seems to be a central feature of concern and one which could readily be undertaken by local health services. Midwives may feel that it is outwith their remit, they may have had limited exposure and lack appropriate information (Cameron *et al.* 2008b), and yet they are well placed to support grieving parents (Mander 2006). Organising tutorials with pathologists or visits to the mortuary and observation of post-mortem may be helpful to increase their knowledge and confidence. In addition specialist midwives from early pregnancy assessment or pregnancy loss units may be able to offer support by visiting other clinical areas.

Bereavement support: practical answers

There is evidence of considerable variation in the way mothers grieve and search for meaning, which challenges any standardised approach, irrespective of practitioner (Genevro 2004). Validating and remembering the loss may assist in this process through photographs, foot and hand prints, locks of hair, shawls/receiving blankets and other mementos, and attending funerals and memorial services (Gensch and Midland 2000; Bartellas and Van Aerde 2003; Mander 2006).

Photographs can help to show the baby to others and do much to provide a personal identity – *it was real, not imagined* – and perhaps then allow greater empathy for the parents. Photography has become easier with the advent of digital photography, which allows instant review of pictures and the opportunity to record a large number prior to any printing. However, picture taking is not always straightforward; for example the baby often looks highly coloured so it is essential to avoid a white background, which would accentuate this. Using a coloured background and low-level flash can help to prevent the pictures looking too harsh. In addition, digital photography can allow changes after taking the picture; a medical illustrations department may be available to do this. Changing pictures from colour to black and white may also reduce the harshness and improve the use of the picture as a memento. It is important to ensure that the baby looks comfortable; the use of small hats and clothes to emphasise the baby's normal features, for example face and hands, and hide abnormalities such as bruising or skin tears, can be helpful. Storage of pictures is now much easier using digital technology and allows parents to access a copy if required, which may be years later.

Hand and footprints are also frequently offered to parents. The use of inkless wipes to obtain these makes the provision easy, clear and clean. Other options for hand and footprints using clay make it less easy to obtain a good print and this will also depend on the size and length of gestation of the baby. Locks of hair may also be taken; the nape of the neck is usually the best place to obtain these. However, care must be taken to ascertain any cultural or religious objections to this form of memento.

Acknowledging the loss

Memorial services can be private, often in the form of a funeral for those babies over approximately 16 weeks or a public memorial service for those under this. These are normally arranged by the health service. Our experience is of offering these services four times a year. Attendance at such events is high and staff also attend. It is valuable that staff attend such services to show concern, acknowledgement and engagement they have with the parents and with the loss of their babies (Macdonald *et al.* 2005). Staff may also find that it can help their own grief process, as often this can be 'disenfranchised' and have no other outlet within the health care organisation.

Gensch and Midland (2000), amongst others, are emphatic in promoting the option to see and hold the dead baby; however, research by Hughes and colleagues (2002) highlights the potential negative outcomes that such a 'forced' choice can have on women in the future, albeit there are questions raised about the research (Mander 2006). As Reynolds (2003) states, blind adherence to the practice of 'mandatory' seeing and holding the dead baby, when it is not supported by research, may be detrimental to women and staff. Parents must be included in decision making and given the opportunity to consider all their options and also given time to make these important choices. Often this may not be feasible but where there is a delay between diagnosis of intrauterine death and delivery this may allow parents to discuss and make choices from the available options.

Experience of dealing with parents suggests that, although there are those who say no they do not want to hold or see the baby and do not want mementos, they often regret this decision and return later to ask if any are available.

Practitioner responses to perinatal death

How then should staff intervene in relation to seeing and holding the dead baby? Carrying out research into effectiveness of seeing and holding the dead baby is, as Harvey and colleagues (2008) point out, problematic as how could parents be randomly allocated to hold or not hold?

You may have your own experiences and thoughts about what is the best approach to holding – do you have any local policy or guidance? Schott and Henley (2008) identify and challenge the discrepancies in one national guideline's recommendations (NICE 2007), which appear to discourage practitioners from encouraging women to hold the dead baby as it is unhelpful. They draw on Sands recommendations (Schott *et al.* 2007) that 'parents should be sensitively offered information and choices and supported in making their own decisions'. How easy it is to make decisions at such a time is open to debate, and Rådestad and Christofferson (2008) are also critical of the Sands guidance, which they consider may prevent parents holding the baby whilst it is soft and warm because of delays in decision making. They also report on a Norwegian study in which, of 40 parents interviewed, 'almost everyone mentioned seeing and holding the baby immediately after delivery as one of the most important things to do' (p. 589). However, it is important to remember that health care is based around informed consent and practitioners cannot force this process even if it means some delay in decision making.

Saflund and colleagues (2004) find similar perspectives from parents in Sweden. Although no measurement of outcomes, such as depression, is undertaken, parents again report the value of holding and spending time with the dead baby. Although we might ask questions related to cultural differences between Scandinavian countries and others (Hebert 1998) there is still a judgement to be made by staff about the approach to take; however, this needs to be based on the individuals concerned rather than a 'one size fits all' approach. Additionally, there may be issues for the midwife or nurse who themselves are struggling with the situation and may be traumatised and need support (Wallbank and Robertson 2008). If you work in midwifery settings, do you have support and opportunity for debriefing sessions?

Culture and religion

Cultural and religious differences are particularly important in relation to perinatal deaths as different rituals and relationships exist. Lovell (2001) identifies that there can be a lack of religious engagement with stillbirth and miscarriage, which may result in parents gaining little spiritual support from this direction even if they themselves are 'religious'. Hsu and colleagues (2004), Chan and colleagues (2003) and Van and Meleis (2003) all provide examples of different cultural, religious and ethnic factors that impact on perinatal death. The extent of such differences is beyond the scope of this chapter but essential to any provision of service. For example, Chan and colleagues (2007) describe the difficulties for midwives in dealing with death and bereavement within a Chinese culture, as it is usually not openly acknowledged and discussed, which may result in emotional challenges for both parents and staff. Hebert (1998) well illustrates the challenges for staff when confronted with a different culture and religion. What she demonstrates is how staff could learn from such encounters; what is apparent is that they may fail to do so, as it can be seen as too different from 'normal' practice.

Recently, the first author cared for two Nigerian women who experienced perinatal loss. Why might this be significant? For some midwives this may be an everyday occurrence; however, many midwives will also work in areas where women from ethnic minority groups are met infrequently. Therefore, at first Elaine assumed that similar attitudes to seeing and holding their babies might be present. However, one mother had Christian faith and one Islamic faith. This resulted in the Christian mother wanting to see and hold the baby and gather mementos and the Islamic mother wanting very little but to ensure that the baby was buried as quickly as possible. These were perhaps clear examples of different cultural and religious issues. However, it is not always so straightforward, as Mander (2006) also points out. Even within these particular cultural and religious faiths there will also be significant variations and it is important not to assume but to seek guidance from the mother and partner. Even within indigenous populations, making assumptions in respect of cultural variation can be erroneous and in addition may miss some other important aspects such as issues of disadvantage or communication difficulties due to sensory impairment (Schott *et al.* 2007). Have you been confronted with different cultural, religious or challenges related to communication? Did you learn from these and did you pass on this experience to others?

Within the available literature there is also a distinctive component related to men. Although it is often considered that men have not been studied in this bereavement context there are a number of papers that explore their perspectives. Janssen and colleagues (1996) highlighted the potential for delayed grief in men and chronic grief because of lessened interventions at all points (Lasker and Toedter 1994). McCreight (2004) and Puddifoot and Johnson (1997) illuminate these through a qualitative study and consider that the present societal, health care organisations and voluntary group processes and procedures do not assist men to grieve and need to be addressed. Puddifoot and Johnson (1997) graphically illustrate the lack of engagement in the health care setting. Alderman and colleagues (1998) illustrate the different experience of grief in male partners and highlight the need for this to be considered more fully. Men often report having to 'stay strong', be stoical for their partners and not cry; this can often be misinterpreted as not grieving, when in fact men report strong feelings about the bereavement, which can persist (Murphy 1998; McCreight 2004). This should dispel the view that, as Athey and Spielvogel (2000) report, men grieve less intensely and for a briefer time. Owing to the stoical approach, men may be overlooked in emergency or clinical situations and sometimes may need time to talk to you away from their partners. It is also, as discussed earlier, valuable for men to accompany their partners to follow-up sessions.

Perinatal death: impact on the family

Irrespective of sex, experience of perinatal bereavement usually occurs within a family context, albeit the structure of the family has changed significantly. Whereas attention has been paid to mothers and some to fathers, less has been to siblings and grandparents who may be equally affected. It is worth remembering that between six and eight people will normally be affected by one death (Nucleus Group 2004) and this may represent the wider family circle. Open visiting may help to promote family support.

Grandparents may themselves have had a perinatal death and the manner in which this was handled would, we assume, have been less empathic than would be expected today. There have been several occasions we are aware of when grandparents, particularly grandmothers, have sought out the midwife to talk about their own losses, which can be heightened by their daughter's or son's loss. Parents may want to have grandparents present and to see and hold the baby but again this will be an individual choice. Additionally, the involvement of other children in the family will be important. Chapters 2 and 9 deal with bereavement in children and the same messages would apply equally to perinatal bereavement. Schott and colleagues (2007) highlight the availability of information from Antenatal Results and Choices (ARC), Miscarriage Association and Sands about talking to children about perinatal loss. They highlight work by Wilson (2001), who identified three aspects of dealing with perinatal loss with siblings/other children:

- recognise and acknowledge the child's grief;
- include the child in family rituals related to the dead baby;
- keeping the baby's memory alive in the family.

Oikonen and Brownlee (2002) reviewed such work and describe the potential benefits of family-based approaches to loss, as grieving usually goes on in some form of family unit and the different 'stories' of each family member can be helpful to share to develop understanding of each other's loss and subsequent support.

The final significant group to be considered in the selected literature is adolescents. Adolescence and bereavement is dealt with more fully in Chapter 2. There are significant factors which could identify this group as at particular risk. Perinatal loss is high in this age group. Welch and Bergen (2000) report that an estimated 15,788 infant deaths may have been to adolescent mothers in the USA in 1994 and that adolescent mothers experienced the second highest stillbirth rate. Adolescent mothers may experience significant levels of grief that may be disenfranchised (Doka 1999) as they are unable to openly express their grief. This may be compounded by feelings of guilt if they had at some stage considered terminating the pregnancy. There may actually be relief, rather than grief, expressed by parents of the adolescent as they cope with the stigma of pregnancy.

I wonder if midwives ever feel relief in these situations as well, that in some way the loss was considered a better outcome for a mother whom we may consider still to be a child herself. However, this may reduce levels of support and follow up for adolescent mothers. Welch and Bergen (2000) contend that on account of the emotional, physical and social changes occurring in adolescents they need specific age-appropriate support. Many services are geared up for adults, which may restrict information and education to assist younger individuals.

Future pregnancy

One of the features of perinatal loss, especially in women who have no children and still wish to begin a family, is the daunting prospect of a future pregnancy. Much of the difficulty around this situation is influenced by the circumstances of the loss, in particular the often poor advice or insensitive comments by others, which often appeal to women to ignore the loss or deny its consequences by minimising its impact – 'never mind try again'. Mander (2006) commences her chapter, 'Future Childbearing after Perinatal Loss', with the view that future pregnancy is a subject that often arises from health care providers. Mander highlights that in her research it was midwives who raised the topic and they were aware of how 'you can have another baby' trivialised the loss.

However, Kohner and Henley (2001) acknowledge that the subject of a future pregnancy is of high priority for many couples who have experienced some form of perinatal bereavement. Many couples, although understanding that a new baby will not lessen the grief they are feeling, feel an intense need for a living child. This may itself add to the emotional strain of a future pregnancy, as they feel guilty for wanting another child (Kohner and Henley 2001). Hughes and Riches (2003) state that complicated and prolonged grief is more commonly seen in the next pregnancy and likens it to a post-traumatic stress disorder. Although there is limited evidence to support this, it is important to consider the extent to which grief may impact on subsequent pregnancies and how support can be offered.

It is also important to remember that for a small number of couples there is no possibility of another pregnancy because of an underlying medical condition. It may also be the case that some couples cannot face the trauma of another possible loss. Many couples fear that the next pregnancy may follow the same path as the last and they may feel that their fears are not sufficiently well recognised by health professionals who focus on the new pregnancy and so offer little emotional support. It is useful to consider what care is provided for future pregnancies in your area and how we as health care providers help couples at this time.

NICE (2008), in its most recent antenatal care guidelines, identifies previous stillbirth or neonatal death as a reason for referral for additional consultant-led care. This gives the parents more opportunity to discuss any implications for the new pregnancy and to discuss future management, which may involve closer monitoring. The RCOG (2006) guidelines for early pregnancy loss recommend early ultrasound scans for women who have undergone recurrent miscarriage. However, there is no guidance on the amount and this may vary between maternity centres. In addition there is no evidence that early pregnancy ultrasounds will assist with existing grief. An ultrasound may, of course, reassure at the time it is performed but does not guarantee a successful outcome, although Chudleigh and Thilaganathan (2004) indicate that crown rump length of > 5 mm in an embryo is associated with lower risk of miscarriage (7 per cent). A further issue may be one of service provision for increased scanning, which may bring with it additional costs for an organisation.

If there is an identified genetic problem then couples may be referred to a genetic counsellor before embarking on another pregnancy. They may also be offered early diagnostic tests to determine the fetal karyotype in this pregnancy. However, it is important that couples are made aware of the risks of miscarriage associated with these tests.

The decision to embark on another pregnancy is a difficult choice for the majority of couples who have experienced pregnancy loss. Health care providers are in an ideal situation to provide support and advice. For some couples the continuing support of their community midwife may be all that is needed in conjunction with consultant-led care. However, for some women and their partners who experience grief that is overly lengthy or deep, the support of specialised perinatal mental health teams (CEMACH 2004) may be appropriate, if available.

Conclusion

The chapter has outlined some of the key issues relating to some of the difficulties surrounding perinatal death, in particular that associated with bereavement support and the form this could take in terms of practical strategies such as taking photographs and obtaining locks of hair for helping to establish the baby's identity. This approach has been shown to be successful in helping family members come to terms with the loss, based on clinical practice where parents do not make the request initially. In order for follow-up bereavement support to be helpful, practitioners should examine their own attitude as well as being aware of the ethical implications related to encouraging parents to see and hold the baby immediately after delivery. Although it is important, it is useful to remind ourselves that health care is based around informed consent and practitioners cannot force this issue. The evidence also encourages caution in relation to consideration of the variance in the way women from different cultures and religious backgrounds respond to the dead child.

Moreover, the chapter has highlighted how the death of a child has significant impact on not only the woman and her partner but also the wider family. The evidence, from a variety of sources, suggests that where parents feel supported and feel that their loss has been acknowledged and recorded their bereavement journey may be less traumatic and more 'natural'. Additionally, providing follow-up opportunites for couples can also assist them in the journey. Finally, although perinatal loss is never forgotten, the arrival of a healthy baby can help to move the couple out of the loss phase and more into the restorative phases associated with grief.

References

Alderman L, Chisholm J, Denmark F and Salbod S. (1998) Bereavement and stress of a miscarriage: as it affects the couple. *Omega: Journal of Death and Dying* 37(4): 317–327.

Athey J and Spielvogel AM (2000) Risk factors and interventions for psychological sequelae in women after miscarriage. *Primary Care Update Obstetrics/Gynaecology* 7(2): 64–69.

Bartellas E and Van Aerde J. (2003) Bereavement support for women and their families after stillbirth. *Journal of Obstetrics & Gynaecology Canada* 25(2): 131–138.

Bowlby J (1969) *Attachment and Loss: Vol. 1. Attachment.* London: Hogarth Press.

Cameron M and Penney G (2003) *Scottish audit of the management of early pregnancy loss.* Aberdeen: Scottish Programme for Clinical Effectiveness in Reproductive Health (SPERCH).

Cameron J, Taylor J and Greene A (2008a) Evaluating professional guidelines for the care of dying previable infants. *Evidence Based Midwifery* 6(4): 136–142.

Cameron J, Taylor J and Greene A (2008b) Representations of rituals and care in perinatal death in British midwifery textbooks 1937–2004. *Midwifery* 24(3): 335–343.

CEMACH (2004) *Why Mothers Die 2000–2002.* London: RCOG Press.

CEMACH (2007) Confidential Enquiry into Maternal and Child Health (CEMACH) Perinatal Mortality. United Kingdom. CEMACH, London,

Chambers HM and Chan FY (2005) Support for women/families after perinatal death. *Cochrane Library*, Issue 2.

Chan, MF, Chan SH and Day MC (2003) Nurses' attitudes towards perinatal bereavement support in Hong Kong: a pilot study. *Journal of Clinical Nursing* 12(4): 536–543.

Chan MF, Lou F-l, Zang Y-l, Chung YF, Wu LH, Cao F-L and Li P (2007) Attitudes of midwives towards perinatal bereavement in Hong Kong. *Midwifery* 23(3): 309–321

Chudleigh T and Thilaganathan B (2004) *Obstetric ultrasound: how, why & when?,* 3rd edn. Edinburgh: Elsevier.

Doka KJ (1999) Disenfranchised grief. *Bereavement Care* 18(3): 37–39.

Friedrichs J, Daly MI and Kavanaugh K (2000) Follow-up of parents who experience a perinatal loss: facilitating grief and assessing for grief complicated by depression. *Illness, Crisis & Loss* 8(3): 296–309.

Frost M and Condon JT (1996) The psychological sequelae of miscarriage: a critical review of the literature. *Australian and New Zealand Journal of Psychiatry* 30(1): 54–62.

Genevro JL (2004) Report on bereavement and grief research. *Death Studies* 28(6): 491–575.

Gensch BK and Midland D (2000) When a baby dies: a standard of care. *Illness, Crisis and Loss* 8(3): 286–295.

Harvey S, Snowden C and Elbourne D (2008) Effectiveness of bereavement interventions in neonatal intensive care: a review of the evidence. *Seminars in Fetal and Neonatal Medicine* 13(5): 341–56.

Hebert MP (1998) Perinatal bereavement in its cultural context. *Death Studies* 22(1): 61–78.

Hsu MT, Tseng YF, Banks JM and Kuo LL (2004) Interpretations of stillbirth. *Journal of Advanced Nursing* 47(4): 408–416.

Hughes P, Turton P, Hopper E and Evans CDH (2002) Assessment of guidelines for good practice in psychosocial care of mothers after stillbirth: a cohort study. *The Lancet* 360(9327): 114–118.

Hughes P and Riches S (2003) Psychological aspects of perinatal loss. *Current Opinion in Obstetrics and Gynaecology* 15(2): 107–111.

Janssen HJ (1997) Grief after pregnancy loss was predicted by length of pregnancy, neuroticism, psychiatric symptoms, and absence of other children. *Archives of General Psychiatry* 54: 56–61.

Janssen HJ, Cuisinier MCJ and Hoogduin KAL (1996) A critical review of pathological grief following pregnancy loss. *Omega: Journal of Death and Dying* 33: 21–42.

Kennell JH, Slyter H and Klaus MH (1970) The mourning response of parents to the death of a newborn infant. *New England Journal of Medicine* 283(7): 344–349.

Kohner N and Henley A (2001) *When a baby dies*. Routledge: Abingdon.

Lasker JN and Toedter LJ (2000) Predicting outcomes after pregnancy loss: results from studies using the Perinatal Grief Scale. *Illness, Crisis & Loss* 8(4): 350–372.

Lilford RJ, Stratton P, Godsil S and Prasad A (1994) A randomised trial of routine versus selective counselling in perinatal bereavement from congenital disease. *British Journal of Obstetrics & Gynaecology* 101(4): 291–296.

Lovell A (2001) The changing identities of miscarriage and stillbirth: influences on practice and ritual. *Bereavement Care* 20(3): 37–40.

McCreight BS (2004) A grief ignored: narratives of pregnancy loss from a male perspective. *Sociology of Health and Illness* 26(3): 326–350.

Macdonald ME, Liben S, Carnevale FA, Rennick JE, Wolf SL, Meloche D and Cohen SR (2005) Parental perspectives of hospital staff members' acts of kindness and commemoration after a child death. *Pediatrics* 116(4): 884–890.

Mander R (2006) *Loss and bereavement in childbearing*, 2nd edn. Abingdon: Routledge.

Murphy FA (1998) The experience of early miscarriage from a male perspective. *Journal of Clinical Nursing* 7(4): 325 –332.

Murray JA, Terry DJ, Vance JC, Battistutta D and Connolly Y (2000) Effects of a program of intervention on parental distress following infant death. *Death Studies* 24(4): 275–305.

NICE (2007) Clinical Guideline 45. *Antenatal and postnatal mental health*. London: NICE.

NICE (2008) Clinical Guideline 62. *Antenatal care: routine care for the healthy pregnant woman*. London: NICE.

Nikčević A (2003) Development and evaluation of a miscarriage follow up clinic. *Journal of Reproductive and Infant Psychology* 21(3): 207–213.

Nucleus Group (2004) Review of Specific Grief and Bereavement Services Department of Human Services Victoria, Melbourne, Australia. http://www.health.vic.gov.au/palliativecare/archive/finalrep_grief.pdf

Oikonen J and Brownlee K (2002) Family therapy following perinatal bereavement. *Family Therapy* 29(3):125–140.

Parkes CM, Stevenson-Hinde J and Marris P (1991) *Attachment across the life cycle*. Routledge: London.

Puddifoot JE and Johnson MP (1997) The legitimacy of grieving: the partner's experience at miscarriage. *Social Science and Medicine* 45(6): 837–845.

Rådestad I and Christoffersen L (2008) Helping a woman meet her stillborn baby while it is soft and warm. *British Journal of Midwifery* 16(9): 588–591.

Rankin J, Wright C and Lind T (2002) Cross sectional survey of parents' experience and views of the post-mortem examination. *BMJ* 324: 816–818.

RCOG (2006) *The Management of Early Pregnancy Loss*. RCOG Guideline No 25. Available at: http://www.rcog.org.uk/womens-health/clinical-guidance/management-early-pregnancy-loss-green-top-25

Reynolds JJ (2003) Stillbirth: to hold or not to hold. *Omega: Journal of Death and Dying* 48(1): 85–88.

Rybarik F (2000) Perinatal bereavement. *Illness, Crisis and Loss* 8(3): 221–226.

Saflund K, Sjogren B and Wredling R (2004) The role of caregivers after a stillbirth: views and experiences of parents. *Birth* 31(2): 132–137.

Schott J, Henly A and Kohner N (2007) *Pregnancy loss and the death of a baby: guidelines for professionals*, 3rd edn. London: Sands.

Schott J and Henley A (2008) Seeing and holding a stillborn baby. *British Journal of Midwifery* 16(9): 593.

Simmons RK Sing G, Maonochie N, Doyle P and Green J (2006) Experience of miscarriage in the UK: qualitative findings from the National Women's Health Study. *Social Science and Medicine* 63(7): 1934–1946.

SPCERH (2003) *Scottish audit of the management of early pregnancy loss*. Aberdeen: Scottish Programme for Clinical Effectiveness in Reproductive Health.

Toedter LJ Lasker JN and Janssen HJEM (2001) International comparison of studies using the Perinatal Grief Scale: a decade of research on pregnancy loss. *Death Studies* 25(3): 205–228.

Turner MJ, Flannelly GM, Wingfield M, Rasmussen MJ, Ryan R, Cullen S, Maguire R and Stronge JM (1991) The miscarriage clinic: an audit of the first year. *British Journal of Obstetrics and Gynaecology* 98(3): 306–308.

Van P and Meleis AI (2003) Coping with grief after involuntary pregnancy loss: perspectives of African American women. *JOGNN: Journal of Obstetric, Gynecologic, and Neonatal Nursing* 32(1): 28–39.

Wallbank S and Robertson N (2008) Midwife and nurse responses to miscarriage, stillbirth and neonatal death: a critical review of qualitative research. *Evidence Based Midwifery* 6(3): 100–106.

Welch KJ and Bergen MB (2000) Adolescent parent mourning reactions associated with stillbirth or neonatal death. *Omega: Journal of Death and Dying* 40(3): 435–451.

Wilson R (2001) Parents' support for their other children after a miscarriage or perinatal death. *Early Human Development* 61(2): 55–65.

Wong MK, Crawford TJ, Gask L and Grinyer A (2003) A qualitative investigation into women's experiences after a miscarriage: implications for the primary healthcare team. *British Journal of General Practice* 53(494): 697–702.

11 Bereavement in care homes

Paul Dempster

Key messages

- Old age is not neatly categorised, nor should it be. Health, mobility and cognisance vary widely and as a result we should not have a single description to describe old age.
- Coping better with bereavement is not necessarily a by-product of ageing.
- Home is a major focus of our lives and deaths.
- There are multiple losses associated with ageing. Although projections show people are less likely to die at home, consideration still needs to be given to home deaths.
- Research is fragmentary about experiences of living (and dying) in care.
- Creating training co-ops may allow smaller businesses to provide training for bereavement care that logistically and financially they otherwise could not afford.

Introduction

This chapter is in four parts. It looks first at where people die and what old age is. Old age is not neatly categorised, nor should it be. Health, mobility and cognisance vary widely and as a result old age should not be applied as a blanket description. The ageing process is multidimensional.

Second, the chapter explores the place of home in older age and its links with care and with subsequent bereavement. It highlights research that shows that homes are a major focus of our lives, a key factor in maintaining independence. With poor health, or a need for specialist terminal care, the home may have to be relinquished, creating a further source of bereavement.

The evidence is fragmentary about experiences of living (and dying) in care. The third part of the chapter highlights research which shows that living and dying in care homes is not necessarily negative (as reflected in the genre of institutionalisation literature popularised by Townsend 1962). In fact it can provide new experiences both for family and for the new resident.

The final part of the chapter examines carers and the culture within the nursing or residential home for the elderly. Workers often adopt the metaphor of caring family to counterbalance the perception of being distant. These sensitive adults look after the care needs of the living and dying. They can often experience multiple bereavements themselves when people die, as specialist staff and relatives leave, and they have often not received adequate training. A small vignette raises some issues for the reader and points out that more needs to be done to recognise the bereavements that workers and residents face on a regular basis.

This chapter can be read in conjunction with Chapter 4, which explored the broader aspects of bereavement for older people.

Where do older people die?

Where older people die will effect and influence the bereavement journey. Empirical studies have been undertaken retrospectively, making comparisons between the late 1960s and 1980s in England (Cartwright 1991) and between the 1980s and 2000s in Wales (Ahmad and O'Mahony 2005); and prospectively up to 2030, for England and Wales (Gomes and Higginson 2008).

Recent figures from Gomes and Higginson (2008) show that deaths are much more likely to occur in institutional care. A much smaller proportion of people die at home. The figures for home deaths are declining, from around 31 per cent in 1974 to 18.1 per cent in 2003. They find that the figures are a little higher for people dying of cancer than from other illnesses, possibly reflecting the important strides forward of hospices and other groups trying to promote dying outwith institutions over the last few decades.

These figures for deaths at home are likely to fall even further. Gomes and Higginson highlight there will be 'more ageing and more deaths in the future' (2008: 39), to the point that deaths will outnumber births by 2030. This has implications for staff in caring institutions, as will be discussed later in this chapter. In addition, the figures do not take into account that people may be admitted briefly to hospital prior to dying, creating a change in the locus of care. Gomes and Higginson (2008) acknowledge that 'Institutional deaths include hospitals but also residential homes and nursing homes; the latter are an increasingly important locus of care and death for older people' (p. 40). These changes of location can create their own problems and influence the bereavement journey, not only for the patient and relatives but also for staff.

What constitutes old age?

A number of aspects become apparent when looking at the literature surrounding older people and care homes. There is no real consensus on what constitutes old age. The concept of 'older person' rejects a simple definition. Similarly, trying to apply blanket concepts relating to ageing, simply by defining chronological age, is unhelpful because physical and mental needs can vary so much. Thus, coping with bereavement is not necessarily a by-product of ageing. Some may even argue that it is not appropriate to define older people as a homogenous group anyway (Bennett *et al.* 1997), as this can lead to ageist stereotyping (Thompson 2002), which if internalised can lead to depression and low self-esteem (McMurray

2005). In the introduction of their paper Townsend and colleagues (2006) highlight two polarisations of thought based on Cole's (1992) discussion of ageing: first the problematic old, seen often as a burden, and, second, the positive active old. They argue that these narrow conceptions of age do nothing to represent the perceptions older people have. Successful ageing had as much to do with being 'acutely aware of losses they had to cope with or would experience in the future' (Townsend *et al.* 2006: 897).

Suffice to say how we represent old age in care settings is often described as a sociological device of institutionalisation (Townsend 1962; Smith 1998), which at times is unhelpful (Ahmedzai *et al.* 2004). The images of decline, ill health, failing and dependency have become a stereotype that is not useful (Bond and Cabrero 2007), although they often predominate. Moss and Moss (2007) argue that many of the issues which present in older age can be negotiated around rather than merely overcome. This means that often older people have a range of choices and options they can make. Thus, the experience of ageing, and indeed of old age, is not always negative.

What is home?

Discussing the context of the care home without mention of the concept of home seems alien. As our needs and circumstances change so do our dwellings (Gott *et al.* 2004). Care homes form one part of possible living opportunities for older people. Currently there is a distinction in the literature, which often focuses attention on one type of establishment. So for example research will concentrate on examinations of the 'care home' or the 'residential home', or 'sheltered housing' or 'palliative care in hospices'.

The literature on care homes needs to be brought closer together with that on other institutional living. Simply mapping the experiences from one place to the other is not acceptable either. They need to form a consolidated whole, whereby the home is seen as experienced living irrespective of type. Too often 'the home' is seen as an instrument of care.

For example, a number of papers and chapters (see Komaromy 2000; Katz *et al.* 2001; Katz and Peace 2003) explore an earlier report, by Katz and colleagues (2000), which examined palliative care provision within a handful of English care homes. This mixed-method study found that homes did not have uniform policies for dealing with bereavement, or in fact for supporting dying residents. The work focuses on palliative care, but tries to overextend findings based on a small qualitative sample resulting in a partial analysis of larger experiences.

The call for a dynamic approach to the literature is borne out by Holman and colleagues (2004), who examined life within care institutions and found that much of the research is fragmentary in that it looks from a single perspective or methodology, which hides aspects of other people's loss within these institutions. Current research provides an incomplete picture. Having examined a wide variety of research they find that often there are divisions within the literature, which result in only partial analysis of larger experiences.

Home as experienced living

Bond and colleagues (1998) define what a home is for older people. They identify three themes, taken from Sixsmith (1990):

- First, home 'provides a major focus in life' (Sixsmith 1990: 204), taking on more significance as other social roles decrease.
- Second, the home is instrumental in maintaining independence.
- Third, homes are a source of attachment, where 'memories' and 'past associations' can be stored and impact on the perception of what the home is.

For Franklin (1996), the home can also remain an economic asset and the dwelling can become the context for service delivery. Indeed where you live may impact on morbidity and health (Shaw *et al.* 2008). Governmental policy reflects the importance placed on the home. It has become politicised. Some cynics, such as Hanford and colleagues (1999) and Wistow (1995), argue that keeping older people at home longer (i.e. care in the community) is for cost-cutting reasons. It is cheaper and puts less pressure on an overburdened system. Less cynical critics (Baldwin *et al.* 1993) argue that a person's home has many benefits in terms of care, including care around death. Ahmedzai (2004) highlights that dying at home does not necessarily mean a good or bad death; it does not carry any stigma, unlike some other settings. Many older people also worry more about the quality of dying, (Steinhauser *et al.* 2000), which involves, for example, having adequate pain relief and family and professional carers available (Shemmings 1998). Leaving a home can be a source of bereavement too.

Thinking about home

I have included a few small exercises throughout this chapter which offer the opportunity for you to think about yourself and your practice. This first exercise aims to get you thinking about what home means to you.

> Take a moment to think about what home is for you. What do you associate with your home? Is it:
> - bricks and mortar; a sleeping place?
> - a holding place of memories good and bad?
> - a family place?
>
> Has the meaning of your home changed?
>
> For what reasons?
>
> What do you associate with going home?
>
> What thoughts and feelings would you encounter if you were never able to return home?

In summary, the dwelling or home constitutes a lived experience wherein a number of interactions past and present occur. You may have heard people use phrases such as 'if only these walls could talk'. The dwelling can in some ways communicate meaning, thoughts and feelings, just as objects or artefacts can. The above exercise sought to get you interpreting what your home means to you. We have all created our own sense of meaning which surrounds the concept of home. This is likely to be stronger if the place has been inhabited for a while (Després 1991).

Living without a home

Could you list a range of words that would describe what it would be like to be without your home?

I have started my own list, which included the following:

- loss of independence;
- losing memories;
- feeling 'uncomfortable', as I cannot 'do my own thing'.

Finally, look over your list and see how that impacts your practice. Has it raised any issues for you and your work?

The home can become a pastoral space, where the memories and actions contained therein (Fänge and Ivanoff 2008) provide a sense of being when other things are counted lost (Finn 2009). These spaces can allow people to continue to interact with the deceased through remembrance; something that 'institutions' find harder to do.

The importance of 'setting' plays a large role in the dying of an older person. In fact Després (1991) indicates the importance of architecture for older people. There are certain motifs and symbols which can actually aid the bereaved, by their familiarity. Imagine losing the concept of 'going home', to that familiar place, surrounded by familiar things. Suffice to say that 'losing one's home' may be an additional loss that is often overlooked.

With infirmity there is less opportunity to 'interact' with the home environment (Fänge and Ivanoff 2008). For example, cleaning and other activities are less likely to be conducted by the home owner. This relinquishing of tasks is part of the journey that older people make towards different types of homes which can better integrate their needs. Giving up a home can cause grief too, not just for the older person, but possibly for the family too.

Gott and colleagues (2004) examined concepts of what a home is from the perspective of older people. Homes have a sense of meaning, which Gott argues may change during the death trajectory. Although older people see the 'home' as an essential part of what constitutes the experience of a good death it is possible that later in the dying trajectory they would prefer to be cared for in a different place. It may be that the influx of carers and other professionals changes what the concept of home is. Similarly, having people present seems to create the setting for a good death.

Finally, Bond and colleagues (2003) suggest that the transfer of care of individuals with dementia to care establishments and their subsequent death can have a positive effect on the carer/bereaved in relation to their health status, psychological well being and activity participation. This would suggest that for some elderly carers the relinquishment to care establishments may be a positive intervention for bereavement. In addition, Ryan (1992) found a comparatively reduced death rate in those who had their loved ones admitted to care establishments, suggesting that relinquishing of care can be a positive event in some older people's bereavement journey.

Care homes as experienced living

Death in institutions may be described as depersonalised, because family members are cared for by professional strangers. This apparently creates fewer burdens on family but also reinforces the idea that 'proper care' cannot be provided at home. To counteract this, workers may adopt the metaphor of 'family' so that 'caregiving becomes more meaningful when professional distance is weakened and residents are humanized' (Moss *et al.* 2003: 293).

Bass and Bowman (1990) suggest that the greater the care-giving strain on an individual prior to bereavement then the greater the strain on the individual after bereavement to manage this issue. To manage this issue they suggest that interventions to support the caregiver should commence before death to relieve the burden of care and that relinquishment of care to care homes is not the only option. By entering into a partnership with the carer to maintain the dying individual at home, perhaps the suggestion of care in the home as being 'improper' as suggested by Moss and colleagues (2003) can be addressed. Social workers and Macmillan nurses have developed complex partnerships with people to provide such care. Further evidence suggests that family carers with considerable workloads were more likely to suffer from depression when hospice stay was short (Kris *et al.* 2006). One wonders if this is because some of the support mechanisms are not fully bonded or in place.

The sensitive adults' experienced living

Shemmings (1998) wonders if the concept of home needs to reflect the desire of people to not be alone when they die. This desire to not be alone has been discussed in a history of death and dying provided by Ariès (1983). Possibly there are further changes that we are now witnessing in care homes where family are being replaced by 'sensitive adults', that is, carers who are present at the death. These carers are sensitised to death and sensitive to the needs of relatives and dying clients; they are able to play a surrogate role, where the family are unable to attend.

Although many people will say that they prefer to 'die at home', what they often go on to say is that they would prefer to 'die with their loved ones around them', failing that they might accept, or tolerate, being cared for by sensitive adults (even though not related to them). Most people would not prefer to die at home if this meant being cold, lonely and forgotten. And even if loved ones are around, it is difficult for dying people to find peace if they feel that their decline is tearing apart those for whom they most care.

(Shemmings 1998: 154)

Shemmings downplays the role that professional carers can have after death, when dealing with bereaved families, which is unfortunate, as some could have a much more central role, even given organisational constraints. Although these 'sensitive adults' provide opportunities to ease the dying, they too must be supported, simply because the fear is they may become desensitised. They may attempt to protect themselves, by 'not getting too close' to a resident or emotionally involved in the first place (Dempster 2006).

The action of preparing for a death can result in a range of adaptations and support for the soon to be bereaved. Thus workers may 'prepare' for and even anticipate a death. This is often dealt with as part of the culture of the home. It has been described as the emotional labour of care (Smith 1992) or may be part of anticipatory grief (see Chapter 5).

In order to address the emotional aspects of care of the bereaved several suggestions have been made. Tudiver and colleagues (1995) identifies that emotional support through regular support group meetings and incorporating health promotion fills many of the bereaved individual's needs; Segal and colleagues (2001) suggests that distress after bereavement is greatly decreased by encouraging the venting of emotions. This venting of emotions helps to refocus on the positive aspects of the lost relationship, which also helps promote adaptation.

Most care homes do not feed into this process (officially) at present; nurses and carers have traditionally been advised to be stoic and see death as part of the job (Ashurst and Ashurst 2007), although I am aware that plenty of venting occurs in staffrooms, and in tea and coffee breaks throughout the country (Dempster 2006).

Do you discuss dying before the death of a resident? Within your work what opportunities are there to:

- grieve over the loss of a resident?
- talk about a death?
- mourn or commemorate a death?
- vent?

Is death a hidden or open aspect of your work?

Is there time set aside to talk or are moments snatched at tea breaks and other times?

Is there a place that is set aside for these conversations?

Do you make use of the building or other activities to enable talk?

Is there anything that could be done better?

Where do you discuss death?

This small exercise asks you to think about when you talk about death, what opportunities you have and the location of these conversations.

Putting aside staff issues for a moment, often little support is available for residents' bereavement needs. Within the care home context, Komaromy and Hockey (2001) found that there is little special provision when an older person is dying. As long as the death is not problematic it is considered natural and is unlikely to give rise to 'problematic emotions'. As they aptly put it: 'contained, controlled and timely deaths were therefore the ideal product of homes in which older people came to accept the "natural" ending of their lives' (Komaromy and Hockey 2001: 75).

Where there is extra provision, for example specialist Macmillan nurses, there is a loss that is not considered. Carers may have developed bonds with these staff. At death, they lose the resident, the family will soon dissipate and the specialist nurses will leave as well. There is a complicated process of compounded loss and bereavement for the worker that has not been fully explored (Dempster 2006). Indeed multiple losses are experienced as all the various 'actors' (i.e. resident, relatives and specialist workers) leave almost simultaneously.

Komaromy and Hockey (2001) found problems of lack of time and resources within homes to devote between the living and dying, highlighting Blakemore's (2005) concern that government funding does not cover much more than the personal care aspect of residential living. Therefore in care homes, where there is constant engagement with death and dying, there is as yet usually no bereavement support given to either staff or residents. In addition it may be unlikely that care homes will seek to follow up the bereaved relatives or others who may have been affected by the death, although in a small number of cases the relatives may continue to visit other residents or to help as volunteers and so contact is maintained.

Against the backdrop of the ideal of a natural death, Komaromy and Hockey (2001) found that home management controlled many aspects of the home and as a result they controlled the ageing bodies within the home. Therefore they are intrinsically involved in the dying of residents and also the bereavement practices contained therein. They also 'set the tone for acceptable emotional demeanour' amongst staff.

Disenfranchised grief

It would seem that in many cases care homes are not (presently) designed to provide bereavement care (as well as they might); they are there to provide care and support for the living and those who are terminally ill (Dempster 2006). It is ironic in an institution that regularly deals with death and dying that it avoids providing bereavement support for staff, relatives and residents. Compare this for example with hospice care, where bereavement is considered a 'natural' component of palliative care (Field *et al.* 2004).

There is a legion of disenfranchised (i.e. voiceless) grievers (see for example Rowling 1995), who are actively prevented from actions of bereavement (Corr 1998; Doka 2002; Attig 2004). In general within health care there is often little acknowledgement of the loss or impact on an individual (Bertman 1991).

Workers in a care home, it would seem, are often torn between feelings that they have in private and those that they exhibit in the home; they may for example try not to show 'too much emotion' within the care home setting, by trying to 'keep a lid' on their public feelings about bereavement by being professional (Dempster 2006).

An example

This example is based on actual events. It will help tease out some of the issues facing workers and residents. A carer outside the room takes up the story:

> It happened in the middle of lunches, there was a death. The other residents were having lunch, and the door to her room was across from the open plan lounge.
>
> One of the carers was very upset, she had got to know the person very well, and she was 'doing the body, giving her a clean and tidy up and that . . .'
>
> The residents all knew what was going on . . . you could see it on their faces they were trying to get on with their lunches. The probably didn't want to eat, but they had to, it was lunchtime! Who was to say it would not be their turn next!
>
> I made a point of sitting with them, even the ones who could eat by themselves. I said, 'come on now, eat your lunch'. I said it just for comfort. We would not talk about it at that time, maybe later, I thought.
>
> And all the while the carer was crying away very loudly.
>
> What was worst was no one told Jean, the cook, for a fortnight that Bella had died, and they had been close. She was in the kitchen crying and just had to get on with it, in the full knowledge she had missed the funeral because no one had told her.

Death at mealtimes brings with it certain strains for workers (especially carers) and residents. The worker above found it difficult, embarrassing even. It is hard enough to deal with mealtimes, which are exceedingly busy, but to have a number of residents sitting feeling the strain was too much in this particular case. Hearing the cries of a familiar member of staff who has clearly broken down is likely to make residents feel compassion. Probably the last thing on anybody's mind would be a cheese sandwich or a bowl of soup at this time! Costello (2006) classifies this type of death as 'problematic' in an NHS setting. We often fail to address such issues within the 'routine' of care home/health care practice.

Offering a diversion by getting people to eat, thus creating moments of silence, seems the best way to get by for the worker serving the food. In fact sometimes that silence can be very loud. The action of non-communication is not always helpful. Creating a distraction means that issues are not being dealt with. As a balance, however, residents may not want to know 'of yet another death', so a careful balancing act is needed. Thoughtful and care-filled responses to death, dying and subsequent bereavement may create better spaces in which older people can grieve and mourn appropriately. Indeed, for residents, this could be a friend and companion who has shared and lived within the home.

The person died in their room. Ironically it was located directly opposite the meal table so it was impossible to hide the fact, given the number of people going in and out of the room, that someone had died. To compound matters, the carer in the room with the dead resident acted in what another worker described as 'an inappropriate manner' and grieved loudly, which other workers thought was excessive. What was it that made her actions inappropriate? Was it the fact that residents were eating? Was it the manner in which she is grieving? Why is the worker expected to be silent? Were the other workers annoyed because it caused a lot of embarrassment? What are the appropriate actions in this type of situation? What are your views?

Discussion with colleagues

The discussion and answers to the rhetorical questions posed above may be different in every workplace.

> You may find that you have policies or ways of doing things within your own workplace. What are these?
>
> Are these written or unwritten?
>
> Discuss the example with your colleagues; what do they think?
>
> Consider the story from the point of view of the worker who was 'noisy'!
>
> Have you come to any conclusions?
>
> Did you consider that the worker may have been recently 'sensitised' by a recent personal loss? Does that change your view of her?

The case is very poignant, and slightly disturbing. Finally, the cook is expected to continue with cooking the evening meal, in the knowledge that she has missed the funeral of someone she had known for 30 years (in social circles outwith the home as well). Staff who are not on shift at the time of the death may be less likely to be informed and there may be an assumption that they do not wish to know as the 'professional distance' is such that it places a distinction between the personal and professional selves.

Concluding questions about practice

What could be done better for the bereaved in care homes?

What can be done to improve communication?

How can space be used positively?

How should staff behave when faced with bereavement?

What can be done for residents?

Does 'just getting on with it' provide opportunities for healthy bereavement?

I concur with Shemmings (1996) that:

> Residential staff are attempting to marry the norms of society, which tend ideologically to accept or even 'welcome' death at the end of a long and useful life, with their experience as workers, which requires them to accept death – and thus loss – among those to whom they have become attached during the course of their work. The act of balancing good and sensitive care for older people with the need to protect oneself from overwhelming feelings is not an easy task.
>
> (Shemmings 1996: 92)

In society we consider the loss of home to be acceptable, even inevitable, when it is hard for a person to 'manage' in the community. However, we do not always translate the 'benefits of home' to other care environments.

Second, there is a train of thought which considers death as acceptable after a 'long and useful life', according to Shemmings (1996) above. In other words death is to be welcomed when a person is old and in pain. We also consider what constitutes a good death. However, the carer in a home is confronted with a strange conundrum. There is a feeling of guilt in accepting death, because, as Shemmings hints, death is the antithesis of their job, which is to care for people. How do they hold that tension together?

Furthermore, the actions of attachment occur within a set location, the (care) home, in which they are employed. Clearly it is hard to be caring and sensitive whilst protecting themselves from the overwhelming feelings of loss. This intellectual struggle faces staff at all different levels. For academics, practitioners and managers, how do we tease apart these issues? Also, how do we provide suitable environments in which to be subjected to loss? If you have answered and thought about the questions in this chapter then you will be well on the way to personally examining these issues.

It is this tension of balancing care on the one hand with protection (of feelings etc.) that is coming to the fore. More research needs to be undertaken to explore how staff and residents cope with bereavement and how they understand death and dying within their living spaces. Although some venting occurs (Segal *et al.* 2001), it is often done in private and there is a culture within the care home where public displays of grief are seen as shameful and emotions should not be talked about (see Riordan and Saltzer 1992).

Training and the workplace

This small exercise gets you to now consider what training and skills are necessary for working with bereaved people. It may be worth discussing your own thoughts with your colleagues and with management. What is available and how can you now effect change in practice?

> What training and skills do you consider important when working with bereaved people?
>
> What do you consider to be vital?
>
> Consider the training at your workplace. List the important factors that make the training suitable for your job.
>
> How could that training be improved?
>
> What is missing?

There is probably a harder question to answer. How do you know what is missing? Often people working with older people have a perception of what would make better care. There may be organisational constraints within the home which limit training, such as finance, time or staff shortages. Another perceived problem may be a lack of up-to-date skills in the first place. The Department of Health (2008) found that many workers in care homes have unmet training needs which may limit the extent to which they may draw on training related to when a patient dies (DoH 2005a).

The Department of Health commissioned a survey to explore the level of bereavement services provided in or by NHS Trusts (DoH (2005b). The research found that support and formal counselling was available for two-thirds of staff, with a lower proportion of bereaved people receiving similar services. The document is available in electronic format at http://www.dh.gov.uk/en/Publicationsandstatistics/Publications/PublicationsPolicyAndGuidance/DH_4115879

Gathering information on what training is provided allows pinpointing of need that can be met by training. Often bereavement research focuses on the outcomes of training (Linn *et al.* 1983, 1989) rather than searching for training needs (see, for example, Froggat 2000a–c). Holland and Peace (1997) found that small private care homes had similar issues with training needs. Training and support remain important factors in the delivery of good care (Sidell *et al.* 1997). Economies of scale are always going to affect smaller homes which do not employ training officers, and courses can be expensive to undertake.

Conclusion

This chapter has sought to open up discussion on what home is and what it means, as it is often the case that the idea of 'home' is seen as integral to care home settings. If this is the case then issues related to death, dying and bereavement, in such establishments, need to consider the meaning of home and how it impacts on loss and grief. The 'professionalisation' or 'institutionalisation' of the care, whilst providing a means by which it can be organised and managed, may conversely limit the extent to which it is humanised and is 'home like' in nature.

It is clear that in many cases care homes rely on a workforce that is transitory and often has limited training. How best to address education and training issues related to death, dying and bereavement is a moot point but one which is in need of addressing so that greater knowledge and understanding is fostered and increasing attention paid to developing a greater understanding through research. The latter is at present lacking and yet it is essential if bereavement care is to be improved and contextualised to care in such settings.

References

Ahmed S and O'Mahony MS (2005) Where older people die: a retrospective population-based study. *Quarterly Journal of Medicine* 98(12): 865–870.

Ahmedzai S, Bellamy G, Clark D, Gott M and Seymour J (2004) Older people's views about home as a place of care at the end of life. *Palliative Medicine* 18(5): 460–467.

Ariès P (2000) Death denied. In: Dickenson D, Johnson M and Katz J (eds) *Death, dying and bereavement*. London: Sage/Open University Press.

Ashurst G. and Ashurst A (2007) Palliative care: the bereavement process. *Nursing and Residential Care* 9(6): 263–265.

Attig T (2004) Disenfranchised grief revisited: discounting hope and love. *Omega* 49(3): 197–215.

Baldwin N, Harris J and Kelly D (1993) Institutionalisation: why blame the institutions? *Ageing and Society* 13: 69–81.

Bass DM and Bowman K (1990) The transition from caregiving to bereavement: the relationship of care-related strain and adjustment to death. *The Gerontologist* 30(1): 35–42.

Bennett G, Kingston P and Penhale B (1997) *The dimensions of elder abuse: perspectives for practitioners*. London: Macmillan.

Bertman SL (1991) *Facing death: images, insights and interventions*. New York: Taylor and Francis.

Blakemore K (2005) *Social policy: an introduction*, 2nd edn. Maidenhead: Open University Press/McGraw-Hill Education.

Bond J and Cabrero R (2007) *Health and dependency in later life*. London: Sage.

Bond J, Coleman P and Peace S (eds) (1998) *Ageing in society: an introduction to social gerontology.* London: Sage.

Bond JM, Michael SC and Davies S (2003) The quality of life of spouse dementia caregivers: changes associated with yielding to formal care and widowhood. *Social Science and Medicine* 57(12): 2385–2395.

Cartwright A (1991) Changes in life and care in the year before death 1969–1987. *Journal of Public Health* 13(2): 81–87.

Cole T (1992) *The journey of life: a cultural history of aging in America.* Cambridge: Cambridge University Press.

Corr CA (1998) Enhancing the concept of disenfranchised grief. *Omega* 38(1): 1–20.

Costello J (2006) Dying well: nurses' experiences of 'good and bad' deaths in hospital. *Journal of Advanced Nursing* 54(5): 594–601.

Dempster PG (2006) Journeying on to a better place? The processes and experiences associated with working around death and dying in care homes for older people. Unpublished thesis, Robert Gordon University, Aberdeen.

Despres C (1991) The meaning of home: literature review and directions for future research and theoretical development. *Journal of Architectural and Planning Research* 8(2): 96–115.

DoH (2005a) *When a patient dies: advice on developing bereavement services in the NHS.* London: Department of Health.

DoH (2005b) *Survey of bereavement care and other support services.* London: Department of Health.

DoH (2008) *End of life care strategy: promoting high quality care for all adults at the end of life.* London: Department of Health.

Doka KJ (ed.) (2002) *Disenfranchised grief: new directions, challenges and strategies for practice.* Champaign, IL: Research Press.

Fange A and Ivanoff SD (2008) The home is the hub of health in very old age: findings from the ENABLE-AGE Project. *Archives of Gerontology and Geriatrics* 48(3): 340–345.

Field D, Reid D, Payne S and Relf M (2004) Survey of UK hospice and specialist palliative care adult bereavement services. *International Journal of Palliative Nursing* 10(12): 569–576.

Finn C (2009) Old junk or treasure? *The Guardian.* date.

Franklin B (1996) New perspectives on housing and support for older people. In: Bland R. (ed.) *Developing services for older people and their families.* London: Jessica Kingsley.

Froggatt K (2000a) Evaluating a palliative care education project in nursing homes. *International Journal of Palliative Nursing* 6(3): 140–146.

Froggatt K (2000b) *Palliative care education in nursing homes.* London: Macmillan Cancer Relief.

Froggatt K (2000c) *Palliative care in nursing homes.* London: Macmillan Cancer Relief.

Gomes B and Higginson IJ. (2008) Where people die (1974–2030): past trends, future projections and implications for care. *Palliative Medicine* 22(1): 33–41.

Gott M, Seymour J, Bellamy G, Clark D and Ahmedzai S (2004) Older people's views about home as a place of care at the end of life. *Palliative Medicine* 18(5): 460–467.

Hanford L, Easterbrooke L and Stevenson J (1999) *Rehabilitation for older people: the emerging policy agenda.* London: Kings Fund.

Holland C and Peace S (1997) *The report of a pilot study of small homes for older people carried out in Bedfordshire, Buckinghamshire and Hertfordshire during 1997.* Milton Keynes: School of Health and Social Welfare, Open University.

Holman C, Meyer J and Cotter A (2004) The complexity of loss in continuing care institutions for older people: a review of the literature. *Illness, Crisis and Loss* 12(1): 38–51.

Katz J and Peace S (2003) *End of life in care homes: a palliative care approach.* Oxford: Oxford University Press.

Katz J, Sidell M and Komaromy C (2000) Death in homes: bereavement needs of residents, relatives and staff. *International Journal of Palliative Nursing* 6(6): 274–279.

Katz J, Sidell M and Komaromy C (2001) Dying in long-term care facilities: support needs of other residents, relatives and staff. *American Journal of Hospice and Palliative Care* 18(5): 321–326.

Komaromy C (2000) The sight and sound of death: the management of dead bodies in residential and nursing homes for older people. *Mortality* 5(3): 299–315.

Komaromy C and Hockey J (2001) Naturalizing death among older adults in residential care. In Hockey J, Katz J and Small N (eds) *Grief mourning and death ritual.* Buckingham: Open University Press.

Kris AE, Cherlin EJ, Prigerson H, Carlson MDA, Johnson-Hurzeler R, Kasl SV and Bradley EH (2006) Length of hospice enrollment and subsequent depression in family caregivers: 13-month follow-up study. *American Journal of Geriatric Psychiatry* 14(3): 264–269.

Linn MW, Linn BS and Stein S (1983) Impact on nursing home staff of training about death and dying. *Journal of the American Medical Association* 250(17): 2332–2335.

Linn MW, Linn BS, Stein S and Stein EM (1989) Effect of nursing home staff training on quality of patient survival. *International Journal of Aging and Human Development* 28(4): 305–315.

McMurray A (2005) Older people. In: Oliviere D and Monroe B (eds) *Death, dying and social differences.* Oxford: Oxford University Press.

Moss SZ and Moss MS (2007) Being a man in long term care. *Journal of Aging Studies* 21(1): 43–54.

Moss MS, Moss SZ, Rubenstein RL and Black HK (2003) The metaphor of "family" in staff communication about dying and death. *Journal of Gerontology: Social Sciences* 58(5): S290–S296.

Riordan RJ and Saltzer SK (1992) Burnout prevention among health care providers working with the terminally ill: a literature review. *Omega: Journal of Death and Dying* 25(1): 17–24.

Rowling L (1995) The disenfranchised grief of teachers. *Omega: Journal of Death and Dying* 31(4): 317–329.

Segal DL, Chatman C, Bogaards J and Becker L (2001)One year follow-up of an emotional expression intervention for bereaved older adults. *Journal of Mental Health and Aging* 7(4): 465–472.

Shaw M, Thomas B, Davey-Smith G and Dorling D (2008) *The grim reapers road map: an atlas of mortality in Britain.* London: Policy Press.

Shemmings Y (1996) *Death dying and residential Care.* Aldershot: Avebury.

Shemmings Y (1998) Death and dying in residential homes for older people. In: Jack R (ed.) *Residential versus community care.* London: Palgrave.

Sidell M, Katz JT and Komaromy C (1997) *Death and dying in residential and nursing homes for older people: examining the case for palliative care.* Buckingham: Open University Press.

Sixsmith AJ (1990) The meaning and experience of 'home' in later life. In: Bytheway B and Johnson J (eds) *Welfare and the ageing experience.* Aldershot: Avebury.

Smith P. (1992) *The emotional labour of nursing.* London, Palgrave.

Smith P (1998) *Death and dying in a nursing home.* Norwich: Social work monographs, University of East Anglia.

Steinhauser KE, Christakis NA, Clipp EC, McNeilly M, McIntyre L and Tulsky JA (2000) Factors considered important at the end of life by patients, family, physicians, and other care providers. *JAMA* 284(19): 2476–2482.

Thompson N (2002) *Loss and grief.* London: Palgrave.

Townsend P (1962) *The last refuge: a survey of residential institutions and homes for the aged in England and Wales.* London: Routledge and Kegan Paul.

Townsend J, Godfrey M and Denby T (2006) Heroines, villains and victims: older people's perception of others. *Ageing and Society* 26(6): 883–900.

Tudiver F, Permaul-Woods JA, Hilditch J, Harmina J and Saini S (1995) Do widowers use the health care system differently? *Canadian Family Physician* 41: 392–400.

Wistow G (1995) Aspirations and realities: community care at the crossroads. *Health and social care in the community* 3(4): 227–240.

Resources

Home death: Future issues and potential reasons for variation in London PPT. http://www.gsttcharity.org.uk/pdfs/gomes.pdf

Commission for social care inspection. http://www.csci.org.uk/

Staying at home. http://www.direct.gov.uk/en/Over50s/HomeAndCommunity/StayingInYourHome/DG_10026849

Choosing a care home (includes links to other sites). http://www.direct.gov.uk/en/HealthAndWellBeing/HealthServices/CareHomes/DG_10031516

Choosing a home: The Alzheimer's society. http://alzheimers.org.uk/factsheet/476. You will find other charities can provide help with this; many have websites and information leaflets, e.g. http://www.hda.org.uk/download/fact-sheets/HD-Care-Home-Checklist.pdf

Help the Aged. http://www.helptheaged.org.uk/en-gb

Age Concern. http://www.ageconcern.org.uk/. Note there are separate sites for Scotland, Wales and Northern Ireland, with a range of regional websites as well.

12 Bereavement and people with learning difficulties

Barry Gault

Key messages

- The chapter stresses the importance of not labelling the person with learning difficulties as being deficient in their ability to grieve.
- Productive enabling work with bereaved people who have learning difficulties requires the abandonment of diagnostic, linguistic and discursive practices which have the effect of transforming them into a category which is separated off from the experience of wider humanity.
- The chapter describes a process of 'diagnostic overshadowing' which often has the effect of provoking treatment responses which ignore past experience and present communication difficulties, and thus make difficult any hope of authentic engagement with the person seeking help.
- The helping process must take account of the fact that, for people with learning difficulties, human loss can often entail multiple losses of place of residence and attachment to the wider community.

Introduction

This chapter will argue that our thinking about bereavement has to reflect developments in the way health and social care practitioners regard the rights and needs of people with learning difficulties. Moreover, in relation to loss and people with learning difficulties it is important to be cognisant of changes in the approach to the planning and provision of services (Scottish Executive 2000; Department of Health 2001). It takes cognisance of an emerging consensus, which emphasises the central importance of listening to the voice of people with learning difficulties. Within the medium of a discussion regarding 'definitions and models', the influence of the 'diagnostic' and the 'social model' of disability will be explored, as well as the implications of this wider commitment to giving people with learning difficulties a voice in the planning and provision of the services which support them. In order to be consistent with this commitment to hearing that voice, I have sought the advice of 'John', who has long experience in the self-advocacy movement and has recently suffered bereavement.

Some recent evidence relating to the question of working with bereavement amongst people with learning difficulties will be reviewed, in the light of this changing and developing view of the manner in which supporting services are organised. The chapter will work towards a model of service provision which takes account of the findings of that evidence.

Definitions and models

Historically, education and social services provision in the UK has made wide use of the term 'learning difficulty' and the health services have tended to use 'learning disability'. In the academic world, there has been a movement towards the term 'intellectual disability' (Gates 2005). I have (Gault 2008) focused on the nature of the relationship between those who use the terminology and the subjects of such use. It is a reflection of the power (principally medical) to socially construct difference in a specific manner (McClimens 2007). Such labels are 'sticky on one side only' (Swain and Cameron 1999: 262), in so far as these labels have the potential for negative consequences. Objective categorisation can have a disempowering effect upon people with particular mental or physical attributes. As an adviser within the self-advocacy movement, I have chosen to use the term 'learning difficulties' because it is less inclined to have the effect of excluding service users from the world of ordinary living. In the context of working with people who have undergone bereavement, my feeling is that the literature is referring to essentially the same people, whatever terminology is utilised.

To promote clarity about working with bereaved people who have learning difficulties, it is important to be explicit about the model of disability which underpins both thought and activity. In much of the literature the identification of those in need of help and support appears unproblematic, in so far as service users are identified in terms of medical or other 'diagnostic' criteria which classify them under certain headings (Barnes 1998). Alternatively, this is explained by the fact that they make use of particular services. Such a pragmatic approach to identification of people with a learning difficulty is often *assumed* rather than set out theoretically. However, it is sometimes the case that the exclusion of people with learning difficulties from 'normal' grieving' is made theoretically explicit. In a discussion of the stages of grief LoConto and Arrington (2007: 549) point out:

> Each of these stages suggests the rationality, intelligence and wisdom assumed to be needed to get through the grieving process. People with mental retardation would not necessarily exhibit this rationality, intelligence or wisdom.

In rejecting such an assumption, I make a distinction between impairment and the physical, social and structural barriers which transform impairment into disability by imposing disadvantage and exclusion upon disabled people. Thomas (2004: 23) adds to this by identifying 'constructionist' processes where:

> Those who wield power through the authority conferred upon them by the status and the legitimacy of their knowledge – doctors, state administrators and legislators – can impose the category 'disabled' upon individuals in their

purview. A person who is socially constructed as 'disabled' may often come, in turn, to construct reflexively her or his identity in the image of the disabled person.

(Roets *et al.* 2007: 327)

In this context, as the chapter outlines using John's story, it touches upon the multiplicity of meanings which can be attached to his experience of bereavement, and his resistance to the assumption of 'clienthood' as a concomitant of his earlier assignment to the category of being a person with a learning difficulty. For him the cultural expectation that his position within the family implies certain obligations was of primary importance. In his particular situation, the fact that he lived relatively independently meant that there was no professional carer or 'diagnostician' who could take power over his role in the arrangement of the funeral. In the past John lived in a small, community-based residential facility. If his mother had died while he lived there, he might well have had to confront the power of professionals to determine what was to be done. In the past, in some institutions, it was not uncommon to conceal the very fact of a parental death from people with learning difficulties on the grounds that it might upset them (Oswin 1991). In order to resist such practice, John would need to be prepared to confront the power of the institution within which he lived.

John's story illustrates how, when the person who has a learning difficulty becomes bereaved, it can have the effect of separating rather than including those who are in need of help. In the short review of literature which follows John's story, the aim will be to draw out some of the themes which serve to counteract this tendency.

John's story

John (a pseudonym which he chose for himself) has been given the label of being a person who has a learning difficulty. John lived independently with minimal support. He had been active in the self-advocacy movement for around 14 years and this gave him confidence in the process of speaking up for himself. His mother died just over a year ago. He agreed to talk to me about the experience of losing his mother in the hope that it would enable those who provide services for people with learning difficulties to understand how to provide help and support. John uses the Scottish dialect which is known as 'Doric', so some of the words he uses may be unfamiliar to a wider audience.

John's mother was in hospital suffering from dementia and the hospital phoned him to let him know that she had 'passed awa in her sleep'. 'At the time she died the hospital staff were 'all around me, and supporting me . . . they were excellent'. Although he knew she was ill he said he 'couldna believe it: ma legs were stiff . . . jist like jelly; I couldna believe it at all'. Although he didn't live with his mum, he was the nearest relative and so the task of arranging the funeral fell to him, with some support from his maternal uncle. He knew that she wanted to be buried next to her husband, his late father. He did, at that time, have an assistant employed by the local authority, but he did not think it was part of her job to get involved in helping him to make the arrangements: he and his uncle saw this as a family matter. When asked later if staff in residential care should be involved in talking things through, he replied 'only if there is no one else to fall back on'.

The feeling of not being able to believe that she was 'awa' lasted up until the funeral, which took place 4 days after she died. The funeral service was quite sad, but John thought it was probably 'fit she wis wintin' hersel ye ken' because his mum was a Christian. I asked if it was what *he* wanted, but he said that he 'didna ken fit ta dee', because he was 'blocked up inside'. When asked if he had anyone to speak to about it, he said he mostly spoke to his uncle, and that helped because he needed to decide what his mum would have wanted. She died on her birthday so John thought it would be good to take flowers to her.

I asked him whether there was anybody to talk to in the few weeks after she died, and he said there 'wisna much fowk gan aboot at that time'. When asked to clarify what he meant he said there wasn't really anyone to talk to about how he was feeling: just his uncle. He was around, but sometimes John would 'miss phone calls on his mobile and a' that; wondering who it was'. He did talk to his assistant and that helped.

When asked if it would have helped to have someone who specialised in grief and loss to talk to, John phrased his answer in terms of finding out how *they* had coped with a loss. He clearly thinks that they need to have suffered a loss themselves in order to know how to help. However, he did think that the opportunity to talk might enable someone who had a learning difficulty to 'move forward'. He said that family members were helpful, but he got a feeling that they were glad it was over and done with, and they did not see much benefit in bringing it up again.

John says he thinks about his mum a lot, especially around the anniversary of her death. He says there are people around in his self-advocacy group but 'there's sae much fowk gan aboot that I dinna like to comment on it'. He means that it is hard to bring it up in a busy and active atmosphere. He did think, however, that if someone had found their voice through the medium of self-advocacy, they were more likely to be able to talk to someone about how they were feeling. He said that his Christian belief, and the fellowship of his church meetings, 'instead of sitting in the hoose', was an important comfort to him.

When asked how professionals and other carers could help he said they should ask themselves how *they* would feel if they had lost someone who was close to them. This sounded to me like a plea for empathy, reciprocity and a recognition that people with learning difficulties are not qualitatively different from anyone else at a time of pain and loss.

Engaging with bereaved people who have a learning difficulty

It was the case in the past, and sometimes still is the case now, that there can be an institutionalised reluctance to engage with people who have a learning difficulty and have suffered a loss. Maureen Oswin, a pioneer in the confrontation of this reluctance, was writing at a time when large numbers of people with learning difficulties were confined within mental handicap 'hospitals'. She identified 'emphatically bad attitudes to people with learning difficulties which has meant that their bereavement problems have been largely ignored, for example they do not have the same feelings as the rest of us' (Oswin 1991: 26)

Even though modern provision has become more community focused, John's story illustrates that professional support networks may find it difficult to engage with those who have suffered bereavement. Also, even when professional helpers do attempt engagement with those who have a learning difficulty, the focus of that help is often skewed by the preconceptions of the professionals involved. In a study of 50 'parent bereaved people with learning disabilities' who were compared with a matched control group of 50 non-bereaved people, there was some evidence of 'diagnostic overshadowing' (Hollins and Esterhuyzen 1997). Professional carers tended to ascribe aberrant behaviour to the 'innate personality of the client' or to the 'learning disability itself'. This leads to a failure to make the links with previous events. It may be, for example, that admission to an institution had prevented contact with loved ones in the period before the bereavement, and that the implications of this loss of contact had not been explored. I have worked, for example, with people who have not been told about the death of a loved one or, if they had been, were not involved in the rituals surrounding death and dying. Understandably perhaps, there has been real confusion as to whether their parent is alive or dead.

Another important issue relates to communication difficulties on the part of clients who have not been able to express their feelings. Problems can occur if someone no longer has contact with the person who was familiar with their method (verbal or non-verbal) or medium of communication. It may require a lot of work on the part of the substitute carers before the person can authentically communicate both the factual information about what has happened to them and the manner in which they interpret or experience events.

The effect of this lack of exploration of past experience and 'diagnostic overshadowing' may be that distress will manifest itself in patterns of *behaviour* rather than in verbal communication. A past student of mine had made fruitless attempts to sit down and talk to a young man who was clearly troubled. The young man remained obstinately silent. An experienced member of staff made the point that, in the large hospital where the young man had lived, you only got called to 'the office' if you were in trouble. He suggested that rather than sitting opposite the young man, the helper should try going for a walk along the beach with him. In no time at all productive communication was established.

This lack of authentic engagement can lead to a display of anxiety, anger and other forms of behavioural disturbance which may be mistakenly thought to constitute 'traumatic grief' (Bonell-Pascual *et al.* 2000; Brickell and Munir 2008). It may be that the person with learning difficulties is going through quite normal reactions to the trauma associated with bereavement, but the lack of engagement with helping resources may lead to unexpressed yearning, searching or profound loneliness. This, in its turn, may result in outcomes that are not satisfactory owing to misdiagnosis and subsequent inappropriate treatment of psychiatric symptoms and behaviours (Dodd *et al.* 2005).

Such inappropriate treatment responses may make an already difficult situation considerably worse. The effect upon one service user was described in the following way: 'Angry, that's how I felt if you want to know, angry, angry, angry' (Dowling *et al.* 2006: 282).

Such a lack of engagement may engender a feeling of loss of control over important life decisions (Read 2003). The decisions that are made about the response to bereavement will profoundly affect the remainder of a person's life. John vividly describes the feeling that other people, be they family or caring professionals, may appear to want the problem to be over as soon as possible. To improve the possibility of successful engagement it is thus important to ensure, through our practice, that people with learning difficulties have a voice in such decisions. By enabling their voice to be heard, there is an increased chance that people with learning difficulties can be supported through the process of normal bereavement and can avoid the distress of traumatic grief.

The helping process

In order to offer effective help, it is imperative that professionals adopt a holistic view which takes into account the familial and wider social context within which a person with learning difficulties has lived and is living. Unless the person offering help is aware of the wider impact of a bereavement, it may be that be that grief which is justified by events is misidentified as being traumatic or pathological. (Brickell and Munir 2008). Unfortunately, the loss of a parent for a person who has a learning difficulty often entails the loss of their home and the loss of familiar geographical and social surroundings (Blackman 2003). There is a sense in which such multiple loss is a penalty for the failure of the supporting services to engage with the wider issue of facilitating the transition of young people with a learning difficulty from dependent to independent living (MENCAP 2002).

One method of ensuring breadth of understanding is to develop a bereavement assessment tool which could be used at the time of bereavement or even in advance of bereavement. Blackman (2008) has piloted the use of such a tool within three multidisciplinary teams. The tool encourages helping professionals to be aware of emotional responses, cognitive understanding, social responses and their impact upon the social and familial network, and it does not underestimate the potential effect of physical changes, such as the health of the person concerned and changes in their geographical living environment. She describes an unanticipated side-effect, in so far as fellow professionals reported an increase in their skills, confidence and knowledge in the area of death and bereavement.

In thinking about the interaction between these multiple factors it is useful to make a distinction between predisposing, precipitating and maintaining factors (Summers and Witts 2003). With regard to predisposition, mainstream attachment theory helps us to understand the degree to which people with a learning difficulty have been supported to become autonomous individuals. The ending of the total exclusion of children with learning difficulties from the education system in the 1970s has meant that fewer such children are now brought up in residential institutions. There is still ambivalence around their inclusion in mainstream education (Rieser and Mason 1992). In the area within which I practise, large-scale residential institutions have been closed and replaced first with smaller community-based institutions and later with a commitment to support people with learning difficulties in the place where they live (Gault 2008). Thus people with learning difficulties may have had a loving and supportive family life combined with a thoughtful transition to independent living, or, alternatively, might have experienced poor emotional nurturing within both their family and residential institutions.

With regard to precipitating factors the circumstances surrounding bereavement play a part in determining future adjustment. John described vividly the shock engendered by the phone call from the hospital, even though he was aware that his mother was ill. It is not difficult to imagine the shock which might be engendered by the sudden loss of a parent who had been a sole carer who had been protective to the extent of not wishing to relinquish any caring responsibilities. One hopes that there are no longer any institutions which would keep the news of the death of a parent from a resident on the grounds that it might upset them (Oswin 1991). However, it is sometimes the case that insecure attachments within a family of origin, combined with precipitating factors such as the lack of an opportunity to take one's leave of a person who is lost, may lead to unresolved ambivalence, guilt and regret (Summers and Witts 2003).

The foundations for the maintenance of memories of the person who has been lost are often laid down immediately after the death (Blackman 2003). It may be that people with learning difficulties take some considerable time to accept the finality of a loss. This is sometimes misinterpreted as a lack of feeling or as denoting ambivalence, but it may take a period of time before their grief is explicitly stated (Read 2003). This may be a reflection of an extended period of cognitive searching (Brickell and Munir 2008), or it may reflect a lack of involvement in funeral rites. It was clear from John's story that being actively involved in the organisation of his mother's funeral was very important to him, especially with regard to meeting what would have been her wishes. It is difficult, however, to intervene directly to promote the inclusion of people with learning difficulties. Funeral directors reported that they tend to react to the wishes of family members (Raji *et al.* 2003) and rarely speak directly to people with learning difficulties. In the same study an Anglican chaplain reported that people with learning difficulties may be excluded because of the stigma attached to them and the fear that they may cause embarrassment by expressing emotion openly. In the period following the loss, commemorative activity such as the acknowledgement of anniversaries and visits to the burial place are important. This will lead to a continuation of life in an atmosphere where it is safe to acknowledge both the sad and the happy events of the past (Read 2003). In the past, bereavement has been conceptualised both in terms of a progression through a number of stages and as an oscillation between the experience of both loss and restoration (see Chapter 1; see also Stroebe and

Schut 1999); thus, for people with learning difficulties the events around and after the bereavement can profoundly affect the nature of this subsequent adjustment.

Methods of helping

Helping 'after the event' of bereavement for people with learning difficulties is usually organised in one of two ways. The first method, which seems to appeal to a commonsense view, involves the provision of an integrated service by already existing carers (professional or informal). The second involves counselling provided by 'mainstream' bereavement counsellors, with some basic training in the issues around learning difficulty, who are often volunteers. The outcome of these alternative methods was examined for a sample of people with learning difficulties who had been randomly assigned to the alternative interventions (Dowling *et al.* 2006). Both quantitative (involving the use of behavioural scales) and qualitative methods of evaluation were utilised. Contrary to initial hypotheses, the counselling intervention resulted in 'measurable gains both clinically and in terms of quality of life'. The integrated carer interventions, on the other hand, were often curtailed for practical reasons or through the withdrawal of carers because they found the emotional demands too difficult. Neither were there any measurable improvements in the mental health or behaviour of the subjects involved.

A 'snapshot' of an action research project, using both demographic data and a focus group approach, also showed that it is quite practical to establish a specialist bereavement and support service; however, in order to overcome the inherited legacy of 'practical, emotional and attitudinal difficulties', issues concerning consent and boundaries, the provision of a written manual regarding good practice with this client group, and the influence of the physical location of the counselling activity need to be specifically addressed (Read 2001). It is also imperative that the *content* of the helping process be creatively organised. Life story books, in a loose leaf format which can be added to during the process of creating them; with the subject choosing where they want to begin and in what order they wish to proceed, can be a powerful tool. Photographs, drawings and objects which have survived from the past can aid the ownership of the reminiscence process (Blackman 2003). Unfortunately, it is often the case that movement between institutions or traumatic loss of a home environment can also mean the parallel loss of such mementoes. It may be that a visit to a particular place or the taste of a favourite dish from the past can evoke ownership of a past experience.

An inclusive approach to helping

John's reticence regarding the involvement of caring professionals in the helping process was well founded, although he seems to have been fortunate that his extended family sought to include him in the rituals of the grieving process. It may be that the culture of the north east of Scotland, where he lives, helped to facilitate this process. There is a sense in which his story underlines the fact that after the event, help is only one aspect of the support needs of people with learning difficulties and that, especially when a loved one is ill over along period of time, our knowledge of anticipatory grief illustrates the need for preparatory work *before* the death of a carer. John was fortunate in so far as he had been enabled to achieve independence from his family of origin. A study of 41 people with a learning difficulty living with elderly carers (usually parents) showed that a great majority of the respondents (73 per cent) were aware that they would some day need to consider alternative forms of housing and support. They wished to gain those independent living skills which would enable them to remain in their homes in advance of the inevitable death of their carers (Bowey and McGlaughlin 2005). An interesting finding of this study concerned the fact that 83 per cent of respondents helped with the practical care of their parents. The parents acknowledged that they were dependent to a great degree on the support of their disabled sons or daughters; and people with learning difficulties were often, in turn, worried about the future care of their ageing parents. It was *not* a simple matter of parents being the carers of their offspring and, accordingly, the roles of 'carer' and 'cared for' were far from distinct. Helping endeavour, both before and after bereavement, has consequently to take account of the loss of the role of carer on the part of people with learning difficulties *as well as* their own need for support.

This lack of recognition of the caring role is symptomatic of the wider disempowerment of people with learning difficulties, and although John was reticent in raising the issue of bereavement within his self-advocacy group, the nature of support within the transition process from family of origin to independence might be an issue for such groups to campaign around. The problem has been well summarised in the following manner:

> In resisting or avoiding discussions of future planning, professionals and carers may be attempting to protect people with learning disabilities from the issue of carer mortality, possibly through a belief that they cannot cope with such a notion or would find it too distressing. However, this is not something from which anyone can be protected.
>
> (Bowey and McLaughlin 2005: 1379)

Conclusion

This chapter has raised issues relating to bereavement and people with learning difficulties and included evidence from the literature as well as practitioners with long experience in working with bereaved people who have a learning difficulty. It has examined such issues from the perspective of service users and providers, and has sought to contextualise those issues in the light of the movement away from institutional care. It has identified an approach which seeks to empower service users. It has become clear that particular diagnostic, linguistic and discursive practices have had the effect of producing treatment responses which ignore the past experience and present communication difficulties of people who have learning difficulties. The outcome may be to sabotage any hope of authentic engagement with the person seeking help. The promotion of an inclusive approach to helping is proposed as an antidote to this tendency. The movement away from an institutional form of provision has produced, and is producing, a generation of people with learning difficulties who will not be prepared to be excluded from the process of grieving, whether they live in the community or are cared for in an institutional setting. Service providers who are cognisant of this movement are already involving service users in the planning of their services. The lesson to be drawn from the literature is that individuals with learning difficulties need to be involved in planning for likely future bereavement and in shaping the helping services which are utilised after the event. In the future, it is likely that specialist bereavement services tailored to the needs of people with learning difficulties will have a more positive outcome than a reliance upon the adaptation of existing 'mainstream' support services.

References

Barnes C (1998) The social model of disability: a sociological phenomenon ignored by sociologists? In: Shakespeare T (ed.) *The disability reader: social science perspectives*. London: Continuum.

Blackman N (2003) *Loss and learning disability*. London: Worth Publishing.

Blackman N (2008) The development of an assessment tool for the bereavement needs of people with learning disabilities. *British Journal of Learning Disabilities* 36(3): 165–170.

Bonell-Pascual E, Huline-Dickens S and Hollins S (1999) Bereavement and grief in people with learning disabilities: a follow-up study. *British Journal of Psychiatry* 175: 346–350.

Bowey L and McGlaughlin A (2005) Adults with a learning disability living with elderly carers talk about aspirations for the future: aspirations and concerns. *British Journal of Social Work* 35(8): 1377–1393.

Brickell C and Munir K (2008) Grief and its complications in individuals with intellectual disability. *Harvard Review of Psychiatry* 16(1): 1–12.

Department of Health (2001) *Valuing people: a new strategy for learning disability for the 21st century*. London: Stationery Office.

Dodd P, Dowling S and Hollins S (2005) A review of the emotional, psychiatric and behavioural responses to bereavement in people with intellectual disabilities. *Journal of Intellectual Disability Research* 49(7): 537–543.

Dowling S, Hubert J, White S and Hollins S (2006) Bereaved adults with intellectual disabilities: a combined randomized controlled trial and qualitative study of two community-based interventions. *Journal of Intellectual Disability Research* 50(4): 277–287.

Gates B (2005) What's in a name? *Journal of Intellectual Disabilities* 9(1): 5–7.

Gault B (2008) Punters and providers in the north of Scotland: a study of shared experiences. Unpublished PhD thesis, Robert Gordon University, Aberdeen. Available at: http://hdl.handle.net/10059/242.

Hollins S and Esterhuyzen A (1997) Bereavement and grief in adults with learning disabilities. *British Journal of Psychiatry* 170: 497–501.

Loconto DR and Arrington PR (2007) Pragmatism and grieving: incorporating Mead and Dewey to understand the grieving of people with mental retardation. *Sociological Spectrum* 27(5): 537–553.

McClimens A (2007) Language, labels and diagnosis: an idiot's guide to learning disability. *Journal of Intellectual Disabilities* 11(3): 257–266.

MENCAP (2002) *The housing timebomb: the housing crisis facing people with a learning difficulty and their older parents*. London: Mencap.

Oswin M (1991*) Am I allowed to cry? A study of bereavement amongst people who have learning difficulties*. London: Souvenir Press.

Raji O, Hollins S and Drinnan A (2003) How far are people with learning disabilities involved in funeral rites? *British Journal of Learning Disabilities* 31(1): 42–45.

Read S (2001) A year in the life of a bereavement counselling and support service for people with learning disabilities. *Journal of Intellectual Disabilities* 5(1): 19–33.

Read S (2003) Bereavement and loss. In: Markwick A and Parrish A (eds) *Learning disabilities: themes and perspectives*. London: Butterworth Heinemann.

Rieser R and Mason M (1992) *Disability equality in the classroom: a human rights issue*. London: Disability Rights in Education.

Roets G, Goodley D and Van Hove G (2007) Narrative in a nutshell: sharing hopes, fears, and dreams with self advocates. *Intellectual and Developmental Disabilities* 45(5): 323–334.

Scottish Executive (2000) *The same as you? A review of services for people with learning disabilities*. Edinburgh: The Stationery Office.

Summers SJ and Witts P (2003) Psychological intervention for people with learning disabilities who have experienced bereavement: a case study illustration. *British Journal of Learning Disabilities* 31(1): 37–41.

Stroebe M and Schut H (1999) The dual process model of coping with bereavement: rationale and description. *Death Studies* 23(3): 197–224

Swain J. and Cameron C (1999) Unless otherwise stated: discourses of labelling and identity in coming out. In: Corker M and French S (eds) *Disability discourse*. Buckingham: Open University press.

Thomas C (2004) Disability and impairment. In: Swain J, French S, Barnes C and Thomas C (eds) *Disabling barriers: enabling environments*, 2nd edn. London: Sage Publications.

13 HIV/AIDS and bereavement

Rachel Unwin

Key messages

- Stigma and discrimination continue to hamper our approach to dealing with HIV/AIDS-related bereavement.
- People who are HIV positive can experience survivor guilt when others die before them.
- Survivor guilt may also arise within the person who has transmitted the infection to another person.
- Owing to the combined effects of HIV/AIDS and poverty in sub-Saharan Africa, the consequences of bereavement are devastating, with increasing numbers of orphans requiring care.
- Support for the bereaved through HIV/AIDS must suit the situation/context and be culturally appropriate.

Introduction

The purpose of this chapter is to examine some of the consequences of HIV/AIDS for bereavement care. Although HIV/AIDs care is not context specific, that is acute care or primary care, it does represent a very specific body of evidence that relates bereavement to issues of stigmatised loss. It is for this reason that the chapter has been included. Additionally, it seeks to illuminate the tragic consequences of HIV/AIDS in Africa, which are significant for the bereaved.

Emerging very strongly from the literature are the global effects of HIV/AIDS with very different responses and approaches to dealing with the consequences. Stigma and discrimination have been and continue to be key features of our response to this pandemic in all countries. The issue of bereavement has been, in many ways, sidelined as efforts to tackle the spread of HIV and change behaviours are pushed to the forefront. Where efforts to deal with the effects of bereavement are made in the West, research has largely focused on individual or group support. In developing countries the stark struggle to meet basic human requirements has taken over as poverty, political instability and the effects of war combine with HIV/AIDS to cause devastation.

It is now well known from the history and background of HIV since the 1980s that certain factors were prominent. In the Western world young people were losing friends and family, and were likely to have experienced many losses (Goodkin and Blaney 1996). For some the number of deaths experienced has been in the hundreds (Leaver *et al.* 2008). In other parts of the world, especially Africa, HIV/AIDS has affected communities on a far larger scale with many children now orphaned (Matshalaga and Powell 2002). The purpose of this chapter is to provide a global perspective to the issue, examine the available evidence relating to bereavement support and identify challenges for the future.

Background to HIV/AIDS

When cases of *Pneumocystis carinii* (now called *P. jirovecii*) and Kaposi's sarcoma were identified in young males in Los Angeles in 1981 it was realised that a previously unrecognised disease was emerging. The Centers for Disease Control began tracking this disease and, following comparisons with researchers in France, the virus causing acquired immune deficiency syndrome (AIDS) was identified and the causative agent was named human immunodeficiency virus (HIV) (Keller and Fleming 1999). It has been estimated that 42 million people worldwide have been infected with HIV, with over two-thirds of this number being in sub-Saharan Africa. Worldwide 22 million people are estimated to have died, which includes half a million in America and around 18,000 in the UK (Averting AIDS and HIV 2008). It is the leading cause of death in South Africa with approximately 40 per cent of deaths being due to HIV/AIDS (Demmer 2007a,b).

Initially, in the West, the consequences of HIV/AIDS were very dramatic in terms of whole communities of young people, especially homosexual men, who were affected and died (Adler 2001). From the time that the HIV virus emerged in the Western world certain groups were targeted for health promotion and educational campaigns. These were homosexuals, drug users and sex industry workers. People who had received contaminated blood products, especially haemophiliacs, were also at risk and transmission from mother to child was found to be possible. Media and advertising campaigns were launched with an almost evangelical fervour, promoting the use of condoms, safe sex, clean needles and the message: 'don't die of ignorance'. Worldwide the focus is still on health promotion to reduce transmission; however, with the use of highly active antiretroviral therapies (HAART) life expectancy has considerably improved for some (Piot *et al.* 2001) and people are now living with HIV for some years, which has also changed the experience of loss and bereavement.

Stigma and discrimination: the hallmarks of HIV/AIDS

The sociologist Erving Goffman (1968) wrote about the nature of stigma, which could result in individuals having a spoiled or tainted identity and lead to prejudice and discrimination from others. Table 13.1 outlines some of the reasons why stigmatisation has become one of the hallmarks of HIV infection and also one of the major barriers to effective support for the bereaved. Mallinson (1999a) reports

Table 13.1 Stigma

HIV/AIDS is a life-threatening disease.

HIV infection is associated with behaviours (homosexuality, drug addiction, prostitution, promiscuity) which are already stigmatised.

Most people become infected through sexual activity.

There has been inaccurate information about how it is transmitted.

The virus has been seen to be as a result of personal irresponsibility.

Religious and moral beliefs have led some people to apportion moral blame to those who are infected with HIV and believe that it is a punishment.

Adapted from AVERTing AIDS and HIV (2008).

that many people have died as a result of AIDS in an atmosphere of shame and social stigmatisation which has left the needs of those bereaved neglected. The links with undesirable and socially unacceptable behaviours are paramount here; the implication being that these behaviours are under our control and therefore there is an element of individual 'blame' when contracting the virus.

The devalued status attached to the HIV-positive person can also be passed on to their closest family and friends and will affect the bereavement support (or lack of it) that may be forthcoming. This will not only affect the bereaved when talking about the HIV/AIDS-related death of someone, but also reduce health-promoting behaviours, test seeking and disclosure (of HIV status) in those with the virus (Steward *et al.* 2008). Sensitive communication skills, confidentiality, continuity of care and a non-judgemental, non-discriminatory approach are all crucial components of an effective health and social care system. These approaches should be applied equally to those affected by HIV/AIDS, including those who are bereaved (Madge *et al.* 2004).

When comparing groups of those bereaved by AIDS or cancer, Kelly and colleagues (1999) reported that the former group had less social support and were more likely to conceal the cause of death to family and friends. This can be illustrated by the case of Jean.

Jean had been married to Jim for 30 years. They had three grown-up children. Jim was an engineer who spent some months of the year working away mostly in Asia. On one of his trips home he became seriously ill. Jean was told that her husband was HIV positive and was showing all the signs that his illness had progressed to AIDS. Jean was shocked but also furious, feeling complete betrayal when she realised that her husband had visited prostitutes on his trips away. She was also concerned that she might be HIV positive herself. Jean chose to help care for her husband until he died some months later. She was adamant, however, that not even family members should know the cause of Jim's death. She tested negative for HIV.

This case study raises a number of implications. Jean cannot talk about her loss to anyone, not even her closest family. She cannot discuss the events surrounding her husband's illness and death because of the feelings of shame engendered. Jean was fortunate in having a supportive family around her. Her children did suspect that their father did not die of a 'tropical disease', but were very conscious of their mother's feelings and did not bring up the subject of how he may have become ill. They supported her by visiting regularly and by helping in whatever way they could. However, they were also grieving for their father and the grandfather of their children. They knew, however, that there were certain issues they could not discuss with their mother or others. These alluded to the precise nature of the illness that their dad died of and how he may have contracted such a disease. Such lack of a right to grieve has been called disenfranchised grief (Doka 2002) and may prevent or limit support within the family.

This tainted or spoiled identity of Jim may be passed to the family members through what could be viewed as no fault of their own and thus they may be seen as victims. This has also been the case for haemophiliacs who were infected with HIV after receiving clotting factor concentrates VIII and IX in the 1970s and 1980s (Eyster 2008). In 1985 alone, over 1,000 people in the UK with haemophilia were diagnosed with HIV. Subsequently there have been around 2,000 deaths. Lord Archer's enquiry in the UK has only just concluded and has strongly criticised the fact that contaminated blood products were given when systems should have been in place to prevent this happening. In France, Fillion (2008) has described this as 'serious iatrogenic damage'. In France, some health ministers and personnel were successfully convicted of negligence. In Japan, Mizota and colleagues (2006) reported extreme anger and resentment towards the authorities that had allowed this to happen. Families of haemophiliacs who had died as a result of HIV felt isolated in their bereavement and unable to discuss their loss.

A collection of over 60 interviews has been compiled by the Haemophilia and Life History project carried out at the University of Brighton and supported by the Lottery Fund (http://www.livingstories.org.uk/) (now housed within the British Library Audio catalogue). This catalogues the differing experiences of people who were infected with HIV as a result of treatment for haemophilia and also the experience of bereavement; for example, the mother who described not only feeling guilty for passing on the genetic material that resulted in her son having haemophilia but also guilt at having administered, by injection, the contaminated blood products which eventually went on to cause his death.

Implications for bereavement care: a grief unspoken

We have already acknowledged in Chapter 1 that bereavement is part of the human condition and as such should be viewed as a 'normal' or 'natural' experience. Many people experience a number of losses in their lives which, given time and support, may even lead to personal growth and enrichment. We have also explored the difficulties that may be encountered by individuals where certain risk factors are present (see Chapters 5 and 6). For those bereaved as a result of HIV/AIDS there may well be factors that will lead to more specific difficulties in acknowledging and expressing grief, particularly due to the nature of the disease and social responses to it.

Not only may disclosing the cause of the loss and talking about it be very difficult or impossible but those who are bereaved may also be living with the knowledge or prospect that they are or may be infected with HIV. Coping with illness and AIDS-related bereavement has been shown to lead to more complicated grief reactions and increased psychological distress (Folkman 1997; Ghebremichael *et al.* 2006). Part of this distress may arise from survivor guilt, as those who are HIV positive continue to live whilst family/friends have died. Caroline Guinness (2001) describes these feelings, having lived with HIV since 1986. She states:

> The psychological effects were strange. Having prepared myself for death I found myself strangely afraid of life. I also had a strong sense of 'survivor's guilt'. I had lost so many close friends and colleagues, and asked myself the question 'why me?'
>
> (Guiness 2001: 110)

Of course, this 'survivor guilt' may arise within the person who has transmitted the infection to another person. For example:

Andrew became infected with HIV through sexual contact with his partner Keith, who occasionally was involved in injecting drugs. Although they usually used condoms they had not done so on a few occasions. Keith discovered that someone he had shared needles with was HIV positive and after much soul searching decided to tell Andrew and suggest that they were both tested. Following testing they discovered that they were both positive. It was Andrew who first showed signs of ill health and although he was prescribed antiretroviral drugs he did not respond well. After various months of complications he died in a local hospice. Keith helped care for him and they had support of a local Body Positive group where they had made many friends. Both sides of the family had become estranged, largely on account of their sexuality, and in bereavement Keith sought support from amongst his circle of friends in the Body Positive group. He felt extreme survivor guilt that it was Andrew and not himself that had succumbed to worsening illness, and he struggled for some time with this.

Conversely, in terms of psychological support for HIV-positive individuals in London, Orr and colleagues (2004) questioned whether services in the city were also meeting the needs of heterosexual men as effectively as homosexual men. In a London clinic they concluded that referrals to the psychological unit were more common for homosexual men. However, they were surprised to find that heterosexual men required more help in bereavement and were referred for outside help. Although there were issues with the sample of men included, Orr and colleagues (2004) do comment that services need to be adept and responsive to meeting the needs of a diverse range of HIV-positive people.

Support for HIV-positive individuals in bereavement: do we know what helps?

When looking at bereavement interventions in general, regardless of the cause of death, there are already many doubts about the need for professional support (also see Chapter 16). In a systematic review, Forte and colleagues (2004) found no rigorous evidence that interventions (group, individual counselling) were effective in 'treating' the bereaved other than pharmacological treatments for depression. Stroebe and colleagues (2005) found no evidence that emotional disclosure facilitates adjustment to loss in normal bereavement. However, some of the work which has been conducted relating to HIV/AIDS bereavement has indicated that individuals who attend supportive group sessions may benefit. Leaver and colleagues (2008) described such benefits for bereaved HIV-positive individuals who attended a group retreat in Ontario. Benefits were categorised in terms of bereavement experience, sexual and social relationships, psychosocial well-being and resiliency.

There has also been research in North America examining the experience of bereaved HIV-positive individuals in relation to immunological and physiological function. This research has attempted to identify whether interventions (group or individual) could affect disease progression. Clinical indicators such as CD4 T-cell counts (as an indicator of immunological function) and the onset of symptoms have been used in addition to indicators of psychological status (Goodkin *et al.* 2001; Center for the Advancement of Health 2003). It is already acknowledged that bereavement itself has negative consequences for physical and mental health in general and increases risk of mortality (Stroebe *et al.* 2007) (see also Chapter 1). However, there appears to be no conclusive evidence to suggest that particular types of support may promote the body's immunological function and thus hold off the progression of illness in HIV-positive individuals.

Other studies looking at the effects of group therapy for bereaved HIV-positive individuals reported that those who scored higher on 'psychiatric distress' seemed to do better when attending a group session (Ghebremichael *et al.* 2006; Sikkema *et al.* 2006). Those who appeared to achieve most benefit were those who could be considered at risk of complicated grief reactions. This could include such factors as a previous history of a mental health problem (including substance misuse), those with reported low self-esteem, those with few social supports and those who had experienced multiple losses.

In order to try and understand how individuals may react differently in bereavement, Goodkin and colleagues (2001) developed a theoretical model generally specific to those bereaved through HIV/AIDS, the 'Stressor–Support–Coping' model. This identified three principal variables relating to psychosocial variables. These variables related to life stressors (S), burden, social support (S) and coping (C). The model was designed to predict who may be likely to experience the greatest psychological distress. So for example if someone had experienced many losses, had minimal social support and had a negative style of coping they would be predicted to demonstrate greater distress. This model has been used in some of the studies looking at the mediating effects of interventions and to predict those who may develop more complicated reactions in bereavement (Goodkin and Blaney 1996). It has been concluded that more research would be needed to validate this model's predictive potential in this area of bereavement. This model also resonates with the more general theories and models of bereavement examined in Chapter 1 or as part of end of life care examined in Chapter 5.

In examining the personal characteristics of those who are bereaved as a result of HIV/AIDS, some studies have identified positive psychological states existing in men caring for partners dying from the disease (Park and Folkman 1997; Bonanno *et al.* 2005; Rogers *et al.* 2005; Cadell 2007). This is in spite of the issue of multiple losses with a consequent reduction in personal and social support. More recent studies have involved groups other than gay men drawing attention to gender differences and it may be that women are at increased risk of complicated grief reactions including thoughts of suicide (Sikkema *et al.* 2004).

Supportive approaches

From the time that HIV/AIDS emerged, the response from those sections of the community most strongly affected has been to form groups and supportive networks. This is perhaps no different from other charities and organisations which have arisen to support people affected by diseases such as heart disease or dementia, for example. Part of the aim of these organisations has been for like-minded people with similar experiences to come together to provide support of various kinds. The drive within HIV/AIDS charities has additionally been to support sections of the community who may be marginalised because of their sexuality or behaviours. Coming together with those who are in a similar position has been the key to this type of support. At the beginning of the epidemic in the 1980s, there was a great deal of misinformation and fear engendered, which led to groups of people feeling very vulnerable and isolated. Before the widespread use of antiretroviral therapies, many people were dying.

In the UK the Terrence Higgins Trust was established as early as 1982, in memory of the first gay men in the UK to die from AIDS. It is now the largest sexual health charity in the UK. There are many other examples of charities that support those who are HIV positive, those caring for partners/family members with AIDS and providing support groups and social networks into bereavement. In the UK almost half of the new diagnoses in 2005 were made in London (Health Protection Agency United Kingdom 2009). For this reason support services for those affected by HIV/AIDS in the UK have developed more strongly in London.

In terms of health and social care responses to HIV/AIDS there are a variety of statutory services that may be involved in support, though how far this would extend to support into bereavement is difficult to tell. Much of the literature in the UK about HIV/AIDS has traditionally been geared towards sexual and mental health issues, prevention of transmission and living with HIV. There has been less mention of support in bereavement. Globally, there is a similar situation. There is a small section on the Joint United Nations Programme on HIV/AIDS (UNAIDS) website, dedicated to psychological care, which mentions bereavement (UNAIDS 2009).

The difficulties of seeking supportive contact in bereavement can be illustrated by the case of Bill and Linda, whose only son, Peter, died in his mid-30s as a result of AIDS.

> Peter was born when Linda was nearing her late 30s and she had almost given up hope of having any children. As a couple they were even more aware of the generation gap between themselves and their son. He told them when he was 24 years old that he was gay and, although this was not what they wanted to hear, they supported him and welcomed any friends of his. His death was devastating to them and they felt that they had no one to speak to other than their local doctor. Despite numerous suggestions by their doctor that counselling might help, Bill and Linda were resistant. They belonged to a generation for whom 'talking about death' was unusual. However, eventually they relented nearly 1 year after Peter had died. They found it an extremely painful process but were amazed themselves gradually at how much relief they felt. The counsellor also put them in touch with another couple in a similar situation. With sensitive handling they began to understand and deal with some of their intense grief.

On a global scale the World Health Organization launched its AIDS strategy in 1987, and this has now been replaced by UNAIDS (Joint United Nations Programme on HIV/AIDS). This has primarily been to educate populations in order to prevent further transmission of HIV/AIDS. However, the former director of UNAIDS, Peter Piot (Piot and Coll Seck 2001), stated that 'HIV related stigma may well be the greatest obstacle to action against the epidemic, for individuals and communities as well as political, business and religious leaders' (p. 1109).

Parker and Aggleton (2003) argue that rather than look at stigma and discrimination in relation to HIV/AIDS as a matter of individual or social psychology, it should be seen in terms of power, inequality and social exclusion. Using human rights legislation to raise resistance to discrimination is one way forward. An example of this is in Mumbai, India, where the Lawyers Collective is raising awareness among young people with HIV of their legal rights as citizens and patients. This has also extended to doctors and other health care workers (Piot and Coll Seck 2001).

Mallinson (1999b) urges those in supportive relationships to remove the 'shame, blame and stigma' (p. 29), in order to facilitate open and trusting relationships. There will be aspects of HIV/AIDS which make this more difficult, but essentially we should be adopting similar compassionate and caring approaches regardless of diagnosis of the deceased.

Caring and compassionate approaches

Annual Aids day is an international commemoration which is now 20 years old. On 1 December each year, countries throughout the world remember in their own way those who have died and reflect on the actions that still need to be taken to ameliorate the effects of HIV/AIDS. Remembering those who have died has become part of many communities' mourning: AIDS memorial quilts in the USA or candlelit ceremonies at which the names of those who have died are read out have become important ways for some to openly acknowledge their losses. Some of these commemorations have attracted 'celebrity' status with people, such as Elton John and Bono of U2, taking on prominent positions to raise awareness and funds for HIV/AIDS charities.

One of the positive aspects of this response has been an attempt to tackle stigma and discrimination where it exists and to focus on living positively with HIV/AIDS. Many services in the UK and the West provide information and support for individuals and groups. For the gay communities who may feel isolated this has also been viewed as creating a sense of 'family' to provide on-going support.

HIV/AIDS and the African context

In terms of the African context and the impact of HIV/AIDS upon bereaved communities, Demmer (2007c) describes this as differing in many ways from a European or North American context as a result of:

* pervasive poverty;
* limited access to anti retroviral (ARV) treatment;
* scarce resources;
* high levels of AIDS-related stigma;
* gender inequality;
* high levels of unemployment;
* crime and violence.

In fact, Demmer (2007a) states that the AIDS epidemic in Africa is on a 'scale far larger, more complex and overwhelming than that witnessed elsewhere in the world' (p. 839). A major issue is the number of children who have been left orphaned especially in sub-Saharan Africa (Kidman *et al.* 2007). Although the care of these children may pass to other family members, this is not always possible. Many orphans live on their own in child-headed households or with grandparents. These bereaved orphans are more likely to come from a poor background and be HIV positive themselves (Cluver and Gardner 2007; Kidman *et al.* 2007). A scene in Malawi is described: 'Outside there were gangs of children living on the streets, orphaned by AIDS. And it seemed that everywhere, any time of day, people were hungry. Living on the inedible . . . banana skins, corn husks, grass seed, eating grass to survive . . .' (Bono 2006: 6).

Although this scenario might not apply to AIDS orphans it illustrates the potential lack of someone to care and provide sensitive, emotional support. Li and colleagues (2007), in a useful review of evidence, indicate that such a lack can result in behavioural problems often expressed as anger and depression.

Stigmatisation and discrimination is an enormous barrier resulting in social isolation and rejection by communities. Not talking about HIV/AIDS is more usual in order to try and escape the negative effects (Wood *et al.* 2006). It has also been identified that where there are attempts to establish bereavement programmes they are more likely to be based on Western approaches to palliative care, which are unlikely to be appropriate. In China, the stigma of being an orphan is considered 'bad fate' and this would affect the subsequent support of children in addition to the link with HIV/AIDS (Zhao *et al.* 2007). Importing the types of interventions carried out for the bereaved, if not appropriate, is unlikely to assist and until some of the differences identified by Demmer (2007a) are addressed then it is difficult to see what might be effective. However, this should not deter engagement with the bereavement issue in these communities albeit with a view to developing context specific interventions.

Conclusion

Where does this leave us when faced with people who have experienced loss through HIV/AIDS? On a global scale different strategies will apply depending on the circumstances. The stigmatising nature of HIV/AIDS is still undoubtedly felt and experienced in most parts of the world and this could be considered one of the key differences from other illnesses. The effects of HIV/AIDS are global. Despite stigma and discrimination continuing to hamper our interventions, it is clear that many HIV-positive people are surviving longer and experiencing the effects of treatment more than the effects of the disease itself. Perhaps this calls for a shift in the way practitioners respond in a compassionate and caring way by understanding need and becoming re-educated about the bereavement needs of people who are HIV positive. Clearly, support for the bereaved through HIV/AIDS must suit the situation/context and be culturally appropriate. It must also be cognisant of the wider issue of how death from HIV/AIDS can impact on a wide range of people, not only the family but those who form the friendship circles and support groups that are so effective in promoting the well-being of those surviving the disease.

References

Adler MW (2001) Development of the epidemic. In: Adler MW (ed.) *ABC of AIDS*, 5th edn. London: BMJ Publishing Group.
Averting AIDS and HIV (2008) *HIV and AIDS stigma and discrimination*. Available at: http:// www.avert.org/aidsstigma.htm (accessed 1 October 2009).

Bonanno G, Moskowitz JT, Papa A and Folkman S (2005) Resilience to loss in bereaved spouses, bereaved parents, and bereaved gay men. *Journal of Personality and Social Psychology* 88(5): 827–843.

Bono (2006). Preface. In: Conroy A, Blackie MJ, Whiteside A, Malewezi JC and Sachs J (eds) *Poverty, AIDS and hunger: breaking the poverty trap in Malawi*, 1st edn. Basingstoke: Palgrave Macmillan.

Cadell S (2007) The sun always comes out after it rains: understanding posttraumatic growth in HIV caregivers. *Health & Social Work* 32(3): 169–176.

Center for the Advancement of Health (2003) *Report on bereavement and grief research*. America: Project on death in America of the Open Society Institute of the Soras Foundation.

Cluver L and Gardner F (2007) Risk and protective factors for psychological well-being of children orphaned by AIDS in Cape Town: a qualitative study of children and caregivers' perspectives. *AIDS Care* 19(3): 318–325.

Demmer C (2007a) Responding to AIDS-related bereavement in the South African context. *Death Studies* 31(9): 821–843.

Demmer C (2007b) Grief is a luxury: Aids-related loss among the poor in South Africa. *Illness, Crisis & Loss* 15(1): 39–51.

Demmer C (2007c) Coping with AIDS-related bereavement in KwaZulu-Natal, South Africa. *AIDS Care – Psychological and Socio-Medical Aspects of AIDS/HIV* 19(7): 866–870.

Doka K (2002) *Disenfranchised grief: new directions, challenges, and strategies for practice*. Champaign, IL: Research Press.

Eyster ME (2008) Coping with the HIV epidemic 1982–2007: 25 year outcomes of the Hershey Haemophilia Cohort. *Haemophilia* 14(4): 697–702.

Fillion E (2008) Clinical relationships tested by iatrogenicity: the case of haemophiliac patients faced with the epidemic of transfusional AIDS. *Social Science and Medicine* 67(9): 1400–1409.

Folkman S (1997) Introduction to the special section: use of bereavement narratives to predict well-being in gay men whose partners died of AIDS: four theoretical perspectives. *Journal of Personality and Social Psychology* 72(4): 851–854.

Forte AL, Hill M, Pazder R and Feudtner C (2004) Bereavement care interventions: a systematic review. *BMC Palliative Care* 3(3): http://www.biomedcentral.com/1472-684X/3/3/.

Ghebremichael MS, Hansen NB, Zhang H and Sikkema KJ (2006) The dose effect of a group intervention for bereaved HIV-positive individuals. *Group Dynamics* 10(3): 167–180.

Goffman E (1968) *Note on the management of spoiled identity*. London: Penguin Books.

Goodkin K and Blaney NT (1996) Bereavement and HIV infection. *International Review of Psychiatry* 8(2/3): 201–217.

Goodkin K, Baldewicz T and Blaney NT (2001) Physiological effects of bereavement and bereavement support group interventions. In: Stroebe MS, Hansson RO, Stroebe W and Schut H (eds) *Handbook of bereavement research: consequences, coping and care*. Washington, DC: American Psychological Association.

Guiness C (2001) Having AIDS. In: Adler MW (ed.) *ABC of AIDS*, 5th edn. London: BMJ Publishing Group.

Health Protection Agency (2009) Last update. Available at: http://www.hpa.org.uk/web/HPAwebfile/HPAweb_C/1287145127922 (accessed 15 June 2011).

HIV Life History and Research Team (2003–2007) Experiences of people living with haemophilia and HIV. Available at: http://www.livingstories.org.uk/categoryaudio_id_45.html (accessed 19 February).

Keller J and Fleming WD (1999) HIV and AIDS: a clinical sociological application of assumptions and principles developed by the International Work Group on Death, Dying, and Bereavement. *Illness, Crisis and Loss* 7(3): 287–309.

Kelly B, Edwards P, Synott R, Neil C, Baillie R and Battisutta D (1999) Predictors of bereavement outcome for family carers of cancer patients. *Psychooncology* 8(3): 237–249.

Kidman R, Petrow S and Heyman S J (2007) Africa's orphan crisis: two community-based models of care. *AIDS Care* 19(3): 326–329.

Leaver CA, Perrealt Y and Demetrakopoulos A (2008) Understanding AIDS-related bereavement and multiple loss among long-term survivors of HIV in Ontario. *Canadian Journal of Human Sexuality* 17(1–2): 37–51.

Li L, Wu Z, Wu S, Zhaoc Y, Jia M and Yan Z (2007). HIV-related stigma in health care settings: a survey of service providers in China. *AIDS Patient Care and STDs* 21(10): 753–762.

Madge S, Matthews P, Singh S. and Theobald N (2004) *HIV in primary care*, 2nd edn. London: Medical Foundation for AIDS and Sexual Health.

Mallinson RK (1999a) Grief work of HIV-positive persons and their survivors. *Nursing Clinics of North America* 34(1): 163–177.

Mallinson RK (1999b) The lived experience of AIDS-related multiple losses by HIV-negative gay men. *Journal of the Association of Nurses in AIDS Care* 10(5): 22–31.

Matshalaga NR and Powell G (2002) Mass orphanhood in the era of HIV/AIDS. *British Medical Journal* 324(7331): 185–186.

Mizota Y, Ozawa M, Yamazaki Y and Inoue Y (2006) Psychosocial problems of bereaved families of HIV-infected hemophiliacs in Japan. *Social Science and Medicine* 62(10): 2397–2410.

Orr G, Catalan J. and Longstaff C (2004) Are we meeting the psychological needs of heterosexual men with HIV disease? A retrospective case controlled study of referrals to a psychological medicine unit in London, UK. *AIDS Care* 16(5): 586–593.

Park CL and Folkman S (1997) Stability and change in psychosocial resources during caregiving and bereavement in partners of men with AIDS. *Journal of Personality* 65(2): 421–447.

Parker P and Aggleton P (2003) HIV and AIDS-related stigma and discrimination: a conceptual framework and implications for action. *Social Science & Medicine* 57(1): 13–24.

Piot P and Coll Seck AM (2001) International response to the HIV/AIDS epidemic: planning for success. *Bulletin of the World Health Organization* 79(12): 1106–1112.

Piot P, Bartos M, Ghys PD, Walker N and Schwartlander B (2001) The global impact of HIV/AIDS. *Nature* 410: 968–973.

Rogers ME, Hansen NB, Levy BR, Tate DC and Sikkema KJ (2005) Optimism and coping with loss in bereaved HIV infected men and women. *Journal of Social and Clinical Psychology* 24(3): 341–360.

Sikkema KJ, Hansen NB, Ghebremichael M, Kochman A, Tarakeshwar N, Meade CS and Zhang H (2006) A randomized controlled trial of a coping group intervention for adults with HIV who are AIDS bereaved: longitudinal effects on grief. *Health Psychology* 25(5): 563–570.

Sikkema KJ, Hansen NB, Kochman A, Tate DC and Difranceisco W (2004) Outcomes from a randomized controlled trial of a group intervention for HIV positive men and women coping with AIDS-related loss and bereavement. *Death Studies* 28(3): 187–209.

Steward WT, Herek GM, Ramakrishna J, Bharat S, Chandy S, Wrubel J and Ekstrand ML (2008) HIV related stigma: adapting a theoretical framework for use in India. *Social Science and Medicine* 67(8): 1225–1235.

Stroebe MS, Schut H and Stroebe W (2007) Health outcomes of bereavement. *The Lancet* 370(9603): 1960–1973.

Stroebe W, Schut H and Stroebe M (2005) Grief work, disclosure and counselling: do they help the bereaved? *Clinical Psychology Review* 25(4): 395–414.

UNAIDS (2009) Uniting the world against AIDS. Available at: http://www.unaids.org/en/ (accessed 22 February 2009).

Wood K, Chase E. and Aggleton P (2006) 'Telling the truth is the best thing': teenage orphans' experiences of parental AIDS-related illness and bereavement in Zimbabwe. *Social Science and Medicine* 63(7): 1923–1933.

Zhao G, Li X, Fang X, Zhao J, Yang H and Stanton B (2007) Care arrangements, grief and psychological problems among children orphaned by AIDS in China. *AIDS Care – Psychological and Socio-Medical Aspects of AIDS/HIV* 19(9): 1075–1082.

14 Bereavement and occupational health

Rosemary Shaw

Key messages

- A holistic approach is essential to the recovery of the bereaved and this should include consideration of the working environment.
- Human resource departments and managers have a very important role and are sometimes the first people to speak to the employee after bereavement.
- Support should be given by colleagues at the funeral, for example by sending flowers and cards and making phone contact. The bereaved person needs to know that their employer and colleagues care for them and this can assist their bereavement journey and return to work.
- The bereaved employee should not be avoided. If appropriate, work colleagues should consider meeting the bereaved employee outwith work, for example for lunch, before the bereaved individual returns to the workplace.
- A phased return to work should be available, tailored to each individual.
- Occupational health staff should be aware of agencies that provide bereavement support in their geographical area.
- The various types of support that need to be available in the workplace for people whose employment is affected by bereavement
- Parental leave may be necessary if children are involved.

Introduction

This chapter will consider the bereavement needs of working people whose employment is affected by bereavement. What support should be available in the workplace for this person and what should be in place to support the bereaved employee returning to work? The role of occupational health staff, line managers, colleagues and human resources in caring for the bereaved employee will be considered. However, from the outset it is important to highlight the paucity of evidence in this area of practice and also the importance of all parts of any employing organisation working together to provide support and care.

These days people from teenage years to late adulthood spend more of their waking hours at the workplace than at home and this is a significant aspect of life. Despite the work–life ratio there is limited evidence of occupational health practice in relating to bereavement support. However, it is still possible to high-light some key elements that may assist the bereaved. If you are reading this then you may be an occupational health practitioner who, like me, is interested in improving practice related to bereavement as it is often a neglected area. As a practitioner, you may have already had a great deal of experience of dealing with the bereaved and supporting their return to work, although in many cases the pro-cess may have been handled by others, for example human resources. Therefore, the occupational health practitioner may not be involved and their role may be unclear, although it may, at least, include the provision of advice and information to the bereaved.

Some people may not consider bereavement to be a health issue and therefore no protocols or procedures may be in place in your occupational health depart-ment to address this, other than for death at work, for which very particular protocols and guidance exist. However, as described in previous chapters, there are health consequences of bereavement that could be ameliorated. My experi-ence as an occupational health nurse and a bereaved person helped me to realise that there are a number of factors that could enhance care in the workplace and which need to be more fully considered in occupational health terms.

Occupational health

Occupational health has changed dramatically since the first factory nurse, Phillipa Flowerday, was employed in 1872. It has also become more specialised and focused on health and safety in the workplace and so it is unlikely that occu-pational health nurses will now, as Flowerday did, visit employees in their own homes. Occupational health and in particular occupational health nurses (OHNs) are now an established part of the nursing profession. OHNs are entered onto the third part of the Nursing and Midwifery Council (NMC) Register, which is related to public health nursing. Similar specialisation occurs in medicine and other health-related professions.

There is a general, worldwide consensus that the twentieth century has seen significant changes in patterns of employment (Aw *et al.* 2007). Technological advances and improvements in communication have also allowed for more con-tinuous production and increased flexible working hours (Arnold 2005). Logically one may assume that the concept of health at work should be of paramount importance to employers to ensure that the workforce is able to deal with such changes. However, it is largely considered to be negative factors such as sickness absence and inability to perform at work that result in referrals to the occupational health departments (Wilkinson 2001).

Occupational health is defined as the science concerned with the effects of work on health and health on work, with the main aim being to prevent ill health from arising (Aw *et al.* 2007). Occupational health services have also largely been associated with the identification and control of hazardous substances in the workplace (Wilkinson 2001), assessing fitness for work and protecting those who may be vulnerable to adverse working conditions.

Assessment of fitness for work after bereavement is equally important and returning to work at the right time can assist recovery, whereas delay could aggravate a sense of uselessness, isolation and lack of confidence. The occupational health practitioner (OHP) can play an important role in the return to work for the bereaved person and this could enhance a positive health culture within the organisation. There is also a need to recognise that, as Bento (1994) points out, there is no place for sadness and grief at work and a need to get over it quickly. This can result in 'disenfranchised' grief where the person is not allowed or given permission to grieve (Doka 2002).

However, as Charles-Edwards (2005) rightly asks, 'Is grief and bereavement any of our business?' in the workplace. Bereavement may be viewed as something that happens outside work, often to others and those who are retired and no longer working. If only this were the case. Significant numbers of employees take leave for bereavement and yet little recognition of its effects are evident. Some never return to work, others are unable to return to their previous jobs, particularly if demanding, and there are those who move to state benefits for financial support (Corden *et al.* 2008). Charles-Edwards (2005) provides one of the few resources which seek to illuminate the problems, challenges and approaches to bereavement in the workplace. However, it does not specifically identify the role of occupational health practitioners.

Should the occupational health practitioner get involved? Occupational health practitioners have been identified as forerunners in protecting and promoting the health and well-being of the working population (Mullally 2003). Although these remain vitally important aspects of the service, the government has called for occupational health nurses to take on a broader public health-oriented focus (Mullally 2003). Bereavement may be considered something which has a public health involvement and, as identified elsewhere, we are now perhaps more aware that bereavement can impact on health. In addition, Dame Carol Black, the national (UK) Director for Work and Health, states that the profession should address non-work-related issues (O'Reilly 2007). This idea is reflected in current occupational health nurse training, which, in the UK, takes the form of a public health degree, rather than a specific occupational health qualification. Although these courses rarely consider bereavement, they may deal with some of the practicalities and responsibilities related to death at work (Health and Safety Executive 2006).

We appear to becoming an increasingly 'death defying' society with a need to consider bereavement as a public health issue as levels of societal support appear to be diminishing (Stephen *et al.* 2009). The workplace has great potential to be supportive and, as a setting for health promotion, provides access to a large number of people known to the bereaved (Department of Health 2003). The role of the occupational health practitioner could be instrumental in developing understanding and approaches to bereavement at all levels by knowing what resources are available locally. This would need to be developed in conjunction with management, employees and particularly human resources (HR) departments, who are normally responsible for, for example, compassionate leave policies. Corden and colleagues (2008) identify how supportive organisations can make a difference, through being understanding, having supportive colleagues, clients and HR departments, being able to have a structured return to work and allowing a flexible work pattern to enable accommodation of 'bad days' and other responsibilities.

Compassionate leave

Human resources is often considered a key department in many larger businesses/ organisations, especially in an economy where there is an increasing shift towards service-based industries. HR accounts for a large proportion of costs as it is considered important to business success.

Arguably, there is a moral right to compassionate leave, but there are differences in the way compassionate leave entitlement is provided. In some organisations the amount of leave may be minimal and may also be unpaid. It is often a decision made by the employee's line manager as to how much leave is required; for example a large company in the oil industry may allow line managers to give up to 4 days off after a bereavement. Should more time be required, the employee would have to visit their GP to be 'signed off work', although the time and medical reason for certification may vary. This flexibility is often highlighted as important so that if 'rightly judged can/will benefit the company as well as the individual' (Charles-Edwards 2005: 163). Although bereavement is not a medical diagnosis, being 'signed off' will allow the bereaved space to grieve, as early return to full-time work may not be in anybody's interest.

Where death is concerned, custom and local practice usually determines a prescribed period of authorised absence for the bereaved, whether paid or unpaid, as compassionate leave. If the contract of employment does not stipulate entitlement for compassionate leave, middle managers often make up their own minds about what is acceptable. What the law does not do is provide a general right to compassionate leave in the event of a death, although an individual company may have contractual provisions or policies. There are also statutory provisions in the Employment Rights Act (HMSO 1996) that should facilitate unpaid leave in the event of the death of a dependant. However, for some employees the death that affects them most may be not a dependant but a friend or colleague. This is always the challenge of dealing with bereavement: the impact of a death is not always directly determinable.

A brief email survey by the author, to occupational health departments in large companies, suggests that most companies give 3–5 days' compassionate leave, with some companies giving up to 6 weeks, including the offer of counselling. These companies giving 3–5 days expect the employee to visit their GP. Should further time off be required, the sickness absence certificate may not state that the reason as bereavement.

Regardless of the length of time and support given to enable staff to come to terms with the death of a loved one, it is clear that there are likely to be stress factors that could undermine the health of the returning employee. Consider the following outline case:

Bill, a 50-year-old project manager with three school-age children, has just lost his wife and wants to return to work after 4 days' absence. What would you recommend if you were working in occupational health at his company? Should he have more time off work to grieve? Would his GP be the only source of support? How much control should Bill have over when he returns to work?

A study by the trade union Amicus (2006) revealed that a safe and healthy workplace, control over the working environment and fairness and dignity at work were among the key elements identified by staff as important in improving the quality of working lives. A common feature was that all bereaved employees eventually returned to work. To assist the needs of those in such circumstances, occupational health departments could be involved in all stages of return to work. After the death of a loved one it is difficult to concentrate and cope with the stresses of coming to terms with a loss, while maintaining work standards, particularly if, like Bill, you also have other personal demands which may need assistance outside the work environment (see assessment of risk in Chapter 5). Although each person's experience of loss and grief is unique there are some common feelings and symptoms often experienced by those who are grieving. These include sadness, betrayal, anxiety, fear, mistrust, irritability, guilt, anger, tension, depression and loss of confidence. Grieving people also often develop physical symptoms such as abdominal pain, headaches, insomnia, fatigue, changes in appetite, increased drug or alcohol use, restlessness, absentmindedness and poor concentration. These responses to and symptoms of grief can significantly impact on a person's ability to function at work and yet may be rarely assessed or considered.

Although some companies may offer counselling services in or outside the workplace these may not necessarily be appropriate (see, for example, Chapter 15). An important part of the return to work is resuming relationships with work colleagues. In-house support from occupational health practitioners could assist in this process, by supporting both the bereaved and their work colleagues. From personal experience the most important aspect when returning to work after a death is the support and help of work colleagues, and yet they are often unsure of what to do.

Returning to work

For some people returning to the workplace is an overwhelming burden whilst they are still grieving. Once back at work, some workers experience reduced work performance caused by lack of concentration and memory, tiredness and sleepless nights, and feelings of sadness and depression. However, grieving workers may often worry that they will lose their job from reduced work performance or because of extra time taken off from work, which may compound their grief.

It may be possible for the bereaved to arrange a visit to the workplace before they return to work just to have a chat with their line manager and relevant colleagues, if only to 'break the ice'. Although coming back to work on a phased return can help some people it is not for all. I remember how helpful it was when colleagues invited me to lunch, outside work, prior to my returning after the death of my husband. It 'broke the ice' and allowed my loss to be discussed in a safe environment rather than in whispers at work or in more public spaces.

When a person returns to work after a death, colleagues can be embarrassed about what to say, if they say anything at all. In general it is useful to find a way to acknowledge their loss openly and as quickly as possible (Charles-Edwards 2005). This should take the form of a private discussion and be as natural as possible, although it is never easy. The offer of practical and emotional support is always worth considering. It may not be needed as friends and family may help at this time. However, work communities may be equally supportive and offer support such as bringing in a meal or offering to take the children to school. Therefore it is important for occupational health departments and practitioners to 'educate' other members of staff on how to support a colleague who is bereaved. Charles-Edwards (2005: 230) provides a checklist for colleagues for when a bereaved person returns to work:

Do
- Respect their reticence and their openness.
- Acknowledge the loss. Care more about the person than your own embarrassment.
- Encourage the person to talk, if they want to.
- Enable people to cry without loss of safety or self-respect.
- Reassure them that very powerful, vivid and unfamiliar feelings and dreams are a normal part of grieving.
- Check whether close colleagues know of the bereavement.
- Check whether the bereaved wants others to be informed (who and how).
- Acknowledge important anniversaries suitably and sensitively (deaths as well as births, weddings, etc.).
- Discourage people from taking major decisions (job change, house move, etc.) early in the bereavement.

Don't
- Pressurise them to get on with work if it is not essential.
- Minimise the impact of the loss.
- Reassure, when what is needed is permission to share grief.
- Limit the time in which support is given.
- Expect bereaved colleagues to be 'back to normal' quickly.
- Let your embarrassment stop you offering support.

Achieving all the dos and don'ts is probably unrealistic but using the items on the checklist may raise awareness and some colleagues may accept and adopt the messages.

Of course, it is also the case that the person who is bereaved may need a similar list as they may expect to just slot back into the workplace and carry on as before. Although for some this may be advantageous, it can often reduce the opportunity to experience and express grief and could contribute to development of complicated grief. Men, in particular, are reluctant to express their feelings but this does not mean they are not experiencing intense grief.

A colleague and I both lost our husbands suddenly in the last 5 years. We both feel that, based on our personal experience, the support we received from work friends and colleagues was paramount in enabling us to return to work. We received flowers and cards and letters of support from work colleagues and offers of help. It made us feel that people whom we spend a lot of time with at work cared and were concerned. Colleagues also attended the funeral of our husbands; some had never met them, but they made it clear that they were there to support us. Again, their support at the funeral was very much appreciated.

We also received assurances that our work was covered and that everyone was aware of the situation. Before our return to work, we were both invited out for lunch with colleagues who were genuinely concerned and wanted to know how we felt; it was a safe environment. We both had a month off work and our line managers allowed us to come back to work on a phased return. When we returned we found it difficult to concentrate and appreciated the shorter days. My colleague had young children and was able to take most of her leave at that time during the school holidays and, in negotiation with human resources, some unpaid leave to allow her to be with the family. Such flexibility assisted both the 'grief work' and the return to work. The continued support that we have from colleagues remains important to us and has enabled us to manage our workload successfully.

However, we both appreciate that not everyone works in a supportive workplace. The role of OHPs in all settings could be to give support and advice to the bereaved and their colleagues and to line managers and HR staff so that managing the bereaved employee and their successful return to work can be more effective.

Death at work

For occupational health practitioners there has been an increasing engagement in health and safety issues at work. Therefore any deaths which occur at work due to lapses in health and safety will inevitably involve them, although this involvement may not necessarily be considered from the bereavement perspective. There are, of course, many practical aspects to consider when someone dies at work. Some of these will depend on the nature of the death but it is good to have some form of strategy in place (for an outline example see Safeworkers website) that, like other organisational policies or guidance, is reviewed on a regular basis. In addition, the Health and Safety Executive (http://www.hse.gov.uk) in the UK provides protocols and guidance about dealing with death in the workplace related to England, Wales and Scotland (see, for example, Health and Safety Executive 2006).

The Chair of the Health and Safety Commission in the UK, Sir Bill Callaghan, in response to a rise in the number of people who died at work in 2006/7 (241

from 217 the previous year), highlighted that 'Behind every one of these numbers was a man or a woman, with a life, friends and family' (Health and Safety
Executive 2009). In addition, it might also be suggested that there will be work
colleagues who will be affected and who may need support, particularly if there
are feelings of guilt from death through suicide or negligence.

Charles-Edwards (2005) draws on work by Mayhew (1997) in relation to some
useful and appropriate responses to sudden death at work:

- Be aware of staff who have suffered other traumas as their experiences of
  distress and grief may be compounded.
- If appropriate, encourage staff to contact home before the event is publicised
  in the media.
- Staff who are absent should be informed of the event so that they do not hear
  of it indirectly or arrive at work without knowing.
- Ensure a co-ordinated and sensitive management response.
- Expect short-term reduced efficiency from staff, including those who may not
  be directly involved.
- Encourage (but do not compel) all staff to return to work the following day.
- Arrange a debriefing, if possible within 48 hours of the incident, preferably
  within 24 hours.

Although some of the issues in the list will be determined by the organisation,
the role of the OHP could be significant. For example, they could be aware of
staff who may be significantly affected by the death, provide a point of listening
and in the future possibly provide counselling for all staff, or refer them on, and
additionally assist in the debriefing session. They may also provide support for the
line manager and senior managers who are dealing with staff and the dead person's relatives and possibly police, health and safety investigators and the media.

Conclusion

Bereavement is an important aspect of a person's life that can, and often does,
impact on their work. It challenges those who are bereaved in returning to their
work following a significant loss. It also challenges those in the workplace, from
workers to senior managers, to address bereavement in an appropriate manner.
How well this challenge is addressed is relatively unknown and how much of
bereavement support is provided by occupational health services is also hidden.

There are therefore a number of challenges and questions for occupational
health services in respect of bereavement. To what extent are occupational health
practitioners knowledgeable about bereavement and its consequences? How is
bereavement viewed in the workplace and incorporated into leave and return to
work patterns? Can workplaces become better prepared to deal with the bereaved
and how can occupational health services assist with this process?

Finally, based on my personal and professional experience it is important to
take care of the bereaved employee and show an interest by asking periodically
how they are. It also needs to be recognised that support should continue.

References

Amicus (2006) Unions and good work: results of an amicus survey on the quality of peoples work experience. Available at: http://www.unitetheunion.org/news__events/archived_news_releases/2006_archived_press_releases/amicus_survey_reveals_secret_o.aspx

Arnold J (2005) *Work psychology: understanding human behaviour in the workplace*. London: Prentice Hall.

Aw TC, Gardiner K and Harrington JM (2007) *Occupational Health*, 5th edn. Oxford: Blackwell Publishing.

Bento RF (1994) When the show must go on: disenfranchised grief in organizations. *Journal of Management Psychology* 9(6): 35–44.

Charles-Edwards D (2005) *Handling death and bereavement at work*. Oxford: Routledge.

Corden A, Hirst M and Nice K (2008) *Financial implications of death of a partner*. Social Policy Research Unit, University of York.

Department of Health (2003) *Taking a public health approach in the workplace: a guide for occupational health nurses*. London: HMSO.

Doka KJ (2002) *Disenfranchised grief: new directions, challenges, and strategies for practice*. Campaign, IL: Research Press.

Health and Safety Executive (2006) *Work related deaths: a protocol for liaison*. Available at: http://www.hse.gov.uk/scotland/workreldeaths.pdf

Health and Safety Executive (2009) Bill Callaghan press release 241 lives lost is unacceptable. Available at: http://www.hse.gov.uk/press/2007/c07011.htm

HMSO (1996) Employment Rights Act. London: HMSO.

Mayhew G (1997) Post-traumatic stress. In Feltham C (ed.) *The gains of listening: perspectives on counseling at work*. Buckingham: Open University Press.

Mullally S (2003) *Taking a public health approach in the workplace: a guide for occupational health nurses*. London: HMSO.

O'Reilly N (2007) OHN tsar Dame Carol Black calls for occupational health practitioners to work more closely with GPs and employers. Available at: http://www.personneltoday.com/articles/2007/05/15/40520/oh-tsar-dame-carol-black-calls-for-oh-practitioners-to-work-more-closely-with-gps-and-employers.html

Safeworkers Website (n.d.) *When an employee dies at work*. Available at: http://safeworkers.co.uk/EmployeeDeath.html.

Stephen AI, Wimpenny P, Unwin R, Work F, Macduff C, Dempster P, Wilcock SE and Brown A (2009) Bereavement and bereavement care in health and social care: provision and practice in Scotland. *Death Studies* 33(3): 239–261.

Wilkinson C (2001) *Fundamentals of health at work: the social dimensions*. London: Taylor & Francis.

Part III

Education, interventions and organisation of bereavement care

15 Professional development for health and social care practitioners

Peter Wimpenny

Key messages

- There is a need to consider how a better understanding of bereavement can be fostered in our society.
- Educational programmes should include supporting students to examine personal loss, to be multiprofessional, where possible, and to consider appropriate cultural values and beliefs.
- Courses or programmes need to consider a wide range of clinical and social contexts as these require specific/targeted input. They should also consider the nature of communication with the bereaved, particularly around the time of death.
- As with other educational provision there is limited evidence demonstrating impact on practice.
- There is an acknowledged challenge to including death, dying and bereavement in educational programmes that could be addressed through nationally driven initiatives, such as the development of principles/guidelines/curricula/cascadable programmes rather than local, variable provision.
- A tiered model of education could provide an appropriate structure through which educational provision could be organised.

Introduction

Increasingly organisations and practitioners are building up their skills and knowledge in bereavement care (Klein and Alexander 2003). The perceived burden of bereavement on services, the development of end of life/palliative care standards, and the increasing amount of evidence related to bereavement are factors that have created this environment.

If we want to enhance care for the bereaved there are a number of ways in which this could be addressed. First, at a societal level we need to become more informed about the nature and impact of bereavement, much like any other public health campaign. This may involve engaging with children through schools. Second, educational provision for those in volunteer roles, who at present provide the majority of bereavement care, particularly in respect of counselling types of interventions. Finally, there is a need for education for those in professional roles and also those who may come into contact with the bereaved in, for example, general hospital settings. This should include nurses, medical staff, social workers, physiotherapists, occupational therapists, volunteers and those who are on information/admission desks, porters and mortuary staff.

Society and bereavement

Through the later decades of the twentieth century, particularly in Western contexts, death, dying and bereavement are topics that have become hidden from everyday life, even though they will be experienced by everyone (Johnson 2004). Perhaps, as Arnason and Hafsteinson (2003) report, we need to encourage discussion of how death, dying and bereavement can be absorbed into wider society in a way that makes them more acceptable. There may be a place for media campaigns and public service broadcasts that mirror other campaigns such as those for smoking, alcohol use, heart disease or mental health. At a national and international level agreed assumptions and principles and national strategies may assist (International Work Group documents, Nucleus Group 2004). In the political context, the desire to see all services working together is frequently expressed and assumes that at present there is limited co-ordinated activity.

It has also been suggested that the societal level of awareness of death, dying and bereavement should be tackled through raising awareness in schools (Stephen *et al.* 2009). This could be either as distinct components or through inclusion in a variety of subjects such as history, social subjects or science (Ribbens-McCarthy and Jessop 2005). Children are often older when they encounter death and bereavement (see Chapter 2) and may have had limited opportunity to discuss this within their families before they reach adolescence. It may also be the case that schools could provide support for pupils (Lowton and Higginson 2003) as they may have better access to resources and be in a position to identify any consequences of bereavement. Teachers may, of course, require additional education and may be reluctant to get involved, although they could, with additional knowledge, become aware of the kind of support that is available and what may help, for example the Seasons for Growth Programme highlighted in Chapter 2.

Future education about bereavement for health and social care professionals should be organised and provided on a national scale. The Centre for Advancement of Health (CAH) (Genevro 2004) review states that there is little evidence available on education and training for health care professionals. Questions such as: is it adequate? what should it cover? when should it be done? and does it make a difference? remain unanswered. This is not to say that there is no evidence available, merely that it is relatively limited and at the lower end of traditional evidence levels. Making clear links between education provision and improved outcomes is difficult to demonstrate. However, when health and social care professionals are asked about bereavement, they often identify a need for further education and training (Stephen *et al.* 2006), often irrespective of setting and culture (Chan *et al.* 2007). This is perhaps not surprising as it is may be only briefly addressed in undergraduate curricula (Stephen *et al.* 2009). There is perhaps an assumption that practitioners will either learn from others or draw on their own experience. Although both of these can be valuable it may be contended that few other aspects of health or social care would be assigned solely to such a personal and experiential approach. The International Work Group on Death, Dying and Bereavement (1991) indicates that education on death, dying and bereavement should be a 'required, distinct and substantive' part of programmes for all health care professionals. A central aspect of such education, and highlighted as challenging and problematic, is breaking bad news.

Breaking bad news and communicating with the bereaved

It is highly probable that the way we communicate and break bad news in the period around death will have an impact on the manner in which those affected will grieve and subsequently adapt. However, it can make us feel extremely uncomfortable and we are often uncertain what to say. I remember very clearly, as a new member of staff in a coronary care unit, accompanying a senior house officer (SHO) to break bad news to a woman whose husband had died soon after entering the unit. I had expected that I could learn from the experience; and I did. The SHO remained standing and said something like 'Hello Mrs Jones, I'm Doctor Evans, your husband is dead', and with that she left the room. Although I could in no way have been as shocked as Mrs Jones, I was left sitting next to her now wondering what to say – I don't remember what it was but it was probably something of little consequence that addressed my need to break the silence. I felt an urge to get out of the room as quickly as possible as well, to ease my discomfort. Why was it so difficult to know what to say and do? And why had nobody rehearsed this with me as they had for wound dressings, making beds, giving injections and so on? The extent to which training or education for communicating in such sensitive periods of time is incorporated into health and social care curricula is probably minimal. It compares badly with much of the technical care skills and associated knowledge acquisition that populate courses.

However, Alexander and Klein (2000) offer some general guidelines and identify that these should be 'used flexibly and tailored to meet the specific needs and circumstances of those who are to be told' (p. 11). In a later paper they identify the influence that attitudes and behaviours of professionals can have on the bereaved; this is particularly the case in the initial phase immediately after the death (Klein and Alexander 2003). The following are provided as a guide:

- *Consider the setting*. Always try to find a quiet room. Avoid interruptions from a pager, mobile phone or colleagues looking for you to go for coffee.
- *Listen*. And, if in doubt about what to say, say nothing. The bereaved will not welcome being talked at and irrespective of your oratory style will not be able to listen in such circumstances. It is best to provide the opportunity for the bereaved to vent feelings and provide opportunity to ask questions. What you need to avoid is, as I had done, beating a hasty retreat back to the safety of the ward or unit office.

- *Tolerate their reactions*. The bereaved are often angry, not necessarily with us, but we must refrain from becoming defensive – 'well we did our best so don't be angry with us!' It is much better to try and normalise their feelings – 'I think I can understand why you are feeling angry and upset at the moment'.

- *Ban the cliché!* Because we feel uncomfortable, insecure and anxious about death-related topics, we sometimes fall back on clichés or euphemisms, learned from films or soaps and by listening to others: 'He's passed on.' Remember that such comments may be hurtful. Or 'He has gone to meet his maker' (reference to God and avoids use of death). The point is to avoid being patronising and unkind by being aware of the potential that your response has; for example do not say 'it's a blessing', as it may not be to the bereaved relative. At the time of a miscarriage or death of a neonate, it is not helpful to say 'you can always try for another baby'. At the same time, minimising the impact can also sound very uncaring: 'well it could have been worse if Jim had died as well'. Often we try to maintain sensitivity to people at the time of death, although at times it is difficult to be aware of the vulnerability of the bereaved.

- *Identify sources of help*. In the immediate period after the death this may be undertaken by the bereaved themselves as they draw on relatives and friends. Having a phone available in the room for the bereaved to use can be extremely helpful. Have good information which contains, for example, contact details for voluntary groups such as Cruse, although we need to be aware that support will not be available immediately from such groups. It should also contain contact details for you, the unit, the spiritual care department or the hospital bereavement service with the addendum that if there are further questions then the bereaved should be encouraged to call. Essentially, we do not know how or the extent to which information is given to the bereaved or indeed the best approach to such provision.

Additionally, if there is reason to suspect that grieving may be difficult because of some of the factors identified earlier in this book you may want to consider contacting primary care staff so that early contact can be facilitated. However, this, in my experience, is unusual and limited connectivity between, for example, secondary and primary care occurs in respect of the bereaved, other than to report the death.

So what if you find yourself in the position of having to take responsibility for communicating to relatives and friends that someone has died? You can of course always seek to delegate the job but this should perhaps be to someone who, for example, knows the family well, is better prepared to speak to the bereaved at that time or knows more about the care and situation leading up to the death, and not to the most junior member of staff. However, we must accept that there is no set approach; each situation will be different.

Alexander and Klein (2000) suggest three questions that may help you to prepare:

1 Am I properly prepared in relation to:
   - Whom I will meet?
   - What information I might need?
   - Where I can speak to the bereaved?
   - How I look (clothes that are stained with blood or other bodily fluids might be distressing for relatives)?
2 Have I thought about how I am going to share the bad news?
   - It is usually helpful to state your name, role and involvement.
   - Find out what they already know and what they want to know.
   - Speak slowly and use pauses to check if what you have communicated has been received. We often tend to speak too quickly when we are anxious and, additionally, the bereaved may be distressed and this will affect attention and memory.
   - In an effort to ameliorate the bad news we can sometimes be less than truthful. If possible don't; it can backfire and people are much more familiar with health-related terminology than you might think.
3 What will I do when I have delivered the bad news? Sharing the news is not just an event but, for the bereaved, the start of a journey that is at this stage somewhat uncertain. The following may be helpful to consider:
   - Allow time for the person(s) to absorb what you have said.
   - Don't leave them alone immediately after the bad news is given and offer for someone to stay with them; this could be you, so make sure others in the clinical area are aware of this.
   - Ensure the bereaved know what will happen next (support with clear concise written information as well), for example seeing the body, collecting the death certificate, post-mortems and taking home belongings. This last is an issue all of its own as it is often the case that staff believe they have to put everything in a bag, even if it is ripped, soiled or the like. In addition the type of bag may be more of a bin liner than one in which possessions may be carried.
   - Establish who else may be available to support the bereaved; this will obviously depend on who is present, the sort of death, the time of death and the assessment of the bereaved. This last is particularly difficult if the death is sudden and unexpected.

If at all possible, opportunities to practise can be valuable, in order to gain a certain framework and confidence in breaking bad news. Ultimately, this will help the bereaved begin their journey, rather than leave them confused, uncertain and still angry. The communication process around death, dying and bereavement is one of the main areas of complaint to the health or public service ombudsman in the UK, often accounting for over 50 per cent of cases. Again it may be that health care professionals need greater support to improve their practice. I remember clearly an elderly man who came onto the medical ward I was working on as a third-year nursing student. He was in the terminal stages of cancer. He was on the ward a number of days and I provided care for him consistently. He died just as visitors were entering the ward and we managed somehow to screen his bed and take his daughters into the 'sister's office'. They were distressed by his death and I was totally useless as I had assumed at that time that because his death was 'expected' and he was deteriorating very quickly that they would be 'pleased' to see he had died peacefully. They were not. It is important to remember not to assume how the bereaved may react to death, whether sudden or 'expected'. Always seek to use an approach like the framework given by Alexander and Klein above and consider what mechanisms are in place to support you.

Professionals and bereavement

The review of evidence by the Center for Advancement of Health (Genevro 2004) reports that, for health care professionals, longer periods of contact with the bereaved before death tend to increase their own feelings of grief. It has therefore been suggested that practitioners may have some degree of disenfranchised grief (Doka 2008; Genevero 2008) as they are not able to 'work through' their grief. A dear colleague, Neil Gordon, once suggested that when he explored death and dying with nurses he found what he called the juke box model whereby once one of the deaths was 'played' it was followed by all of the others. A similar feature is noted by Shanafelt and colleagues (2003) when unresolved emotions related to death and dying are shelved, and if not resolved build up and eventually 'overflow' with personal and professional consequences. Therefore, it might be suggested that support as well as education should be available for health and social care professionals. Who should provide such support is rarely formally identified although healthcare chaplains have often been assigned to, or adopted, such a role (Mowat 2008) whilst many practitioners will also use colleagues, friends and family. You may want to consider if there is any identified means of support for you in your work area. Whom do you talk to about deaths and your own needs?

The CAH review (2003) indicates that health care workers who receive education on death and dying are more comfortable in dealing with grief and bereavement, although this does not necessarily mean they are less anxious. Most professional groups have identified a need for further educational provision, including GPs and community nurses (Johnston *et al.* 2001; Barclay *et al.* 2003), acute care practitioners (Douglas *et al.* 2002), physiotherapists (McAteer and Murray 2003), medical students (Field and Wee 2002) and social workers (Kramer 1998). In addition, Wass (2004) identifies the need for paramedics to undertake education, as they are often faced with acute and traumatic death and dying. Even dental schools (Johnson and Henry 1996) are now more likely to include some education, on death, dying and bereavement in the undergraduate programme.

Although these are mainly uniprofessional approaches, there is no doubt that education on bereavement could, and perhaps should, be undertaken within the increasing approach of interprofessional learning as it is high on the list of all professional groups (Llamas *et al.* 2001) and not just within palliative care settings.

Provision of education

One of the key factors identified for education is the need to ensure that the course or programme addresses the experiences and needs of the participants (International Work Group on Death, Dying and Bereavement 1991; Gould 1994; Papadatou 1997; Douglas 2002; Wass 2004). Specific groups, within the broad range of health and social care professionals, may require specific training/education. Papadatou (1997) seeks to highlight specific need for this training in respect of children's deaths, Ng and Li (2003) for those working in learning disability settings, and DiMarco and colleagues (2002) and Thomas and Kohner (1994) for those who deal with perinatal deaths. Although there will of course be common themes in bereavement across all areas of practice, it appears appropriate to suggest that any educational provision needs to be specifically focused within the context of the practitioner's work. The International Work Group on Death, Dying and Bereavement (1991) and Doorenbos and colleagues (2003) also support the principle that any education should be interdisciplinary in nature, examining the different professional perspectives whilst at the same time seeking similarities.

Wass (2004) contends that the inadequacy of educational preparation threatens the quality of bereavement interventions and suggests that consensus on the knowledge, skills and personal understanding required is necessary. A recent Scottish policy document (*Shaping Bereavement Care*, Scottish Government Health Department 2010) identified a number of core components for educational programmes (Table 15.1).

Such core components could cut across a variety of contexts and provide the basis for development of educational provision.

Several papers describe specific educational initiatives (Gould 1994; Thomas and Kohner 1994; Papadatou 1997; Kramer 1998; Di Marco *et al.* 2002; Douglas *et al.* 2002; Matzo *et al.* 2002; McAteer and Murray 2003). Particular approaches to teaching have been described in the literature: use of humanities, such as literature, poetry, drama, music, art (McAteer and Murray 2003), metaphor (Gould 1994), volunteer parents (Thomas and Kohner 1994), illustrative case histories (Matzo *et al.* 2002) and videos (Thomas and Kohner 1994; Matzo *et al.* 2002). Only anecdotal evidence exists to support the effectiveness of any of these approaches but it appears that an eclectic mix of provision may be the most beneficial.

Table 15.1 Core components of educational programmes

Emphasis on the *normality of grief*

Considering bereavement care in three stages: before the death, around the time of death and following the death

Communication skills, including the management of distress

Recognition of risk factors in grief and awareness of applicability, accessibility and limitations of assessment tools

Theories and models of grief and the nature of grief

Self-awareness and reflection

Curriculum content and teaching

Curriculum content in this area, in most health-related programmes, may have increased and the approach to teaching death, dying and bereavement positively changed since the 1980s. However, in UK medical schools it is still often associated with palliative care education (Field and Wee 2002) and viewed as challenging to deliver (Fuller 1999), factors which are still present (Billings *et al.* 2010). In social work programmes death, dying and bereavement may be spread throughout courses, which may leave practitioners feeling ill-prepared as insufficient attention is paid to awareness of personal experiences and specific knowledge and skills (Kramer 1998).

Nursing education is also deficient in dealing with this topic, although nursing schools in the USA have sought curriculum change for bereavement but often draw on bereavement models that may be inappropriate in all settings, or now outdated (Coolican *et al.* 1994). However, there is a paucity of literature relating to the situation in the UK. A national US programme for nurses, End-of-Life Nursing Education Consortium (ELNEC), was developed to assist nurses in dealing with death, dying and bereavement and evaluated by Ferrell and colleagues (2005). The cascade process used initiated change at faculty level that appeared to impact on educational provision (a similar medical programme had also been developed). Significant improvements in students' knowledge were demonstrated in six out of nine modules. However, 0 per cent improvement in knowledge was reported for the grief and loss module. Grief and loss was also unique in being the only module where mastery improvement was not significant. The authors (Ferrell *et al.* 2005) suggest this is because responses may have been influenced more by personal experience than by knowledge. You might want to consider where and how you gained your knowledge about bereavement. How much do you rely on personal experience of bereavement and loss to know what may be appropriate to provide to others?

However, exploring the personal dimension of bereavement and experiential learning are often viewed as crucial components of bereavement-related education and are highlighted in several other educational initiatives (Gould 1994; Thomas and Kohner 1994; Papadatou 1997; Kramer 1998; Matzo *et al.* 2002; McAteer and Murray 2003; Wass 2004). This is an interesting perspective as it has implications for future educational provision and should be investigated further. Can knowledge and understanding increase if no account is taken of personal experiences and how might these be managed? Teaching bereavement (including grief and loss) acontextually, as though it were formal knowledge, may be inappropriate, although facilitating groups where personal experiences may be brought to the surface requires a skilled facilitator and these may be thin on the ground (Fuller 1999).

Some on-line US programmes exist that may help volunteers and practitioners (http://itrs.scu.edu/fow/), although these may be more related to death and dying than bereavement. This may also be the case for the UK-based Open University course on Death and Dying (http://www3.open.ac.uk/courses/bin/p12.dll?C01K260), although reports of increasing impact related to bereavement and bereavement care are reported (Silverdale and Katz 2003, 2005). Addressing the personal experiences of bereavement and providing bereavement care can still be raised in such programmes, although the level of facilitator and group support may be less overt and students may opt out of any exercises which encourage reflection on difficult or personal bereavement experiences.

It may also be the case that bereavement education should always be undertaken in conjunction with education on death and dying, as influencing practitioners to facilitate a 'good death' can clearly impact on the bereaved. The Department of Health in England and Wales has funded a range of initiatives aimed at developing and implementing bereavement training including some on-line developments. These initiatives appear to cover a range of perspectives, from that related to post-mortem guidelines to general grief and bereavement courses in a variety of local settings. Again, the extent to which bereavement and bereavement care can stand alone and where its boundaries lie is important to consider.

Table 15.2 details the content of some of the courses identified. As can be seen, the content related to bereavement is often combined with other aspects of death and dying that may involve the practicalities of dealing with death through an examination of death and bereavement in specific contexts through to an examination of sociological explanations. It would appear that educational provision for bereavement and bereavement care includes some of the broader understandings related to death and dying.

Cultural factors and education

A small amount of education-related literature highlights the need to ensure inclusion of cultural factors in education. Matzo and colleagues (2002) discuss cultural considerations in the context of the ELNEC programme, outlined above. They identify culture as including ethnicity, race, gender, age, differing abilities, sexual orientation, religion and spirituality, socio-economic factors and place of residency. In addition cultural competence is seen as a key factor. Dowd and colleagues (1998) perceive the need for a more 'relevant' cultural model for death, dying and grief education that deals with communication, space, social organisation, time, environmental control and biological variation. The above highlight how complex the issues surrounding death, dying and bereavement can be and the extent to which these have been adequately addressed in educational provision.

From a slightly different perspective Doorenbos and colleagues (2003) argue for the inclusion of anthropological, ethical and sociological content into end of life programmes. They argue that students need to have their awareness raised of impact of culture on death, dying and grief (anthropology), how ethical and moral factors affect any care and the context of spiritual and religious factors (sociology). Again this illustrates the difficulties of separating out death and dying from bereavement and also the extent to which there are broader fields of study that may add to understandings.

On a more practical note Hunt (2002) outlines the use of a 3 × 3 bereavement table to assist volunteers and professionals of different cultures, races and faiths to identify key areas of bereavement across the time span from 'immediate', through

Table 15.2 Some identified educational programmes to assist volunteers and practitioners

Curriculum topics	Type of course	Teaching strategies	Reference
Grief theory, phases of bereavement, role of clergy, cultural and religious beliefs and perinatal loss, children's responses to perinatal loss, losses in early pregnancy, strategies for care, parent reflections	One-day conference – perinatal loss	Lecture, small group presentations, role play case presentations, panel presentations	DiMarco *et al.* (2002)
Pregnancy and parenting tasks, grief theory, grief counselling, parent panel, miscarriage, ectopic pregnancy and infertility, cultural and religious perspectives, strategies for care, communication skills, children and death, role of the funeral director, parent support groups, role of the clergy, physician perspective, telephone follow up, getting started, care for the caregiver	Three-day conference – perinatal loss	Lecture, small group presentations, role play case presentations, panel presentations	DiMarco *et al.* (2002)
Attitudes towards death and dying, symptom relief in advanced terminal disease, analgesics for chronic pain, analgesics for cancer pain, communication with family members of dying patients, grief and bereavement, psychological aspects of dying, social contexts of dying, euthanasia, communication with dying patients, the experience of dying, certification of death, advanced directives, end of life hydration, religious and cultural aspects of dying, end of life nutrition, relating to patients with AIDS, neonatal issues, other physical therapy	Undergraduate medical education – themes across courses in UK medical schools	Seminar/small group discussion, role play, clinical case discussions, hospice visit, lecture, video/film, use of dying patient to address class, simulated patients	Field and Wee (2002)

Content	Course	Teaching methods	References
Nursing care at end of life, pain, symptom management, ethical/legal issues, communication, grief, loss, bereavement, quality care at the end of life, death Patient, family and nurse, nurse's role, the grief process, loss, mourning, grief and bereavement, cultural considerations, anticipatory grief, normal grief, complicated grief, risk factors, complicated reactions including disenfranchised grief, children's grief, stages and tasks of grief, factors affecting grief process, grief assessment, bereavement interventions, grief interventions, completion of bereavement process	End of Life Nursing Education Consortium Undergraduate Faculty Training Program	Lecture, use of literature, exemplars and case studies, role modelling, experiential learning, cumulative loss exercises, reflection, facilitated discussion	Matzo *et al.* (2003), Ferrell *et al.* (2005)
Paediatric hospice philosophy and principles of care, research and applications, chronic and life-threatening illness in childhood, factors affecting individual and family coping and adjustment, symptom control and management during terminal phase, psychological and spiritual care of the dying child and support of family, symbolic and creative methods of interaction with dying and bereaved children, grief process (parental and sibling bereavement) cultural aspects, impact of caring for a dying child and grieving families on professionals, stress management and prevention of burnout, ethical issues, developmental psychology; crisis intervention, counselling skills, systematic theory and applications to families facing illness and death	600-hour training programme on home-based palliative care for children dying of cancer	Class attendance, supervised clinical practice, participations in a sensitivity group, journal keeping, lectures, discussions, case presentations, simulations, role play	Papadatou (1997)
Society and death and dying; end of life care in practice; grief and bereavement, decision making at end of life	Distance learning module offered by the Open University in the UK	On-line learning, core text books specifically written for the course and other audiovisual resources	Silverdale and Katz (2003, 2005)

Table 15.3 Bereavement table

	Immediate	After several months	After a couple of years
Felt			
Shown			
Allowed/expected			

Source: Hunt (2002).

'after several months' to 'after a couple of years'. This is shown in Table 15.3 and seeks to encourage students to identify feelings and demonstrations of grief across a broad time line from immediate to 2 years after the death.

Such a simple tool may be a helpful aid to teachers in seeking to open up bereavement and to illuminate the diversity that exists among individuals, sexes and cultures.

The organisation of education for grief and bereavement

Organising education for health and social care practitioners requires consideration of who might need what type of programme. Offering only one type or level may reduce the likelihood of impact and assume that everyone needs the same irrespective of role.

Stephen and colleagues (2006) proposed a tiered model of educational provision (Figure 15.1).

This model is not unique to bereavement care and can be seen in other settings, for example health care-associated infection (West *et al.* 2006) and is commensurate

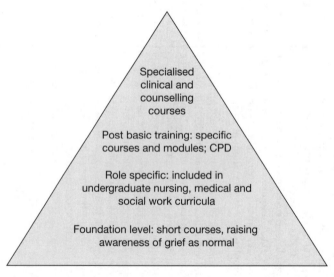

Figure 15.1 Tiered model of educational provision.

with that produced by O'Driscoll (2004) and described in Walsh and colleagues (2008). The model above seeks to illustrate the need for education from the fundamental level for those who have limited but important contact with the bereaved (for example hospital porters, reception and mortuary staff), through those with direct contact (for example nurses, midwives and medics) to those in specialist roles (senior nurses, medics and specialists) and skilled practitioners who provide services addressing complicated grief reactions (for example psychologists, counsellors and psychiatrists). There may, of course, be some development across these boundaries but such tiers could be a helpful model in planning provision at a local or national level.

Such a tiered model can fit the premises in the NICE (2004) guideline which highlights levels or components of support required, from the general level, requiring all bereaved to receive appropriate support and information, to the specialist level, where there is need for interventions for those who have complicated or prolonged grief (Figure 15.2).

Shaping Bereavement Care (Scottish Government Health Department 2010) seeks to put these into a framework for education and training within health care settings that would enable consideration of the numbers of staff involved at each level and how provision fits to a knowledge and skills framework (Department of Health 2004).

Component 1 – Core education and training for all staff: core principles – e.g. grief is normal, theories of grief, communication skills – self-awareness and how to respond to extreme distress.

Component 2 – Skills training for staff exposed to bereavement on a regular or deeper basis: e.g. initiating end of life conversations; informing family/carer of death; providing practical and psychological support

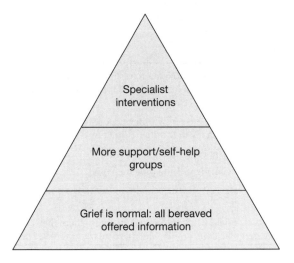

Figure 15.2 Tiered levels of support for bereaved, from NICE (2004).

> Component 3 – Specialist education and training for specialist staff: e.g. Core
> Dimension 1 Communication – management of complex grief; specialised
> training for staff's particular requirements.

It may also be argued that providing such education and training for staff will
increase morale and retention and have an impact on service as all staff will be
more able to offer support, not just those in specialist services (Charles-Edwards
2009). However, at present the quality of available education and training is
variable and likely to be driven by specialists or those with particular interests or
personal experiences. Moreover, it may be argued that provision of 'good practice' could be maintained with better education and training provision for staff
(Mackenzie and McCallam 2009), particularly in identified areas of practice.

The availability of support to practitioners raises concern because of its importance in ensuring staff are able to provide good-quality care, whilst at the same
time being able to access support. This could be provided either informally by
peers or through local debriefings. It can also be formal, for example as provided
by significant event analysis, clinical supervision and formal counselling.

The Shaping Bereavement Care group (Scottish Government Health
Department 2010) identified a number of principles that can be recommended in
respect of support, alongside education and training, for those who are involved
in providing bereavement care (Table 15.4).

Do you know what training, education and support are available in your own
area of practice? Do they cover all the components/levels and principles described
above? How could you influence this if these are not available?

Finally, it may also be argued that service provision for the bereaved could
mirror this tiered training and educational model as is described in the next chapter. The value of these tiered models is that they also represent the number of
people involved at each level with the numbers decreasing as the levels are scaled.
This is important, as it is essential to focus types of education, training and support on where they will have most impact.

Table 15.4 Principles of support

Management should recognise their obligation to support staff both through their involvement in the death of a patient and in their support of people who have been bereaved or when experiencing a personal loss
A supportive culture needs to be created within each organisation to facilitate staff coping with bereavement especially in traumatic situations
Time allowed for debriefing should become the norm
Links with spiritual care departments should be increased
A resource list of where to access support should be available for managers and staff alike
Particular consideration should be given for staff in areas where they are exposed to death and dying on a regular basis or following particularly traumatic deaths

Source: Scottish Government Health Department (2010).

Conclusion

Professional development in bereavement care is not easy or straightforward, as this chapter has sought to indicate, and will depend on a number of factors. For example, where we work and the personal nature of our own losses and experience can be so strong that they may either enhance or reduce our abilities to provide effective and appropriate care to the bereaved. It is clear that education, training and support are key features of professional development and these can have an impact both personally and professionally.

There are some fundamental aspects of practice in this area, such as breaking bad news, preparation of self and dealing with distress, that, although challenging, can be developed in all of us. In addition the provision of education, training and support related to bereavement care appears, at present, to be uncertain of what to include, although useful courses and resources exist locally and nationally. Determining need in each area and providing access to appropriate education, training and support could go some way to reducing the negative impacts on staff whilst at the same time enhancing care to the bereaved.

References

Alexander DA and Klein S (2000) Bad news is bad news: let's not make it worse. *Trauma* 2(1): 11–18.

Arnason A and Hafsteinson SB (2003) The revival of death: expression, expertise and governmentality. *British Journal of Sociology* 54(1): 43–62.

Barclay S, Wyatt P, Shore S, Finlay I, Grande G and Todd C (2003) Caring for the dying: how well prepared are general practitioners? A questionnaire study in Wales. *Palliative Medicine* 17(1): 27.

Billings ME, Engelberg R, Randall Curtis J, Block S and Sullivan AM (2010). Determinants of medical students' perceived preparation to perform end-of-life care, quality of end-of-life care education, and attitudes toward end-of-life care. *Journal of Palliative Medicine* 13(3): 319–326.

Chan MF, Lou F-L, Zang Y-L, Chung YF, Wu LH, Cao F-L and Li P (2007) Attitudes of midwives towards perinatal bereavement in Hong Kong. *Midwifery* 23(3): 309–321.

Charles-Edwards D (2009) Empowering people at work in the face of death and bereavement. *Death Studies* 33(5): 20–36.

Coolican MB, Stark J, Doka KJ and Corr, CA (1994) Education about death, dying, and bereavement in nursing programs. *Nurse Educator* 19(6): 35–40.

Department of Health (2004) *The NHS Knowledge and Skills Framework (NHS KSF) and the Development Review Process*. London: Department of Health.

DiMarco M, Renker P, Medas J, Bertosa H and Goranitis J (2002). Effects of an educational bereavement program on health care professionals' perceptions of perinatal loss. *Journal of Continuing Education in Nursing* 33(4): 180–186.

Doka KJ (2008). Disenfranchised grief in historical and cultural perspective. In: Stroebe MS, Hansson RO, Schut H and Stroebe W (eds) *Handbook of bereavement research and practice: advances in theory and intervention*. Washington, DC: American Psychological Association.

Doorenbos AZ, Briller SH and Chapleski EE (2003) Weaving cultural context into an interdisciplinary end-of-life curriculum. *Educational Gerontology* 29(5): 405–416.

Douglas M, Pemberton S and Hewitt B (2002) Addressing bereavement issues through education. *Nursing Times* 98(42): 36–37.

Dowd SB, Poole VL, Davidhizar R and Giger JN (1998) Death, dying and grief in a transcultural context: application of the Giger and Davidhizar Assessment Model. *Hospice Journal* 13(4): 33–47.

End-of-Life Nursing Education Consortium (ELNEC) (n.d.) Available at http://www.aacn.nche.edu/ELNEC/about.htm (accessed 16 June 2011).

Ferrell B, Virani R, Grant M, Rhone A, Malloy P, Bednash G and Grimm M (2005) Evaluation of the End-of-Life Nursing Education Consortium (ELNEC) undergraduate faculty training program. *Journal of Palliative Medicine* 8(1): 107–114.

Field D and Wee B. (2002) Preparation for palliative care: teaching about death, dying and bereavement in UK medical schools 2000–2001. *Medical Education* 36(6): 561–567.

Fuller J (1999) Teaching medical students about bereavement is hard [Letter]. *BMJ* 319(7216): 1071.

Genevro JL (2004) Report on bereavement and grief research. *Death Studies* 28(6): 491–575.

Genevro J (2008) A grief apart? loss and bereavement in healthcare staff. Presentation at Pathways Through Grief Conference, Dundee.

Gould JB (1994) 'A picture is worth a thousand words': a strategy for grief education. *Death Studies* 18(1): 65–74.

Hunt J (2002) The nine-cell bereavement table: a tool for training. *Bereavement Care* 21(3): 40–41.

International Work Group on Death, Dying and Bereavement (1991) A statement of assumptions and principles concerning education about death, dying, and bereavement for professionals in health care and human services. *Omega* 23(3): 235–239.

Johnson K (2004) Grief in North America, a death denying society. *International Journal of Palliative Nursing* 10(9): 435.

Johnson HA and Henry RG (1996) Death, dying, and bereavement education in dental schools. *Journal of Dental Education* 60(6): 524–526.

Johnston G, Davison D and Reilly P (2001). Educational needs in palliative care: a survey of GPs and community nurses. *European Journal of General Practice* 7(3): 99–103.

Klein S and Alexander DA (2003) Good grief: a medical challenge. *Trauma* 5(4): 261–271.

Kramer BJ (1998) Preparing social workers for the inevitable: a preliminary investigation of a course on grief, death, and loss. *Journal of Social Work Education* 34(2): 211–228.

Llamas KJ, Llamas M, Pickhaver AM and Piller NB (2001) Provider perspectives on palliative care needs at a major teaching hospital. *Palliative Medicine* 15(6): 461–470.

Lowton K and Higginson I (2003) Managing bereavement in the classroom: a conspiracy of silence? *Death Studies* 27(8): 717–741.

McAteer MF and Murray R (2003) The humanities in a course on loss and grief *Physiotherapy (London)* 89(2): 97–103.

Mackenzie J and MacCallum J (2009) Preparing staff to provide bereavement support. *Paediatric Nursing* 21(3): 22–24.

Matzo ML, Sherman DW, Mazanec P, Barber MA, Virani R and McLaughlin MM (2002). Teaching cultural considerations at the end of life: End of Life Nursing Education Consortium Program recommendations. *Journal of Continuing Education in Nursing* 33(6): 270–278.

Matzo, ML, Sherman DW, Lo K, Egan K, Grant M and Rhome A (2003). Strategies for teaching loss, grief, and bereavement. *Nurse Educator* 28(2): 71.

Mowat H (2008) *The potential for efficacy of healthcare chaplaincy and spiritual care provision in the NHS (UK): a scoping review of recent research.* Aberdeen: Mowat Research.

Ng J and Li S (2003) A survey exploring the educational needs of care practitioners in learning disability (LD) settings in relation to death, dying and people with learning disabilities. *European Journal of Cancer Care* 12(1): 12–19.

NICE (2004) *Improving supportive and palliative care for adults with cancer: the manual.* London: National Institute for Clinical Excellence. Available at: http://www.ipos-society.org/about/federation/EnglandNICEGuidelinesSupportiveCare2004.pdf (accessed 16 June 2011).

Nucleus Group (2004) *Review of specific grief and bereavement services: final report.* Melbourne: Department of Human Services, Victoria. http://www.health.vic.gov.au/palliative-care/archive/finalrep_grief.pdf (accessed 16 June 2011).

O'Driscoll, S (2004) Responding to bereavement in the acute care setting: a journey in service development. In Cruz L (ed.) *Making sense of dying and death.* Oxford: Inter-Disciplinary Press.

Papadatou D (1997) Training health professionals caring for dying children and grieving families. *Death Studies* 21(6): 575–600.

Ribbens-McCarthy J and Jessop J (2005) *Young people, bereavement and loss.* London: National Children's Bureau.

Scottish Government Health Department (2010) *Shaping bereavement care.* Edinburgh: SGHD.

Shanafelt T, Adjei A and Meyskins FL (2003) When your favourite patient relapses: physician grief and well-being in the practice of oncology. *Journal of Clinical Oncology* 21(13): 2616–2619.

Silverdale N and Katz J (2003) Changes in attitudes and practice toward dying people after completion of a UK based distance learning death and dying course. *Illness, Crisis and Loss* 11(2): 183–196.

Silverdale N and Katz J (2005) The impact of a distance learning death and dying course: an analysis of student self-reported changes. *Nurse Education Today* 25(7): 509–518.

Stephen AI, Wimpenny P, Unwin R, Work F, Macduff C, Dempster P, Wilcock SE and Brown A (2006) Bereavement and bereavement care: consultation and mapping of practice. Robert Gordon University, Aberdeen. Available at: http://www4.rgu.ac.uk/nursing/research/page.cfm?pge=41757 (accessed 16 June 2011).

Stephen AI, Wimpenny P, Unwin R, Work F, Macduff C, Dempster P, Wilcock SE and Brown A (2009) Bereavement and bereavement care in health and social care: provision and practice in Scotland. *Death Studies* 33(3): 239–261

Thomas J and Kohner N (1994). The death of a baby: training for staff in bereavement care. *Care of the Critically Ill* 10(2): 73–74.

Walsh T, Foreman M, O'Driscoll S, McCormack M and Curry P (2008) Bereavement support in an acute hospital: an Irish model. *Death Studies* 32(8): 768–786.

Wass H. (2004) A perspective on the current state of death education. *Death Studies* 28(4): 289–308.

West BJM, Macduff C, McBain M and Gass J (2006) *An evaluation of the development and implementation of the NHS Education for Scotland Cleanliness Champions Programme.* Aberdeen: Robert Gordon University.

16 Interventions, organisation of care and on-going support for the bereaved

Peter Wimpenny

Key messages

- The majority of bereaved people do not necessarily need or benefit from interventions such as counselling.
- Co-operation and co-ordination of accredited training and care from professionals is needed to meet the increased need for understanding grief, to recognise abnormal grief and to utilise counselling skills appropriately.
- Standards may be helpful to assist health and social care professionals and others to work together in a co-operative manner.
- Programmes for bereavement care should provide a continuum of care spanning primary, secondary and tertiary prevention.
- Further research into the efficacy of support in relation to age, gender, timing and mode of death is required.
- Services should provide a focus of care for high-risk and high-distress individuals.
- High-risk groups often benefit most from interventions and the results of therapy to people with psychiatric disorders following bereavement are often good. However, high-risk men appear to benefit from different interventions from high-risk women.
- Pharmacological treatment of depression during bereavement is beneficial without necessarily influencing the experience of grief. However, there is limited evidence for or against the use of anxiolytics.
- Care and services for the bereaved can be patchy and inconsistent and would benefit from some form of co-ordinated approach between all sectors.

Introduction

It is estimated that between four and eight people will be directly affected by one death (The Nucleus Group 2004; Wimpenny *et al.* 2007; SGHD 2010). How professionals intervene to assist these is an important question to address and may influence service provision. For example:

- Do all bereaved people need help?

- Do all health and social care professionals need counselling skills to deal with the bereaved?
- Who should co-ordinate activity for the bereaved?
- Is provision already adequate and how would we know?
- When should intervention occur and in what way?

This chapter seeks to address these questions by examining some of the available evidence on interventions and co-ordination.

The loss of someone can involve what Bowman (2000) calls 'shattered dreams', when people struggle to make sense of what has happened and experience more than just the loss of the person. The health and social care professional dealing with this may find it particularly challenging, as we have already discussed elsewhere, in all contexts of care. In the first instance there is a need, if possible, to develop a relationship with the bereaved before death, and also to use skills of breaking bad news and communication. There is often an immediacy of bereavement care that requires a range of practical and emotional engagement that will depend upon the circumstances of the death.

The period immediately surrounding and following death is particularly significant and it is worth repeating that the bereaved will remember clearly the manner in which staff were 'present' and how they communicated. A compassionate approach that is sensitive to the needs of the individuals involved has already been identified as having a positive impact on the subsequent bereavement journey and is something that should be reinforced (see, for example, Department of Health, Social Services and Public Safety, Northern Ireland 2009). Interventions to address this early period must also include any context-specific requirements, for example those related to acute care, maternity or children, and take account of any anticipatory grief, as discussed in Chapter 5.

Individual interventions

At the root of all strategies to assist the bereaved is the desire to help individuals deal with the physical, emotional, social and practical challenges which may arise following the loss of a loved one (Schut *et al.* 2001). At an individual level, there are a variety of strategies from counselling through various types of group therapy to social support (Forte *et al.* 2004). Despite many care options, from health, social, statutory and voluntary bodies, there remains a lack of consensus as to what constitutes an optimal type of support (Forte *et al.* 2004). These views are echoed by others (Allumbaugh and Hoyt 1999; Schut *et al.* 2001; Center for the Advancement of Health 2003; Schut and Stroebe 2005) and also in respect of interventions specific for children (Currier *et al.* 2007).

In addition, studies into the efficacy of bereavement interventions suffer from a lack of rigorous methodology. Forte and colleagues (2004) included 74 studies in their review and noted methodological problems in study design, replication, theoretical heterogeneity and variations between studies. These hamper the ability to draw firm conclusions. One of the problems with studies that have been conducted in this field relates to the recruitment of participants who may not have sought bereavement interventions themselves. Such studies may result in no effect or a negative one. The timing of interventions may also be significant, with interventions in the early period of loss affecting and possibly diminishing the natural social support of family and friends. In their earlier review of the efficacy of different individual interventions, Schut and colleagues (2001) conclude that, based on the evidence to date, 'the more complicated the grief process appears to be, or to become, the better the chances of interventions leading to positive results' (p. 731).

Stages/levels of intervention

Schut and colleagues (2001) distinguish between primary, secondary and tertiary interventions. The focus for primary intervention is all bereaved people; secondary interventions relate to people who are at higher risk of developing problems; and tertiary intervention would be for those who have developed problems. This appears a useful categorisation to use when considering the provision of interventions for the bereaved. Schut and Stroebe (2005) use the same categorisation in an update of the 2001 review and reach broadly similar conclusions that routine intervention for bereavement is not supported in research, although it is more effective for those with more complicated forms of grief. However, they do highlight that primary, secondary and tertiary interventions for children may be more effective.

Schut and Stroebe's (2005) review illustrates the paucity of good-quality research into the effectiveness of interventions, and the message is again a need for well-designed studies. Practitioners are often confronted with such messages and whereas it is imperative that research be carried out they may ask the question 'what should I do in the meantime?' There is no easy answer, and there are many different factors to be taken into account, such as the degree of effectiveness of the intervention, its appropriateness within the particular context, its feasibility in practice, the competency of the provider and how meaningful it might be for the bereaved.

If you are providing care for the bereaved in the period of time surrounding death, which has been alluded to throughout this book in different contexts, a compassionate and informed approach is invaluable in helping the newly bereaved. This may be something as simple as expressing your sadness at the loss or touching the person who is bereaved. These are simple acts which require practitioners to take the important step of engaging with the bereaved. Often this demonstrates a willingness to help and do more than just feeling sorry for their situation. Such gestures will be remembered and can make an important impact on the bereavement journey.

One primary intervention that may be useful later on is to enable the bereaved to tell their 'story'. This has been called 'death review' by some (Parry 1994), and incorporates the need people have to describe the circumstances of the death. This process of describing and adding meaning and emotion to what happened may be repeated frequently in the early stages. Where the person has good family or social networks this process will be accepted and the bereavement journey will be facilitated. However, if these social and familial networks are inadequate, then the risk of complicated grief may increase.

The key risk factors for bereavement, discussed in the end of life chapter (Chapter 5), highlight that, although it is not possible to quantify such factors or know which combinations may be significant, they can be helpful to determine individual needs. Some risk factors may be 'obvious', such as type of death, previous mental health problems, age and relationship with the deceased. Other factors may also affect bereavement; for example, it is often reported that men (see Chapter 3), in particular, have problems expressing their emotions (Crossland 1998) and so may not receive the same support as they are perceived to be 'coping'. However, not talking about grief should not be confused with not grieving. When considering interventions for men who have developed problems then, for example, combining therapy, which promotes verbalisation with art therapy in a cross-modality grief therapy programme, has been shown to be more beneficial than 'conventional' therapy alone in those with complicated grief (Schut *et al.* 1996). However, the key message here is that interventions must be tailored to the needs of the individual.

Interventions which reach out to the bereaved and show a desire to engage in a meaningful way are of the essence here. Some practitioners may have limited skills in terms of their intervention abilities although they may have a desire to help. Spending time with the bereaved actively listening to their story is being helpful; you may decide that the person is lost for ideas or unclear about the type of help they require. Mallon (2008) points out that the personal needs a person has at the time of loss are for love, support and companionship. The thing they want most, the return of their loved one, is not possible. The majority of bereaved people often require sound information and someone who is willing to listen and able to provide advice and help, including knowing how to access other specialist services such as counselling agencies, which form part of secondary approaches.

Counselling

It is difficult to generalise about the provision of counselling for people who are bereaved, given the variety of individuals and professionals involved from the voluntary and statutory sector (Machin 1998; Parkes 2000; Gallagher *et al.* 2005). It is also difficult to conclude who will most benefit from counselling. Parkes (2000) concluded from recently published studies, and years of experience in the field, that people who have suffered especially traumatic and unexpected types of loss and are vulnerable in other ways may benefit from counselling, as may those who do not have other support from families and friends. Therefore, if we consider the provision of services it seems appropriate that, as this group of bereaved will be fewer but require more support, it be undertaken by those with specific qualifications in bereavement counselling (see Chapter 15 on levels of education and training).

One of the most widely recognised organisations in the UK for bereavement support/grief interventions in the UK is Cruse. Cruse provide volunteers who undertake a validated programme for bereavement counselling and on-going support. However, the service provided is normally for those who have been bereaved for some weeks, rather than in the early phase. In addition it is a 'reach in' service – that is, the bereaved contact Cruse – and so relies on their willingness and ability to do so. The support from Cruse and other groups can be valuable although, given its voluntary nature, there may not always be the coverage required in all geographical areas, although general counselling services will normally be available.

Bereavement groups

In addition to one-to-one counselling there are a variety of bereavement groups offered by voluntary and statutory services. One of the difficulties of assessing the value of such groups is that most studies have looked at the experience of those attending, who are self-selecting, and may be more likely to express positive views (Thuen 1995; Thuen and Sandvick 1998; Zonnebelt-Smeenge and De Vries 2003). However, there are benefits from people coming together who are in similar situations, including sharing and normalising experiences and offering support to others (Hopmeyer and Werk 1994). Furthermore, there is variation in the running and leadership of groups from professional/counsellor to volunteer/lay person and therefore there may be variation in effectiveness.

Thuen (1995) describes setting up the Norwegian Bereavement Care Project and the survey conducted to look at the views of support group members. Although recognising the limitations of the sample the authors found that the social and emotional support offered by groups was the most valuable and the style of leadership crucial in influencing the groups. Groups may also be most beneficial for those later in their bereavement journey and perhaps for some particular sections of the bereaved community, such as men or older people, who may have less opportunity or desire to discuss their feelings elsewhere.

Professional approaches

Despite initiatives to support people to die at home 55–60 per cent of deaths still occur in general hospitals (Genevro 2004; SGHD 2010). This increases the need for health professionals to understand the grief and loss associated with death and be skilled in fundamental communication (Youll and Wilson 1996) (see Chapter 15 on education). Therefore, Parkes (2000) suggests health and social care professionals have not only the opportunity but the responsibility to assess bereavement risk in family members before or at the time of death, although there are considerable challenges and barriers to such assessment. Even within palliative care settings where assessment, formal and informal, has often been part of care provision (Relf *et al.* 2008), there remains concern about the reliability of tools, the completion process, the skills of those using them and the intrusive nature of the process at a time when it may not be appropriate to assess (see debate between Relf *et al.* 2009 and Agnew *et al.* 2010) (see also Chapter 5 for further information on risk assessment). It must be remembered that most care staff in general health and social care settings will not have engaged with assessment of the bereaved. With the concerns surrounding this process, at present the best approach may be to ensure that the bereaved are given enough information and opportunity to 'reach in', if and when they need support.

Building appropriate assessment of risk into health and social care settings is challenging but could hold potential for better identification of those at risk and appropriate provision of support. It has been well documented that bereavement following a sudden death is one such risk factor, and health professionals could target such high-risk individuals (Potocky 1993; Youll and Wilson 1996; Parkes 2000). In assessing the risk factors and symptoms of high-risk individuals, Potocky (1993) states there were no standardised definitions of high-risk or high-distress individuals for professionals. However, Parkes (2000) identifies these individuals as people who have unusual or unexpected types of loss or who are vulnerable.

Earlier, Raphael (1977) identified four independent characteristics of individuals who experience morbid grief when their spouse dies: a low level of social support during the crisis; moderate level of social support coupled with particularly traumatic circumstances of the death; an ambivalent relationship with the spouse; and a concurrent life crisis at the time of the death. Such individuals who are identified as being at high risk are more likely to benefit from counselling (Parkes 2000). Individuals who do not have such risk factors, Potocky (1993) suggests, are likely to experience normal grief and will not need professional help, although this is a general assumption; however, all bereaved people may benefit from better information and a means by which 'reaching in' may be better facilitated and co-ordinated.

Interventions for prolonged or complicated grief

For the 5–10 per cent of people who do not adapt 'normally' to their loss, the grief process can become problematic, resulting in a reduced quality of life. Although many terms have been used to describe this, there is a perspective emerging in the literature that this should be identified as prolonged or complicated grief (Prigerson *et al.* 2009). This is covered more fully in the chapter on mental health and bereavement (Chapter 6) as it is within this field that provision of interventions will be most appropriate. However, it is worth highlighting some key features of prolonged or complicated grief and interventions.

The common variables for complicated grief seem to be that the intensity of the grief reaction is either too much or too little and the duration is too long or too brief, in conjunction with other risk factors such as nature of the loss, cultural expectations, involvement of personality factors and unresolved earlier losses (Marwit 1996).

Jacobs and Prigerson (2000) indicate that a range of different psychotherapies (cognitive behavioural therapy, crisis intervention, brief dynamic psychotherapy, behaviour therapies, group therapy, other interpersonal psychotherapy group, individual therapy) have shown some evidence of effectiveness and may be appropriate but should be tailored to meet the individual's needs, particularly those identified as at high risk. They also identify the contribution of self-help groups in their review (as do Zisook and Shuchter in 2001, with the older work of Vachon and colleagues in 1980 identified as significant) and indicate that studies suggest such groups can be just as effective if the group has leadership and has been screened for suitability and if training for interventions has occurred. Furthermore, it is estimated that 80 per cent of bereavement care is now provided by the voluntary sector (London Bereavement Network 2001) and, therefore, it appears appropriate to propose that the quality of care provided by self-help and voluntary groups be strengthened.

Cognitive behavioural therapy (CBT), in the current health care environment (managed health care and push for 'brief' psychotherapy), is viewed as ideal for treating individuals with complicated grief (Matthews and Marwit 2004). However, this is not necessarily supported by those who work in bereavement care, and it is acknowledged that a need for further empirical support exists in this context and the possibility of using it in conjunction with other interventions. It is also acknowledged that CBT, in general, has been shown to be effective in treating anxiety (including post-traumatic stress disorder) and mood disorders.

There is a strong association of complicated grief with anxiety and depression and it is considered a key factor in atypical grief reactions. Bonanno and Kaltman (2001) identify that all forms of depression and anxiety reduce over time in the bereaved, although they may be resistant to time in about 15 per cent of widows and widowers. The diagnostic (DSM-IV Diagnostic and Statistical Manual for Mental Disorders) convention was to wait for 2 months after the death before diagnosis of depression is made, although Zisook and Shuchter (2001) contest this time period as illogical and believe that it delays appropriate diagnosis. In a review of the evidence for treatment of depression during bereavement, they conclude that better assessment and adaptation of interventions should occur to identify and support those at risk more accurately (this could also include prophylactic treatments). Treatment should consist of a combination of education, psychotherapy and pharmacotherapy.

Reynolds and colleagues (1999) (cited in Zisook and Shuchter 2001) identified the combination of medication (nortriptyline) and psychotherapy as associated with the highest rate of treatment completions. The type and duration of treatment would appear to be best based on individual requirements. A more recent randomised controlled trial (Shear *et al.* 2005) highlights some benefit for complicated grief treatment over standard interpersonal psychotherapy, although both interventions show improvement. The message is again that a combination of interventions may work best.

Generally, prescribing of anxiolytics for those who are bereaved has been considered inappropriate (for example see the *British National Formulary*, http://bnf. org/bnf/index.htm) although no evidence appears to exist of a detrimental effect on bereavement, other than that associated with the medication itself. Warner and colleagues (2001) found no evidence of a positive or negative effect of benzodiazepines on the course of bereavement within the first 6 months after death. The amount and extent of prescribing is also unknown, although Gold and colleagues

(2008) identified that approximately half of obstetricians endorse use of sedatives, such as benzodiazepines, for acute grief following perinatal death and there seems limited concern about their use in older people (Cook *et al.* 2007). The key message from this mirrors that for other interventions whereby each individual circumstance should be assessed for need.

Organisation of services

Service provision for the bereaved could possibly reflect the tiered educational model seen in the previous chapter (Chapter 15) so that the delivery of bereavement care could be seen in the same manner (Figure 16.1).

The model in Figure 16.1 is again reflected in the Beaumont Bereavement Care Model described by Walsh and colleagues (2008). The value of these tiered models is that they also represent the number of people involved at each level with the numbers decreasing as the levels are ascended. This is important for strategic development as the model provides some degree of scale to the level of service provision. A model, such as this, may be appropriate to build policy or a national framework for bereavement care, although it will probably require a high level of co-ordination, possibly from a central body, such as a regional health care organisation or government department. Co-ordination at regional and national level has begun to occur in parts of the UK and may exist in other parts of the world. It appears important to the development of services that they be available equitably, irrespective of the place of death and irrespective of cultural or spiritual needs and socio-economic status.

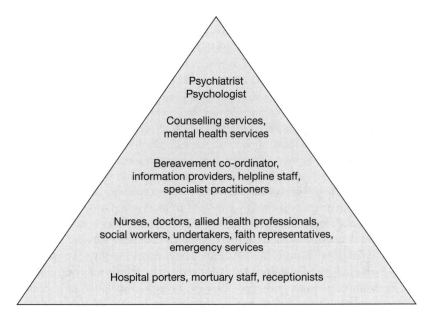

Figure 16.1 Tiered provision of service provision for the bereaved.

Little appears to have been undertaken to determine levels of need related to bereavement within different socio-economic groups. There may be increased levels of grief in areas of disadvantage (Richardson and Pearson 1995). Deaths in these communities will occur at a younger age and additionally involve more deaths of young people, reflecting the health and social care problems related to, for example, addiction and crime (Personal communication and stories from Faith in Community Scotland: http://www.faithincommunityscotland.org/homepage/welcome-to-faith-in-community-scotland/). Therefore it may be assumed that the impact of death will be greater within families and communities in areas of disadvantage. In addition the economic impact of bereavement in such communities may be extensive. Allen (2007) suggests that bereavement organisations often focus on and provide services for the middle class and highlights how Cruse has changed from offering relief for hardship and deprivation among widows and children to promoting well-being and coping with loss (Arnason and Hafsteinsson 2003). He goes on to suggest that the bereavement process can also initiate increased heroin use and also that other areas of life such as criminality may deteriorate as a consequence. It may therefore be the case that the 'inverse care law' (Tudor-Hart 1971) applies equally to bereavement care although this has not been illuminated.

Concerns may exist about the resource implications for health and social care organisations of providing on-going support to the bereaved, irrespective of setting, for those who might be identified as at risk. There is the potential that this will only help to medicalise or pathologise grief. On the other hand, such resources could be set against health gain for those at risk, particularly when there is evidence of health risks and increased morbidity and mortality for the bereaved (Stroebe *et al.* 2007; Boyle *et al.* 2011).

Furthermore, irrespective of setting or type of death, it is estimated that between four and eight people will be directly affected by one death (The Nucleus Group 2004; Wimpenny *et al.* 2007; SGHD 2010). Even if only 5–10 per cent of these develop complicated grief it is a significant number. This also assumes that the 90–95 per cent have no other needs. Looking across the bereavement journey highlights the divisions that may exist between different service provision. Additionally, there may be inequitable distribution and quality of services (NICE 2004), which may compound any fragmentation of services. Figure 16.2 seeks to provide an overview of some of these divisions and where they might exist. It is clear that in some cases there is involvement of professionals and others throughout, from before death to the period surrounding death and immediately beyond, although the extent of this is variable.

Some services are only providing care and support at a particular time, albeit this is at a crucial period. It may be the case that the boundaries between the stages prevent any development of an integrated or co-ordinated service, particularly between the statutory health and social care components and the voluntary sector. However, this may not represent all situations where local links may be functioning well, for example between midwifery services and groups such as Sands (Stillbirth and Neonatal Death Society) or between cancer services and local cancer groups or between social care and carers' support groups. Such engagement is a necessary

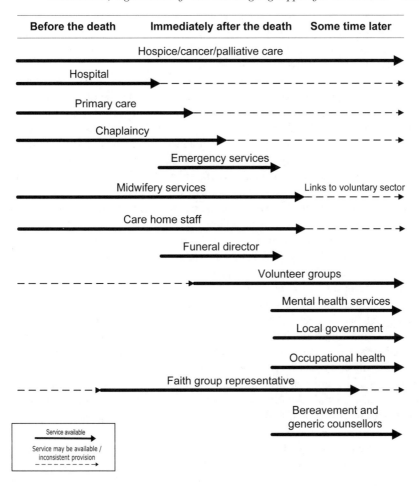

Figure 16.2 Stage(s) of involvement in bereavement care.

part of the co-ordination of bereavement care, although the extent of linkages is unknown and probably reliant on individuals within the systems rather than any robust referral or communication mechanisms.

Figure 16.2 also questions the extent to which voluntary agencies may wish to be involved or be able to engage with all the stages and how support for such engagement may be fostered. There are a considerable number of voluntary organisations/groups that provide information and support for the bereaved. Although some of these will have national coverage and quality assurance processes related to those who provide support, it may be the case that not all groups will do so.

Hospice services often describe providing pre-bereavement support, which may include assessment of how the family will react to the death and other practical aspects such as financial review. They also support the family at the time of the death and continue that care for as long as required after the death. There are also services, such as that provided to women and families after miscarriage, that provide care before and at the time of death but may link into external support networks that will take over at a later stage.

For hospitals, in general (including cancer services), the service provided to the bereaved is less clear and the level of involvement may be determined by the length of time the person was in hospital. Providing pre-bereavement support for families will not be possible if the death is unexpected, for example in an accident and emergency department. The level of follow up of the bereaved from hospital staff is also an area that appears to be underdeveloped. However, some practitioners are beginning to consider the needs of bereaved families in acute care settings (see Chapter 8). Evaluation of such services will be necessary to determine the value of these initiatives for use in other areas. It is also difficult to determine the extent to which primary care staff follow up the bereaved, even after they have cared for dying individuals in their own homes. Again this highlights a lack of information about the burden of bereavement care in the community.

There is clear faith-based support (often chaplaincy) for the bereaved, particularly at the time of death and immediately afterwards. However, the extent to which this is a continuation of pre-bereavement care is largely unknown in an increasingly secular society. Obviously there are links to funeral directors, who play an important role in the journey, although this is usually confined to the period immediately after death. The level of involvement of providers of faith-based support with other service providers is unclear. In addition, other non-religious groups such as humanists are becoming increasingly involved in funeral services and may also become involved in pre-bereavement care as spiritual care departments seek to provide spiritual care to those of all faiths and none.

Voluntary services also become involved with the bereaved at different stages depending on the nature of the service. Some will carry out bereavement care as a continuation of their involvement with the family, for example those organisations which provide support for carers. Others, such as Cruse, will provide a service only at a much later stage in the bereavement journey. Some voluntary sector providers describe their role as supplementary to that of statutory providers. This type of provision adds to the variety and choice of support services made available to the bereaved. However, for the bereaved it may be difficult to know who will be available and when.

Mental health services will have limited engagement with the issue of bereavement until people show signs of mental ill health such as clinical depression and anxiety. The incorporation of complicated grief into mental health diagnoses may, in the future, provide a means by which interventions can be organised. As identified in Chapter 14, the involvement of those working in occupational health is also important to consider as many bereaved will still be of working age. Involvement of occupational health services happens only after the death and the degree of support available will vary considerably.

The above review of services, from before death to sometime later, highlights the potentially fractured nature of bereavement care although this may be little different from other aspects of health and social care. Although this illustrates gaps between services it also highlights the range of support which already exists. What appears to be missing is the way in which the different groups communicate and collaborate to ensure appropriate bereavement care is available. For, as the book has alluded to on several occasions, the majority of people will work through their grief in a normal or natural way but may need initial support, advice and good information from well-informed and prepared staff.

Conclusion

The need for on-going intervention with all bereaved people is not required. At present there is limited evidence for the effectiveness of a range of interventions. However, it is clear that for health and social care organisations and practitioners there is a need for greater engagement prior to, at the time of and immediately after death, as the consequences of doing nothing may be long lasting.

How might we seek to enhance the organisation of available services to address this so that appropriate support is available to those who need it? The provision of a local geographically based co-ordinator may be a valuable step as they could determine available resources and seek to identify gaps in the journey from before bereavement. Where, within health and social care, such a person may reside is an important consideration. If hospital based, will co-ordination relate primarily to hospital-based care and not extend beyond? If in community-based care will this just look towards co-ordination of voluntary groups and services?

The provision of good-quality information for the bereaved could also be addressed. There is a considerable range of material in use, some of which is of high quality; however, there is probably an equivalent amount of 'third-generation' photocopies with information that is outdated and inaccurate. There is also, within health and social care services, considerable overlap of effort that could be harnessed more appropriately.

Standards for bereavement care could be another way of providing benchmarks for provision so that care can be measured. Until recently, little had been provided in such a form and so it was difficult to know where the level of service and provision should lie. These could be linked to educational provision across health and social care settings so that those providing care at appropriate points feel confident in engaging with the bereaved.

References

Agnew A, Manktelow R, Taylor BJ and Jones BL (2010) Bereavement needs assessment in specialist palliative care: a review of the literature. *Palliative Medicine* 24(1): 46–59.

Allen C (2007) The poverty of death: social class, urban deprivation, and the criminological consequences of sequestration of death. *Mortality* 12(1): 79–93.

Allumbaugh DL and Hoyt WT (1999) Effectiveness of grief therapy: a meta-analysis. *Journal of Counseling Psychology* 46(3): 370–380.

Arnason A and Hafsteinsson SB (2003) The revival of death: expression, expertise and governmentality. *British Journal of Sociology* 54(1): 43–62.

Bonanno GA and Kaltman S (2001) The varieties of grief experience. *Clinical Psychology Review* 21(5): 705–734.

Bowman T (2000) Bereavement and shattered dreams: exploring the connections. *Bereavement Care* 19(1): 3–5.

Boyle PJ, Feng Z and Raab GM (2011) Does widowhood increase mortality risk? Testing for selection effects by comparing causes of spousal death. *Epidemiology* 22(1): 1–5.

Cook JM, Biyanova T and Marshall R (2007) Medicating grief with benzodiazepines: physician and patient perspectives. *Archives of Internal Medicine.* 167(18): 2006–2007.

Crossland C (1998) Working with widowed men. *Bereavement Care* 17(2): 19–20.

Currier JM, Holland JM and Neimeyer RA (2007) The effectiveness of bereavement interventions with children: a meta-analytic review of controlled outcome research. *Journal of Clinical Child and Adolescent Psychology* 36(2): 253–259.

Department of Health, Social Services and Public Safety, Northern Ireland (2009) *Northern Ireland Health and Social Care Services Strategy for Bereavement Care.* Available at: http://www.dhsspsni.gov.uk/nihsc-strategy-for-bereavement-care-june-2009.pdf   (accessed November 2010).

Forte AL, Hill M, Pazder R and Feudtner C (2004) Bereavement care interventions: a systematic review. *BMC Palliative Care* 3(3): 20. Available at: http://www.biomedcentral.com/1427-684x/3/3/

Gallagher M, Tracey A and Millar R (2005) Ex-clients' evaluation of bereavement counselling in a voluntary sector agency. *Psychology and Psychotherapy* 78(1): 59–76.

Genevro JL (2004) Report on bereavement and grief research. *Death Studies* 28(6): 491–575.

Gold KJ, Schwenk TL and Johnson TRB (2008) Sedatives for mothers of stillborn infants: views from a national survey of obstetricians. *Journal of Women's Health* 17(10): 1605–1607.

Hopmeyer E and Werk A (1994) A comparative study of family bereavement groups. *Death Studies* 18(3): 243–256.

Jacobs S and Prigerson H (2000) Psychotherapy of traumatic grief: a review of evidence for psychotherapeutic treatments. *Death Studies* 24(6): 479–495.

London Bereavement Network (2001) *Project standards for bereavement care in the UK.* London: London Bereavement Network.

Machin L (1998) Grief counselling in context: multiple roles and professional compromise. *British Journal of Guidance and Counselling* 26(3): 387–397.

Mallon B (2008) *Dying, death and grief: working with adult bereavement.* London: Sage.

Marwit SJ (1996) Reliability of diagnosing complicated grief: a preliminary investigation. *Journal of Consulting and Clinical Psychology* 64(3): 563–568.

Matthews LT and Marwitt SJ (2004) Complicated crief and the trend toward cognitive-behavioural therapy. *Death Studies* 28(9): 849–863.

NICE (2004) *Improving supportive and palliative care for adults with cancer: the manual.* London: National Institute for Clinical Excellence. Available at: http://www.nice.org.uk/nice-media/pdf/manual.pdf (accessed 15 June 2011).

The Nucleus Group (2004) *Review of specific grief and bereavement services.* Carried out on behalf of Metropolitan Health and Aged Care Services Division, Victoria, Australia. Available at: http://www.health.vic.gov.au/palliativecare/archive/finalrep_grief.pdf (accessed 15 June 2011).

Parkes CM (2000) Counselling bereaved people: help or harm? *Bereavement Care* 19(2): 19–21.

Parry JK (1994) Death review: an important component of grief resolution. *Social Work in Health Care* 20(2): 97–107.

Potocky M (1993) Effective services for bereaved spouses: a content analysis of the empirical literature. *Health and Social Work* 18(4): 288–301.

Prigerson HG, Horowitz MJ, Jacobs SC, Parkes CM, Aslan M, Goodkin K, Raphael B. Marwit SJ, Wortman C., Neiymeyer RA, Bonanno B, Block SD, Kissane D, Boelen P, Maercker, A, Litz, BT, Johnson, JG, First, MB and Maciejewski, PK (2009) Prolonged grief disorder: psychometric validation of criteria proposed for DSM-V and ICD-11. *PLoS Medicine* 6(8), published 4 August (doi 10.1371/journal.pmed. 1000121).

Raphael B (1977) Preventive intervention with the recently bereaved. *Archives of General Psychiatry* 34(12): 1450–1454.

Relf M, Machin L and Archer N (2008) *Guidance for bereavement needs assessment in palliative care.* London: Help the Hospices.

Relf M, Machin L and Archer N and Payne M (2009) Debate on bereavement needs assessment in palliative care. Letters. *Bereavement Care* 28(1): 46–49.

Reynolds CF, Miller MD, Pasternak RE, Frank E, Perel JM, Cornes C, Houck PR, Mazumdar S, Dew MA and Kupfer DJ (1999) Treatment of bereavement-related major depressive episodes in later life: a controlled study of acute and continuation treatment with nortriptyline and interpersonal psychotherapy. *American Journal of Psychiatry* 156(2): 202–208.

Richardson S and Pearson M (1995) Dignity and aspirations denied: unmet health and social care needs in an inner-city area. *Health and Social Care in the Community* 3(5): 279–287.

Schut H and Stroebe MS (2005) Interventions to enhance adaptation to bereavement. *Journal of Palliative Medicine* 8(S1): S140–S147.

Schut H, de Keijser J, van den Bout J and Stroebe MS (1996) Cross-modality grief therapy: description and assessment of a new programme. *Journal of Clinical Psychology* 52(3): 357–365.

Schut H, Stroebe MS, Van Den Bout J, Keijser J and Terheggen M (2001) The efficacy of bereavement interventions: determining who benefits. In Stroebe M, Hansson RO, Stroebe W and Schut H (eds) *Handbook of bereavement research: consequences, coping and care.* Washington, DC: American Psychological Association.

SGHD (2010) *Shaping bereavement care.* Edinburgh: Scottish Government Health Department.

Shear K, Frank E, Houck PR and Reynolds CF (2005) Treatment of complicated grief: a randomized controlled trial. *JAMA* 293(21): 2601–2608.

Stroebe MS, Schut H and Stroebe W (2007) Health outcomes of bereavement. *The Lancet* 370(9603): 1960–1973.

Thuen F (1995) Satisfaction with bereavement support groups: evaluation of the Norwegian Bereavement Care Project. *Journal of Mental Health* 4: 499–510.

Thuen F and Sandvik O (1998) The Norwegian Bereavement Care Project: an evaluation of the first twelve years. *Bereavement Care* 17(2): 24–25.

Tudor-Hart J (1971) The inverse care law. *The Lancet* 297(7696): 405–412.

Vachon ML, Lyall WA, Rogers J, Freedman-Letofsky K and Freeman SJ (1980) A controlled study of self-help intervention for widows. *American Journal of Psychiatry* 137(11): 1380–1384.

Walsh T, Foreman M, O'Driscoll S, McCormack M and Curry P (2008) Bereavement support in an acute hospital: an Irish model. *Death Studies* 32(8): 768–786.

Warner J, Metcalfe C and King M. (2001) Evaluating the use of benzodiazepines following recent bereavement. *British Journal of Psychiatry* 178(1): 36–41.

Wimpenny P, Unwin R, Dempster P, Grundy M, Work F, Brown A and Wilcock S (2007) A literature review on bereavement and bereavement care: developing evidence-based practice in Scotland. *Bereavement Care* 26(1): 7–10.

Youll J and Wilson K (1996) A therapeutic approach to bereavement counselling. *Nursing Times* 92(16): 40–42.

Zisook S and Shuchter SR (2001) Treatment of the depressions of bereavement. *American Behavioural Scientist* 44(5): 782–797.

Zonnebelt-Smeenge SJ and De Vries RC (2003) The effects of gender and age on grief work associated with grief support groups. *Illness, Crisis and Loss* 11(3): 226–241.

Index

A&E (accident and emergency) 56, 127–31
ACT (Association of Children's Palliative
   Care) 140, 141, 148, 149
adaptation 14, 29, 31–2, 39, 101–2, 113,
   141, 148, 181
adolescence 23–5, 29, 45, 145, 169–70,
   228
aging and loss 56–9
ambiguous loss 99
anticipatory grief 73–5, 80, 149, 181, 199
assessment of the bereaved 5, 26, 29, 38–9,
   65–6, 71, 73, 74, 81–3, 85, 126, 144,
   147, 160, 163, 196, 231, 233, 248–50
assessment tool 83
attitudes and reactions to death 92
attachment 8–9, 23, 27, 41, 45, 62, 76–7,
   161, 178, 185, 191, 196–7

bereavement counselling 11, 66, 75,
   116–17, 244–8
bereavement support groups 248
breaking bad news 132, 133, 229–32

care pathway for dying children 148
CBT (cognitive behavioural therapy) 105,
   250
CCU (coronary care unit) 132–3
changed identity 63
children's understanding of death 20,
   149–51
CLOC (Changing Lives of Older Couples)
   64
complicated grief 42, 65, 71, 81, 82, 85,
   86, 91 92–4, 96, 97, 103, 115, 126, 142,
   160, 161, 162, 206, 207, 221, 239, 247,
   249–51

commemoration 29, 210
community nurses 117, 232
community Macmillan nurses 117
compassionate leave 218
conjugal bereavement 40, 60, 62, 75, 76;
   see also spousal bereavement
continuing bonds 13, 42, 62–3
counselling 28, 29, 73,79, 84, 163, 186,
   198, 207, 209, 218, 219, 244, 247–8,
   249; *see also* bereavement counselling;
   grief counselling
Cruse 66, 230, 247, 248, 252
cultural factors and education 235
curriculum content 234–5

death anxiety 12, 42
death at work 221–1
death defying 217
death review 246
denial 10, 12, 32, 64, 75, 94, 100, 101,
   105, 113, 119, 143, 147, 153
diagnostic overshadowing 195
disenfranchised grief 37, 57, 128–9,
   182–3, 205, 217, 232
dual process model (DPM) 9–10, 48, 59,
   142
DSM (Diagnostic and Statistical Manual
   of Mental Disorders) categories 42, 93,
   95, 96, 248
dying at home 39, 75, 82, 92, 139, 140,
   143, 152–2, 175, 176, 178, 181, 248,
   254

education and professionals 11, 28, 71, 84,
   123, 127, 128, 133, 142, 152, 160, 227
educational provision for professionals 233

family loss 39
family unit 37
follow-up bereavement care 71, 82, 83,
    84–6, 123, 125, 126, 127, 128, 129,
    130, 131, 132, 133, 154, 160, 163–5,
    168, 182, 254
future pregnancy 170–1
funerals 9, 20, 39, 40, 41, 62, 75, 81, 92,
    98, 113, 114, 119, 149, 153, 154, 165,
    193, 197, 215, 221, 254

gender stereotypes 47
Gold Standard Framework (GSF) 117,
    134
'good enough' memory 141, 149, 156
GP (general practitioner) 63, 80, 115–6
grandparents 144, 147–8, 153, 169, 210
grief counselling 13; *see also* bereavement
    counselling; counselling
grief work 8, 9, 11, 12, 13, 48, 49, 221

holding the baby 166, 167, 168
hope 12, 80, 100,101,102, 141, 143
hospice 2, 39, 40, 72, 73, 74, 81, 84, 85,
    139, 152, 176, 177, 180, 183, 251
hospital deaths – children 151–2
higher education 29

ICU/ITU (intensive care unit/intensive
    treatment or therapy unit) 124, 131–2,
    151, 162
information for the bereaved 19, 20, 21,
    22, 25, 36, 41, 46, 61, 66, 77, 84, 86,
    101, 102, 104,120, 123, 126, 128, 129,
    132, 133, 134, 139, 141, 148, 160, 165,
    167, 216, 230, 239, 248, 249, 251, 253,
    255
interventions 46–7, 65, 66, 103, 104, 111,
    154–6, 162, 164, 198, 207

last offices 103, 125, 128
Liverpool Care Pathway (LCP) 124
loneliness 11, 41, 44, 55, 57, 59, 61–2, 63,
    112, 113, 195

medicalisation of grief 8, 111
mementoes 29, 165–6, 198
'memoir' 153
Miscarriage Association 162, 169
mortality: and bereavement 41, 60, 252;
    carer 199, 205; own 119
multiple loss 59, 91, 96, 97, 98, 175,182,
    191, 194, 207–8

NICE: guideline antenatal care: routine
    care for the healthy pregnant woman
    170; guideline for antenatal and
    postnatal mental health 167; guideline
    for palliative care: 71, 82–4, 86, 239,
    252; guideline on the treatment and
    management of depression in adults
    105

organ donation 128, 149
organ retention 1, 151

parents' response to the death of a child
    141–4
parental bereavement 44
pet death/loss 27–8
policy and bereavement 133–4, 178, 186,
    233
post mortem 131, 134, 165
post traumatic stress disorder (PTSD) 45,
    95–6
professionals and bereavement 232

RCN/BAAEM guidelines 128
religion 7, 92, 102, 129, 153, 167–8, 235
risk factors 44, 81–2, 91, 94, 164, 206, 247,
    249
rituals 7, 19, 20, 62, 92, 94, 100, 118, 129,
    152–4, 166, 169, 195, 198

sacred space 155–6
SANDS (Stillbirth and Neonatal Death
    Society) 162, 167, 169, 252
school 28–9
school nurse 29
'Shaping Bereavement Care' 233, 239
shattered dreams 245
sibling death/bereavement 25–6, 139,
    144–5
social death 75
society 118–19, 185, 228–9
socioeconomic class 251, 252
soul pain 139, 150, 155
SPIKES protocol 73
spiritual care 80, 167, 230, 240, 254
spousal bereavement 40–42
stigma 27, 43, 77, 81, 82, 97, 118, 169,
    178, 197, 202, 203–5, 211
stressor–support–coping model 207
sudden death 45, 77, 222, 249; *see also*
    unexpected death
suicide 26–7, 45, 77, 97, 103, 208, 222
survivor guilt 202, 206

teenagers 24, 27; *see also* adolescence

unexpected death 40, 82, 94, 96, 98, 112, 115, 116, 117, 118, 123, 125, 247, 249, 254; *see also* sudden death

viewing the body 125, 128, 132
viewing human remains 100–1

witnessing resuscitation 123, 125, 128, 129, 132

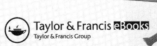